ID	internal diameter
Ig	immunoglobulin
IS	immediate spin
IU	international unit
LDH	lactate dehydrogenase
LISS	low-ionic-strength saline
LIP	low-ionic Polybrene
MCAD	middle cerebral arterial flow by Doppler
MIRL	membrane inhibitor of reactive lysis
MMA	monocyte monolayer assay
MSDS	manufacturer's safety data sheet
MW	molecular weight
NBF	neutral-buffered formalin
NeuAc	N-acetylneuraminic acid
NSAID	Nonsteroidal anti-inflammatory drug
OD	optical density
p	probability
PBS	phosphate-buffered saline
PBV	predicted blood volume
PCH	paroxysmal cold hemoglobinuria
PCR	polymerase chain reaction
PDR	Physicians' Desk Reference
PEG	polyethylene glycol
PNH	paroxysmal nocturnal hemoglobinuria
PNP	ρ-nitrophenol phosphate
RBC	Red Blood Cell (FDA component name) or red cell
RhIG	Rh Immune Globulin
RT	room temperature
SET	salt-EDTA-Tris
SDS	sodium dodecyl suplphate
SG	specific gravity
SNS	sterile normal saline
SOP	standard operating procedure
TE	Tris-EDTA
UDP	uridine diphosphate
vol/vol	volume/volume
WAIHA	warm autoimmune hemolytic anemia
WBC	White Blood Cell
WHO	World Health Organization
wt/vol	weight/volume

Judd's Methods in Immunohematology
THIRD EDITION

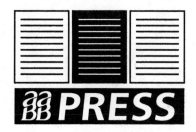

Other related publications available from the AABB:

Technical Manual, 16th edition
Edited by John D. Roback, MD, PhD; Martha Rae Combs, MT(ASCP)SBB;
Brenda J. Grossman, MD; and Christopher D. Hillyer, MD

Transfusion Service Manual of Standard Operating Procedures, Training Guides, and Competence Assessment Tools, 2nd edition
By Lucia M. Berte, MA, MT(ASCP)SBB, DLM, CQA(ASQ)CMQ/OE

Guidelines for Prenatal and Perinatal Immunohematology
Developed for the Scientific Section Coordinating Committee by W. John Judd, FIBMS, MIBiol

Serologic Problem-Solving: A Systematic Approach for Improved Practice
Edited by Sally V. Rudmann, PhD, MT(ASCP)SBB

To purchase books or to inquire about other book services, including chapter reprints and large-quantity sales, please contact our sales department:
- 866.222.2498 (within the United States)
- +1 301.215.6499 (outside the United States)
- +1 301.951.7150 (fax)
- www.aabb.org>Bookstore

AABB customer service representatives are available by telephone from 8:30 am to 5:00 pm ET, Monday through Friday, excluding holidays.

Judd's Methods in Immunohematology
THIRD EDITION

W. John Judd, FIBMS, MIBiol
Department of Pathology
University of Michigan
Ann Arbor, Michigan

Susan T. Johnson, MSTM, MT(ASCP)SBB
BloodCenter of Wisconsin
Milwaukee, Wisconsin

Jill R. Storry, PhD, FIBMS
Skåne Regional Blood Center
and
Department of Laboratory Medicine
Section for Haematology and Transfusion Medicine
Lund University
Lund, Sweden

AABB Press
Bethesda, MD
2008

AABB
8101 Glenbrook Road
Bethesda, Maryland 20814-2749

ISBN NO. 978-1-56395-266-1
Printed in the United States

Library of Congress Cataloging-in-Publication Data

Judd, W. John.
    Judd's methods in immunohematology / W. John Judd, Susan T. Johnson, Jill R. Storry—3rd ed.
      p. ; cm.
    Rev. ed. of: Methods in immunohematology / W. John Judd. 2nd ed. 1994.
    Includes bibliographical references and index.
    ISBN 978-1-56395-266-1
    1. Immunohematology—Methodology. I. Johnson, Susan T. II. Storry, Jill R. III. Judd, W. John. Methods in immunohematology. IV. AABB. V. Title. VI. Title: Methods in immunohematology.
    [DNLM: 1. Blood Grouping and Crossmatching—methods. 2. Blood Group Antigens—immunology. QY 415 J92m 2008]

RB45.5.J83 2008
615'.39—dc22

                               2008034440

Table of Contents

Table of Contents

Table of Contents

Preface

Sixteen years have elapsed since the publication of the last edition of *Methods in Immunohematology*. Much has changed since then, especially the manner in which standard operating procedures (SOPs) are written. This third edition, now called *Judd's Methods in Immunohematology,* substantially conforms to the guidelines for SOP development promulgated by the Clinical and Laboratory Standards Institute. This adaptation required complete reformatting of the previous text and would not have been accomplished without the dedication and diligence of my coauthors, Jill Storry and Susan Johnson, and I thank them.

This new edition contains 143 procedures and 12 process documents, along with flow diagrams to guide the user in the appropriate management of patients and samples. The entire text is also available electronically to permit incorporation into institutional SOPs. All of the procedures from the second edition have been retained, despite the fact that many are no longer performed because of safety concerns (eg, elution techniques using organic solvents). By retaining procedures that may be considered obsolete by most clinical laboratory personnel, we hope to ensure they will not be lost to posterity; indeed they may be useful to research investigators.

This third edition would not have been possible without the goodwill of Peter Issitt, PhD, FIBMS, FIBiol, of Montgomery Scientific Publications for releasing the copyright to AABB, and the interest of Laurie Munk, AABB Publications Director, in acquiring said copyright. The authors thank Judy Fueger, MT(ASCP)SBB, Lead Technologist of the Immunohematology Reference Laboratory at the BloodCenter of Wisconsin, for her expertise and guidance on information mapping. Some procedures have been adapted with permission from BloodCenter of Wisconsin Quality System Documents. Finally, my coauthors and I are indebted to Jay Pennington of the AABB Publications Department for his patience, guidance, and sheer hard work in managing the publication of this book. He has been a pleasure to work with.

W. John Judd, FIBMS, MIBiol
Emeritus Professor
University of Michigan Medical School
September 2008

Editorial Comments

Every effort has been made to ensure the accuracy of information presented in this book. However, neither the authors nor AABB Press can accept responsibility for errors that may result from use of the included procedures. It is the responsibility of each laboratory using this book to validate each procedure, using known samples, at the first use of each method. Once it is established that the method produces the expected results, appropriate controls should be incorporated at each subsequent use.

The references cited in this text are those used as the basis for a given procedure, as noted. They may not always be the original reference to a method, and the method given may vary from the referenced procedure.

For the purposes of this book, no distinction is made between the terms *red cells* and *Red Blood Cells* (or *RBCs*, the proper component name for red cells concentrated by the removal of most of the plasma from sedimented or centrifuged whole blood). *RBCs* is used throughout to stand for both in the interest of abbreviating these often recurrent terms.

Where a specific time or temperature is mentioned, or where a specific concentration of an RBC suspension is mentioned, some variance from the stated figure is acceptable and, from a practical standpoint, necessary. Acceptable variances are given below by topic.

Temperature

- 4 C: 2 C to 8 C.
- Room temperature (RT): 20 C to 25 C.
- All other temperatures: ±1 C.

Incubation Times

In many instances, incubation times are somewhat arbitrary. When a procedure requires use of specific incubation times (eg, enzyme treatment of RBCs), every effort should be made to adhere to that incubation time. In other instances, the following serve as guidelines for acceptable deviations from the stipulated times:

- <10 minutes: ±1 minute.
- ≥10 minutes to 20 minutes: ±2 minutes.
- ≥20 minutes to 60 minutes: ±5 minutes.
- >60 minutes: ±10 minutes.

Cell Suspensions

Every effort has been made to give a range for RBC suspensions used in serologic tests; a variance of ±1% from the stated range is acceptable. For packed RBCs, the hematocrit should be 90%. The following volumes of saline or PBS added to 0.1 mL packed RBCs provide percent suspensions for serologic testing:

- 10 mL = 1%.
- 5 mL = 2%.
- 3.3 mL = 3%.
- 2.5 mL = 4%.
- 2 mL = 5%.

Centrifugation Times and Force

Because not all laboratories use the same equipment, specific times for centrifugation and the required acceleration of gravity (*g*) are not specified for most methods. Each laboratory must, therefore, establish values for each function on the basis of available equipment. In these methods, the phrase "centrifuge as for hemagglutination tests" has been used, and it equates to centrifugation at $1000 \times g$ for 15 seconds. For washing RBCs, centrifugation equivalent to 1 minute at $1000 \times g$ is required. In other instances, centrifugation is used to pack red cells or remove particulate matter; this requires centrifugation equivalent to 5 minutes at $1000 \times g$.

Note: Equipment and materials that are commonly available in immunohematology laboratories (eg, Pasteur pipettes, serologic centrifuges) have been omitted to conserve space. For the same reason, reagent formulae and storage parameters are given in Appendix A, rather than in each method involving their use.

About the Authors

W. John Judd, FIBMS, MIBiol, is Emeritus Professor of Immunohematology in the Department of Pathology at the University of Michigan in Ann Arbor. He received his training in the United Kingdom and came to the Department in 1974 as Director of the Blood Bank Reference Laboratory, one of the few transfusion service reference laboratories in the country that is accredited by the AABB.

He has made significant worldwide contributions to the study of lectins and the streamlining of blood bank testing practices. Having presented over 250 lectures throughout the United States, Europe, Japan, Australia, and Saudi Arabia, he has also authored numerous scientific articles and chapters in textbooks as well as the AABB *Guidelines for Prenatal and Perinatal Immunohematology*.

He has been an active member of both the AABB—having served on its Board of Directors from 1989 to 1993—and of the Michigan Association of Blood Banks (MABB). He is a recipient of the AABB's Ivor Dunsford and John Elliot Awards and served as president of the MABB in 1985/1986.

Professor Judd is now retired. He and his wife Jane now reside in the warmer (than Michigan) climes of the coastal Carolinas.

Susan T. Johnson, MSTM, MT(ASCP)SBB, is Director of Clinical Education and Immunohematology at BloodCenter of Wisconsin in Milwaukee. She has worked in the Immunohematology Reference Laboratory for 25 years, developing a special interest in autoimmune hemolytic anemia, particularly drug-induced immune hemolytic anemia. During this time, she has also been involved with the Specialist in Blood Banking Program as Director. She enjoys mentoring students, helping them with their research projects, and teaching blood group serology.

Ms. Johnson received her undergraduate degree in medical technology at the University of Wisconsin—Madison, where she also played on the women's Division I basketball team. She attended the Specialist in Blood Bank Technology program at the American Red Cross Blood Services—Badger Region (Madison, WI) in 1982 and went on to earn her master's degree in transfusion medicine at Marquette University (Milwaukee, WI) in 2001.

Ms. Johnson has been a member of AABB since 1982 and has served on many AABB committees. Having chaired the Immunohematology Reference Laboratory Program Unit that developed the first edition of *Standards for Immunohematology Reference Laboratories*, she is currently a member of the Molecular Testing Standards Program Unit, which is developing the first edition of *Standards for Molecular Testing for Red Cell, Platelet, and Neutrophil Antigens*. She has also served as an AABB assessor for many years, visiting hospitals and blood centers around the world.

Ms. Johnson enjoys numerous opportunities to speak at educational programs throughout the United States, Italy, and India. Her newest interest is in teaching blood banking to eager students in India. Through the Indian Immunohematology Initiative, she has traveled to India several times in recent years to facilitate wet workshops on pretransfusion testing and antibody identification.

Outside of blood banking, her passion is her family—her husband Dan and son Conor. She is an avid "soccer mom," "taxi service," and music enthusiast who especially loves the sounds of the oboe. She also shares her love for basketball by coaching an eighth-grade girls' team.

Ms. Johnson is grateful for the opportunity to participate in this edition of *Judd's Methods in Immunohematology* and considers it an honor to work with her coauthors.

Jill R. Storry, PhD, FIBMS, is the Coordinator of Special Serology at the Skåne Regional Blood Center in Lund, Sweden and a Research Fellow in the Department of Laboratory Medicine of the Section for Haematology and Transfusion Medicine at Lund University. Her career has followed a somewhat peripatetic course from its start in 1979 at the Salisbury (now Harare) and District Blood Centre in Zimbabwe. After completing medical laboratory technology training while working at the National Blood Service in Bristol, England in 1983, she earned a Fellowship of the Institute of Biomedical Sciences (FIBMS) in 1985 and a master of science degree in applied immunology in 1990.

Dr. Storry moved to the United States for "one year's experience" to join the American Red Cross National Reference Laboratory for Blood Group Serology in Rockville, MD, in 1990. Three years later, she joined the New York Blood Center's Immunohematology Laboratory, where she stayed until 2003, meanwhile gaining her PhD from the University of the West of England in 2000.

"Unlike Groucho Marx," Dr. Storry has said, "I am a member of all transfusion medicine societies that will admit me," namely the AABB, British Blood Transfusion Society (BBTS), International Society of Blood Transfusion (ISBT), and Swedish Society for Transfusion Medicine. Having served on several AABB committees, she currently serves on the ISBT Working Party on Terminology for Red Cell Surface Antigens. She is the recipient of the BBTS Margaret Kenwright and Race and Sanger Awards, as well as the AABB Sally Frank Award. She has been invited to speak at many national and international meetings and has authored over 60 scientific articles and chapters.

Interested in everything having to do with blood groups, Dr. Storry has been obsessed with serology ever since the magic of the first antiglobulin test she performed during a high school vacation. It is her wish that the next generation of blood bankers glean as much pleasure from blood group serology as she has, and she hopes that this edition of *Judd's Methods in Immunohematology* will continue to inspire immunohematologists to "look a bit further."

Dr. Storry is grateful for the opportunity to participate in this edition and has found great pleasure in working with her coauthors.

Section I. Routine Tube Methods

Policies and procedures adopted by transfusion service laboratories for routine ABO and Rh typing and antibody detection undoubtedly vary from institution to institution. The inclusion of specific procedures in this section is not an indication that they are the preferred or only ones to use. Indeed, for antibody detection, some may use the polyethylene glycol (PEG) technique described in Section II rather than the low-ionic-strength saline (LISS) additive method that has been provided. Others use three reagent RBC samples (not two) and/or include the autologous RBCs. These and other decisions, such as use of polyspecific anti-human globulin (AHG) serum instead of anti-IgG, or adoption of an immediate-spin cross-match, are within the purview of transfusion service directors.

The techniques outlined in this section are generic versions of routine manual (test-tube) procedures in use at one author's institution. They have been included because the results obtained by these or similar studies prompt performance of many of the subsequently described tests. Also addressed is the grading and scoring of serologic reactions, a fundamental of good serologic practice, along with a method to ensure uniformity of such grading and identify inadequate washing of RBCs for antiglobulin testing. The latter is intended as part of the ongoing competency assessment of staff performing the procedures described throughout this book.

When performing these studies with commercially prepared reagents, it is imperative that manufacturers' directions be followed. For further information on pretransfusion testing requirements, the interested reader is referred to the sources listed below.

Suggested Reading

Code of federal regulations. Title 21 CFR Parts 606 and 660. Washington, DC: US Government Printing Office, 2008 (revised annually).

Judd WJ. Modern approaches to pretransfusion testing. Immunohematology 1999;15:41-52.

Price TH, ed. Standards for blood banks and transfusion services. 25th ed. Bethesda, MD: AABB, 2008 (or current edition).

Roback J, Combs MR, Grossman B, Hillyer C, eds. Technical manual. 16th ed. Bethesda, MD: AABB, 2008 (or current edition).

I-A. Typing for ABO and Rh

Purpose

To provide instructions for ABO and Rh typing of human blood:

- Pretransfusion testing.
- Perinatal testing.

Background Information

ABO blood types are determined by the presence or absence of A and/or B antigens on RBCs, and by the presence or absence of anti-A and/or anti-B in the serum.

Rh-positive and Rh-negative phenotypes are determined by the presence or absence of D antigen on RBCs.

In adults, there is a reciprocal relationship between the A and/or B antigens on RBCs and A and B antibodies in the serum/plasma; for example, if A antigen is absent on the RBCs, anti-A is expected to be present in the serum/plasma.

Operational Policy

Samples from infants less than 6 months old will not regularly contain expected anti-A or anti-B; therefore, only RBC ABO typing is required.

For Rh typing of patient samples, only direct tests with anti-D are required.

When Rh typing is performed for newborns of Rh-negative females (to determine maternal RhIG candidacy) or allogeneic blood donors, the method for Rh typing must be capable of detecting weak expression of D antigen. See Procedure I-D.

When agglutination occurs in routine tests, reactions ≥2+ are expected; observation of weaker reactions necessitates further study before valid conclusions can be made. See Section XIII and Procedure I-D when weak or discrepant findings are encountered.

A negative test result with either anti-A or anti-B must be obtained before valid conclusions can be made regarding the Rh status of the RBCs. In the absence of such a negative result, repeat the test with anti-D in parallel with an inert Rh control reagent (eg, 6% BSA).

For electronic crossmatching, two concordant ABO types are required: one type on a current sample and one historical type, or both on a current sample. When practical, the two blood types on a current sample should be performed by different technologists using different manufacturers' reagents.

A second Rh type, incorporating an inert Rh control reagent and following reidentification of the sample, shall be performed on all patients without a historical record.

Limitations

Unwanted Positive Reactions:

- Auto- or alloantibodies.

- Contaminated reagent or sample.

Additional Reactivity:

- Anti-A_1 in an A_2 or A_2B individual.

- Passive antibody.

- Antibody to a reagent constituent.

- Acquired-B phenomenon.

- B(A) phenomenon.

Note: T and Tn polyagglutination should not cause a typing discrepancy with currently available monoclonal typing reagents.

Unwanted Negative Reactions:

- Omission of reagent or test sample.

- Contaminated or inactive reagent.

- Contaminated sample (eg, excess soluble blood group substance from a ruptured ovarian cyst).

- Anti-A and/or anti-B prozones.

Missing Reactivity:

- Leukemia.

- Minor cell population (eg, transplant, genetic chimera).

- Non-ABO-type-specific RBC and plasma infusions.

- Newborn sample.

- Impaired immune response.

Sample Requirements

Clotted or EDTA-anticoagulated blood as a source of serum/plasma and RBCs.

Note: If used for pretransfusion testing and the patient has been transfused with RBCs or has been pregnant within the preceding 3 months, or if the history is uncertain or unavailable, the sample must be obtained within 3 days of scheduled transfusion.

Note: Wording in reagent manufacturers' product circulars may impose further limitations on the age and type of samples used for ABO and Rh typing.

Equipment/ Materials

Anti-A and anti-B: only monoclonal products are currently available in the United States.

Anti-D: low-protein, monoclonal IgM anti-D blended with polyclonal or monoclonal IgG anti-D.

RBCs: 3%-5% suspensions of reagent group A_1 (pool of 3 donors) and B RBCs (pool of 3 donors); all donors should be Rh negative.

Quality Control

Daily, for each lot of reagents in use, demonstrate that:

- Anti-A agglutinates (4+, score 12) group A_1 reagent RBCs, but not group B reagent RBCs.

- Anti-B agglutinates (4+, score 12) group B reagent RBCs but not group A_1 reagent RBCs.

- Anti-D agglutinates (3+ to 4+, score 10-12) Rh-positive RBCs (group O, R_1R_1 RBCs from Procedure I-B) but not Rh-negative RBCs (group A_1 or B reagent RBCs).

- Alternatively, document daily that all samples from previously tested patients react according to the blood type of record and that all discrepancies with prior results and between RBC and serum/plasma ABO types were resolved.

Note: Discrepancies between RBC and serum/plasma results must be resolved before the ABO type can be concluded. See Section XIII.

Procedure

Use the following steps to perform the procedure:

Step	Action
1.	Dispense 1 drop of anti-A into an appropriately labeled 10 or 12 × 75-mm test tube. Set up similar tubes for anti-B and anti-D.

2.	Remove approximately 0.4 mL of serum/plasma from the test sample with a Pasteur pipette, and dispense 2-3 drops into 2 appropriately labeled 10 or 12 × 75-mm test tubes.
3.	Prepare a 3%-5% suspension of test RBCs in saline, and add 1 drop to each tube containing antiserum. Mix gently.
4.	To 1 tube of test serum/plasma, add 1 drop of A_1 RBCs; add 1 drop of B RBCs to the other tube.
5.	Gently mix the contents within each tube: • Centrifuge. • Examine the RBCs macroscopically for agglutination and hemolysis. • Grade and record the results.
6.	Interpret the blood type as follows:

If RBCs react...			And serum reacts...		Then type is...
Anti-A	Anti-B	Anti-D	A_1 RBCs	B RBCs	
0	0	≥2+	≥2+/H	≥2+/H	O Rh+
0	0	0	≥2+/H	≥2+/H	O Rh−
≥2+	0	≥2+	0	≥2+/H	A Rh+
≥2+	0	0	0	≥2+/H	A Rh−
0	≥2+	≥2+	≥2+/H	0	B Rh+
0	≥2+	0	≥2+/H	0	B Rh−
≥2+	≥2+	≥2+	0	0	inconclusive
≥2+	≥2+	0	0	0	AB Rh−

If...	Then...
inconclusive	repeat using an inert control reagent.
mixed-field or different reactions are observed	see Section XIII.

Note: If discrepant reactions are observed and transfusion is necessary before resolution, only group O RBCs shall be issued. If sample is from a blood donor, discrepancies shall be resolved before release.

References

Code of federal regulations. Title 21 CFR Parts 606 and 660. Washington, DC: US Government Printing Office, 2008 (revised annually).

Price TH, ed. Standards for blood banks and transfusion services. 25th ed. Bethesda, MD: AABB, 2008 (or current edition).

Roback J, Combs MR, Grossman B, Hillyer C, eds. Technical manual. 16th ed. Bethesda, MD: AABB, 2008 (or current edition).

Effective Date

Approved by:	Printed Name	Signature	Date
Laboratory Management			
Medical Director			
Quality Officer			

I-B. Testing for Unexpected Antibodies: LISS Additive Procedure

Purpose

To provide instructions for testing for unexpected antibodies:

- Pretransfusion testing.
- Perinatal testing.

Background Information

Antibodies to RBC antigens may cause direct agglutination or complement-mediated lysis of RBCs, or they may coat RBCs with IgG and/or C3.

Direct agglutination and/or lysis can be observed following centrifugation of RBC/serum mixtures.

Antibody coating may be accelerated in a low-ionic environment—hence the use of LISS.

RBCs incubated with serum/plasma in the presence of LISS at 37 C are washed to remove unbound globulins and tested with AHG. Agglutination by AHG indicates that the RBCs are coated with globulins.

Note: Detection of C3 coating antibodies is not required when performing routine pretransfusion and prenatal testing.

Operational Policy

Only two reagent RBC samples are required (R_1R_1 and R_2R_2).

One RBC sample should be Jk(a+b–).

Neither should carry strong expression of Bg antigens.

DO NOT READ TESTS MICROSCOPICALLY because unwanted positive reactions may occur.

Limitations

Unwanted Positive Reactions:

- Overcentrifugation of tests.
- Microscopic examination of tests.
- Contaminated or inactive reagents.
- Improper sample.
- Antibody to a reagent constituent.

Unwanted Negative Reactions:

- Failure to wash RBCs adequately.

- Interrupted testing.

- Use of wrong reagent.

- Loss of activity of AHG reagents.

- Failure to add AHG to the test system.

- Too heavy or too light a cell suspension.

- Omission of RBCs or patient's serum or plasma.

Sample Requirements

EDTA-anticoagulated whole blood as a source of plasma and red cells. Serum should be used if detection of complement-binding antibodies is required.

Note: If used for pretransfusion testing and the patient has been transfused or pregnant within the preceding 3 months, or if the history is uncertain or unavailable, the sample must be obtained within 3 days of scheduled transfusion.

Equipment/ Materials

6% BSA.

AHG: anti-IgG; need not be heavy-chain specific.

IgG-coated RBCs.

LISS additive reagent (obtain commercially).

RBCs: 3%-5% suspensions of phenotyped group O, R_1R_1 and R_2R_2 RBCs.

Note: As defined in the Code of Federal Regulations, RBCs used in pretransfusion testing to detect unexpected antibodies must carry the following antigens: D, C, c, E, e, K, k, Fy^a, Fy^b, Jk^a, Jk^b, Le^a, Le^b, M, N, S, s, and P_1.

Weakly (2+) reactive antibody (eg, dilute human IgG anti-D).

Quality Control

Daily, for each lot of reagents in use, demonstrate that the weakly reactive antibody reacts appropriately with the reagent R_1R_1 and R_2R_2 RBCs.

Daily, for each lot of reagents in use, demonstrate that 6% BSA does not react with the reagent R_1R_1 and R_2R_2 RBCs.

Confirm all negative reactions with IgG-coated RBCs (see Step 8 below).

Procedure Use the following steps to perform the procedure:

Step	Action
1.	For each sample to be tested, add 2 drops of serum/plasma to 2 appropriately labeled test tubes.
2.	Add 2 drops of LISS additive to both tubes.
3.	Add 1 drop of R_1R_1 RBCs to 1 tube, and 1 drop of R_2R_2 cells to the other tube.
4.	Mix and incubate at 37 C for 15 minutes: • Centrifuge. • Dislodge the cell buttons gently. • Examine macroscopically for agglutination. • Grade and record the results.
5.	Wash each tube three to four times with saline and completely decant the final wash supernate.
6.	To the dry cell buttons, add 2 drops of anti-IgG: • Mix and centrifuge. • Dislodge the cell buttons gently. • Examine macroscopically for agglutination. • Grade and record the results.
7.	Interpret the reactions as follows: **If agglutination is…** / **Then…** present at Step 4 and/or Step 6 — test result is positive: • Subject samples to antibody identification studies. • See Section VIII. absent at both Steps 4 and 6 — proceed with Step 8.
8.	Add 1 drop of IgG-coated RBCs to all tubes with negative antiglobulin results: • Mix gently. • Centrifuge. • Examine macroscopically for agglutination. • Grade and record the results.

9.	Analyze the reactions of the IgG-coated RBCs as follows:	
	If agglutination is…	**Then…**
	present	test is complete.
	absent	test is invalid: • Repeat Steps 1-8. • Consider cell washer problem or inactive AHG.

References

Code of federal regulations. Title 21 CFR Parts 606 and 660. Washington, DC: US Government Printing Office, 2008 (revised annually).

Löw B, Messeter L. Antiglobulin tests in low-ionic strength salt solutions for rapid antibody screening and crossmatching. Vox Sang 1974;26:53-61.

Price TH, ed. Standards for blood banks and transfusion services. 25th ed. Bethesda, MD: AABB, 2008 (or current edition).

Roback J, Combs MR, Grossman B, Hillyer C, eds. Technical manual. 16th ed. Bethesda, MD: AABB, 2008 (or current edition).

Effective Date

Approved by:	**Printed Name**	**Signature**	**Date**
Laboratory Management			
Medical Director			
Quality Officer			

I-C. Crossmatching by LISS Antiglobulin

Purpose   To provide instructions for antiglobulin crossmatching:

- Pretransfusion testing when clinically significant unexpected antibodies are present.

Background Information   An antiglobulin crossmatch is required for patients in whom clinically significant unexpected antibodies are detected in Procedure 1-B.

Operational Policy   Units selected for antiglobulin crossmatching should lack the antigen(s) corresponding to the clinically significant antibodies known to be present (currently or by history) in the patient's serum. However, antigen-negative units need not be selected for patients with antibodies to M, Le^a, Le^b, and P$_1$ antigens. Also, see Procedure VIII-E.

DO NOT READ TESTS MICROSCOPICALLY because unwanted positive reactions may occur.

Limitations   Unwanted Positive Reactions:

- Overcentrifugation.
- Microscopic examination of tests.
- Septicemia in a patient or bacterial contamination of a specimen.
- Improper sample.
- Antibody to a reagent constituent.
- Positive DAT results on donor RBCs.
- Polyagglutination of donor RBCs.

Unwanted Negative Reactions:

- Failure to wash RBCs adequately.
- Interrupted testing.
- Use of wrong reagent.
- Loss of activity of AHG reagents.
- Failure to add AHG to the test system.
- Too heavy or too light a cell suspension.
- Omission of RBCs or patient's serum or plasma.

Sample Requirements

EDTA-anticoagulated whole blood as a source of plasma and red cells. Serum should be used if detection of complement-binding antibodies is required.

Note: If used for pretransfusion testing and the patient has been transfused or pregnant within the preceding 3 months, or if the history is uncertain or unavailable, the sample must be obtained within 3 days of scheduled transfusion.

Equipment/ Materials

AHG: anti-IgG; need not be heavy-chain specific.

Donor RBCs: 3%-5% saline suspension (washed or unwashed). Shown to lack the antigen(s) corresponding to the clinically significant antibodies known to be present (currently or by history) in the patient's serum.

IgG-coated RBCs.

LISS additive reagent (obtain commercially).

Quality Control

Confirm all negative reactions with IgG-coated RBCs (see Step 8 below).

Procedure

Use the following steps to perform the procedure:

Step	Action
1.	For each unit to be tested, add 2 drops of serum/plasma to an appropriately labeled test tube.
2.	Add 2 drops of LISS additive to each tube.
3.	Add 1 drop of 3%-5% RBCs to the appropriately labeled tube.
4.	Mix and incubate at 37 C for 15 minutes: • Centrifuge. • Dislodge the cell buttons gently. • Examine macroscopically for agglutination. • Grade and record the results.
5.	Wash each tube three to four times with saline and completely decant the final wash supernate.

6.	To the dry cell buttons, add 2 drops of anti-IgG: • Mix and centrifuge. • Dislodge the cell buttons gently. • Examine macroscopically for agglutination. • Grade and record the results. **Note:** Samples yielding positive reactions in either Step 4 or Step 6 are incompatible and should not be released for transfusion without the approval of the medical director. Investigation into the cause of the incompatibility may be warranted.
7.	Add 1 drop of IgG-coated RBCs to all tubes with negative antiglobulin results: • Mix gently. • Centrifuge. • Examine macroscopically for agglutination. • Grade and record the results.
8.	Analyze the reactions of the IgG-coated RBCs as follows:

If agglutination is...	Then...
present	test is complete.
absent	test is invalid: • Repeat Steps 1-8. • Consider cell washer problem or inactive AHG.

References

Code of federal regulations. Title 21 CFR Parts 606 and 660. Washington, DC: US Government Printing Office, 2008 (revised annually).

Löw B, Messeter L. Antiglobulin tests in low-ionic strength salt solutions for rapid antibody screening and crossmatching. Vox Sang 1974;26:53-61.

Price TH, ed. Standards for blood banks and transfusion services. 25th ed. Bethesda, MD: AABB, 2008 (or current edition).

Roback J, Combs MR, Grossman B, Hillyer C, eds. Technical manual. 16th ed. Bethesda, MD: AABB, 2008 (or current edition).

**Effective
Date**

Approved by:	Printed Name	Signature	Date
Laboratory Management			
Medical Director			
Quality Officer			

I-D. Weak D Testing Procedure

Purpose
To provide instructions for testing apparent Rh-negative (by direct testing) RBCs for weak expression of D antigen:

- Apparent Rh-negative donor blood.

- Apparent Rh-negative infants of Rh-negative females, to determine maternal RhIG candidacy.

Background Information
Weak D phenotypes arise from missense mutations to regions of *RHD* encoding the transmembrane portion of the D antigen. Weak D phenotypes:

- Result from less than normal amount of D antigen inserted into the RBC membrane.

- Usually do not make anti-D if exposed to normal Rh-positive RBCs.

- Ideally, should type as Rh-positive with high-affinity IgM monoclonal anti-D.

Also, the expression of D antigen may be weak when an *RHCe* gene is on the chromosome opposite *RHD* (trans effect)—eg, in the *DCe/Ce* genotype.

Partial D phenotypes arise from hybrid genes and missense mutations to regions of *RHD* encoding parts of D external to the RBC membrane. Partial D phenotypes:

- Some react weakly or not at all in direct tests with anti-D.

- May make antibody to missing part of D.

- If transfused, should receive Rh-negative RBCs.

- If pregnant, are candidates for RhIG.

Both weak and partial D phenotypes can evoke the production of anti-D in Rh-negative recipients.

Operational Policy

Run a concurrent test with an inert Rh control reagent.

Do not use polyspecific AHG when testing clotted blood samples because C3 coating of RBCs may result in unwanted positive test results.

DO NOT READ TESTS MICROSCOPICALLY because unwanted positive reactions may occur.

Samples from patients who are pregnant or who are potential transfusion recipients and react weakly (≤2+) in direct tests with anti-D will not be subjected to weak D testing.

Apparent Rh-negative donors whose RBCs give weak or doubtful reactions in the test for weak D shall be considered Rh positive.

Newborns whose RBCs give weak or doubtful reactions in the test for weak D shall be considered Rh positive for the purpose of maternal RhIG candidacy.

Limitations

Unwanted Positive Reactions:

- Positive DAT.
- Contaminated reagent or sample.
- Use of wrong reagent.

Unwanted Negative Reactions:

- Omission of reagent or test sample.
- Contaminated or inactive reagent.
- Use of wrong reagent.
- Failure to wash RBCs adequately before adding AHG.

Sample Requirements

Clotted or EDTA-anticoagulated blood as a source of RBCs.

Note: Wording in reagent manufacturers' product circulars may impose further limitations on the age and type of samples used for Rh typing.

Equipment/ Materials

Low-protein anti-D reagent formulated with polyclonal or monoclonal IgG anti-D, blended with monoclonal IgM anti-D. Alternatively, use a high-protein reagent formulated with polyclonal IgG anti-D.

Inert Rh control reagent of a protein content approximating that of the anti-D, as supplied by the manufacturer. For low-protein anti-D, 6% BSA may be used as the inert control reagent.

AHG: anti-IgG; need not be heavy-chain specific.

IgG-coated RBCs.

Quality Control

Confirm all negative reactions with IgG-coated RBCs (see Step 10 below).

Procedure

Use the following steps to perform the procedure:

Step	Action
1.	Dispense anti-D into an appropriately labeled 10 or 12 × 75-mm test tube, according to the manufacturer's directions.
2.	Similarly, dispense the Rh control reagent.
3.	Prepare a 3%-5% suspension of test RBCs in saline and add 1 drop to each tube containing antiserum; mix gently.
4.	Incubate at 37 C according to the manufacturer's directions: • Centrifuge. • Dislodge the cell buttons gently. • Examine macroscopically for agglutination. • Grade and record the results.
5.	Interpret the direct tests as follows:<table><tr><td>**If reaction with anti-D is…**</td><td>**And reaction with control is…**</td><td>**And sample is from…**</td><td>**Then the Rh type is…**</td></tr><tr><td>≥2+</td><td>negative</td><td>anyone</td><td>positive</td></tr><tr><td><2+</td><td>negative</td><td>recipient or prenatal patient</td><td>negative</td></tr><tr><td>positive</td><td>negative</td><td>donor, or infant of Rh– woman</td><td>positive</td></tr><tr><td>positive or negative</td><td>positive</td><td>anyone</td><td>inconclusive</td></tr></table>Also see Table I-D-1.

6.	Wash the RBCs three to four times with saline.
7.	Add anti-IgG according to the manufacturer's directions: • Centrifuge. • Dislodge the cell buttons gently. • Examine macroscopically for agglutination. • Grade and record the results.
8.	Interpret the tests for weak D on donors and infants of Rh– women as follows:

If reaction with anti-D is...	And reaction with control is...	Then the Rh type is...
positive	negative	positive.
positive	positive	unable to be concluded: • Discard if donor unit. • Repeat test with acid-treated RBCs if infant of Rh– woman (Procedure IV-K).
negative	negative	negative

Also see Table I-D-1.

9.	Add 1 drop of IgG-coated RBCs to all tubes with negative antiglobulin results: • Mix gently. • Centrifuge. • Examine macroscopically for agglutination. • Grade and record the results.
10.	Analyze the reactions of the IgG-coated RBC as follows:

If agglutination is...	Then...
present	test is complete.
absent	test is invalid: • Repeat Steps 1-10. • Consider cell washer problem or inactive AHG.

References   Code of federal regulations. Title 21 CFR Parts 606 and 660. Washington, DC: US Government Printing Office, 2008 (revised annually).

Flegel WA, Wagner FF. Molecular biology of partial and weak D: Implications for blood bank practice. Clin Lab 2002;45:53-9.

Price TH, ed. Standards for blood banks and transfusion services. 25th ed. Bethesda, MD: AABB, 2008 (or current edition).

Roback J, Combs MR, Grossman B, Hillyer C, eds. Technical manual. 16th ed. Bethesda, MD: AABB, 2008 (or current edition).

Effective Date

Approved by:	Printed Name	Signature	Date
Laboratory Management			
Medical Director			
Quality Officer			

Table I-D-1. Interpretation Recommendations for Direct and Indirect Tests with Anti-D

	Direct Tests			Test for Weak D	
Results with Anti-D	**≥2+***	**<2+**	**0**	**positive***	**negative**
Transfusion candidate	Rh+	Rh–	Rh–	Not indicated	
Prenatal patient	Rh+	Rh–	Rh–	Not indicated	
Newborn of Rh– woman[†]	Rh+	Test for weak D		Rh+	Rh–
Blood donor	Rh+	Test for weak D		Rh+	Rh–

*When the control test for autoagglutination is nonreactive.

[†]When testing to determine the need for maternal Rh immune globulin therapy.

I-E. Crossmatching by Immediate-Spin

Purpose

To provide instructions for performing an immediate spin (IS) crossmatch:

- Detection of ABO incompatibility between donor and recipient when unexpected antibodies are absent in the recipient, either currently or by history.

Background Information

High-titer IgG anti-A and/or anti-B may fix C1 (the first component of human complement) to RBCs, and this can sterically hinder agglutination. Unwanted negative reactions resulting from this phenomenon can be prevented by using EDTA-anticoagulated plasma for IS crossmatching or by suspending donor RBCs in EDTA-saline. EDTA chelates ionized calcium (Ca^{++}), which is essential for the integrity of the C1 molecule.

Operational Policy

IS crossmatching shall be limited to samples from patients who lack unexpected antibodies.

DO NOT READ TESTS MICROSCOPICALLY because unwanted positive reactions may occur.

Limitations

Unwanted Positive Reactions:

- Auto- or alloantibodies.
- Contaminated samples.
- Polyagglutination.
- Polycarboxyl-dependent antibody.
- Passive antibody.

Unwanted Negative Reactions:

- Omission of RBCs or test sample.
- Contaminated sample.
- Weakly reactive anti-A and/or anti-B.
- Newborn sample.
- Weakly expressed A and/or B antigens on donor RBCs.

Sample Requirements Clotted or EDTA-anticoagulated whole blood as a source of serum or plasma.

> **Note:** If the patient has been transfused with RBCs or has been pregnant within the preceding 3 months, or if the history is uncertain or unavailable, the sample must be obtained within 3 days of scheduled transfusion.

Equipment/ Materials Normal saline if EDTA-anticoagulated plasma is used for the IS crossmatch.

EDTA-saline if serum is used for the IS crossmatch.

A_1 and B reagent RBCs.

ABO-compatible donor RBCs.

Quality Control Perform serum/plasma ABO typing tests concurrently with the IS crossmatch.

Procedure Use the following steps to perform the procedure:

Step	Action	
1.	**If using...**	**Then...**
	serum	prepare a 3%-5% EDTA-saline suspension of test RBCs (each donor sample; A_1 and B controls) in appropriately labeled test tubes.
	plasma	prepare a 3%-5% saline suspension of test RBCs (each donor sample; A_1 and B controls) in appropriately labeled test tubes.
2.	In appropriately labeled 10 or 12 × 75-mm test tubes, add 2-3 drops of serum or plasma and 1 drop of each of the appropriate RBC suspensions.	
3.	Gently mix the contents within each tube: • Centrifuge. • Dislodge the cell buttons gently. • Examine macroscopically for agglutination. • Grade and record the results.	

4.	Interpret the results of the IS crossmatches as follows:		
	If donor RBCs are…	**And controls are…**	**Then…**
	nonreactive	in accord with patient's ABO type	tests are valid: • Issue blood for transfusion.
	reactive	in accord with patient's ABO type	suspect cold-reactive auto- or alloantibodies: • Crossmatch by Procedure I-C.
	nonreactive	not in accord with patient's ABO type	tests are invalid: • Confirm RBC ABO type of patient and donor. • Blood may be released if ABO compatible.
	reactive	not in accord with patient's ABO type	do not release units: • Issue group O RBCs. • Investigate problem.

References Code of federal regulations. Title 21 CFR Parts 606 and 660. Washington, DC: US Government Printing Office, 2008 (revised annually).

Judd WJ, Steiner EA, O'Donnell DB, Oberman HA. Discrepancies in ABO typing due to prozone: How safe is the immediate-spin crossmatch? Transfusion 1988;28:334-8.

Price TH, ed. Standards for blood banks and transfusion services. 25th ed. Bethesda, MD: AABB, 2008 (or current edition).

Roback J, Combs MR, Grossman B, Hillyer C, eds. Technical manual. 16th ed. Bethesda, MD: AABB, 2008 (or current edition).

**Effective
Date**

Approved by:	Printed Name	Signature	Date
Laboratory Management			
Medical Director			
Quality Officer			

I-F. Grading and Scoring Serologic Reactions

Purpose

To provide instructions for grading and scoring serologic reactions:

- All hemagglutination tests performed in test tubes.

Background Information

Grading of serologic reactions can be standardized among technologists in an effort to attain uniformity and reproducibility of test results.

Numerical values (scores) may also be assigned to the observed reactions to quantify antigen expression.

Moreover, the requirement that certain reactions (eg, results of tests with anti-A, -B, and -D in Procedure I-A) be of a certain grade (strength) before a test is deemed positive is a recommended quality control measure.

Operational Policy

Do not use +++, ++, +, or − designations, since these can be easily altered.

DO NOT READ TESTS MICROSCOPICALLY because unwanted positive reactions may occur.

Limitations

Unwanted Positive Reactions:

- Overcentrifugation of tests.

Unwanted Negative Reactions:

- Shaking tests too vigorously.

Sample Requirements

Centrifuged hemagglutination tests, in 10 or 12 × 75-mm test tubes.

Equipment/ Materials

Illuminated concave mirror.

White background.

Quality Control

See individual methods.

Procedure   Use the following steps to perform the procedure:

Step	Action
1.	Remove a single tube from the centrifuge head and examine the supernate for hemolysis over a white background. **Note:** Serum surrounding the centrifuged RBC buttons must be inspected for hemolysis. Hemolysis must be regarded as a positive sign of an antigen-antibody reaction if the pretest serum was not hemolyzed and no hemolytic agent was added to the test.
2.	Record the degree of hemolysis if present.
3.	Hold the tube firmly between thumb and forefinger over an illuminated concave mirror.
4.	Adjust the tube so that the RBC button is closest to the mirror.
5.	Dislodge the cell button gently.
6.	Observe the way the RBCs leave the cell button. **Note:** The characteristics of the agglutination should be noted. Loose, "stringy," mixed field, or refractile agglutinates should be recorded as they provide valuable clues in the investigation of aberrant findings.
7.	Interpret reactions as follows: <table><tr><th>If agglutination and/or lysis is...</th><th>Then...</th></tr><tr><td>observed</td><td>grade and score reactions according to Table I-F-1.</td></tr><tr><td>not observed</td><td>the test result is negative; the reaction grade and score are both 0 (zero).</td></tr></table>

References   Marsh WL. Scoring of hemagglutination reactions. Transfusion 1972;12: 352-3.

Roback J, Combs MR, Grossman B, Hillyer C, eds. Technical manual. 16th ed. Bethesda, MD: AABB, 2008 (or current edition).

Effective Date

Approved by:	Printed Name	Signature	Date
Laboratory Management			
Medical Director			
Quality Officer			

Table I-F-1. Grading Serologic Reactions

Grade	Score	Appearance
4+	12	COMPLETE AGGLUTINATION: No unagglutinated RBCs
3+^s	11	Intermediate between 3+ and 4+
3+	10	STRONG REACTION: a few detached masses of agglutinated RBCs; no unagglutinated RBCs
2+^s	9	Intermediate between 2+ and 3+
2+	8	MODERATE REACTION: Large agglutinates in a sea of smaller agglutinates; few unagglutinated RBCs
1+^s	6	Intermediate between 1+ and 2+
1+	5	WEAK REACTION: Many agglutinates of up to 20 RBCs with some smaller agglutinates and unagglutinated RBCs
1+^w	4	Intermediate between ± and 1+
±	3	GRANULAR REACTION: Scattered small agglutinates with many unagglutinated RBCs
w	2	TRACE REACTION: Small agglutinates of 3-4 RBCs with many unagglutinated RBCs
0^r		ROUGH REACTION: RBC button does not disperse smoothly; edge of button appears "rough"; characteristic of some antibodies to Knops-system antigen
0	0	NO REACTION
MF^s		MIXED-FIELD STRONG: Large complete agglutinates with a small number of unagglutinated RBCs
MF		MIXED-FIELD: Moderate-sized agglutinates together with unagglutinated RBCs
MF^w		MIXED-FIELD WEAK: Few clumps of agglutinated RBCs, but the majority of RBCs unagglutinated
H^s		STRONG HEMOLYSIS: Few or no intact RBCs seen
H		MODERATE HEMOLYSIS: Some intact RBCs present
H^w		TRACE HEMOLYSIS: Many intact RBCs present

I-G. Intralaboratory Competency Testing: IAT Reading and Grading Procedure

Purpose

To provide instructions for demonstrating problems in routine antiglobulin testing:

- Cell washer malfunction.
- Standardization of reaction grading between technologists.
- Technologist proficiency documentation and retraining.

Background Information

The following procedure is suggested for identifying two potential sources of error in antiglobulin testing:

- Washing of RBCs before testing with AHG.
- Grading of hemagglutination reactions.

Other potential variables are eliminated as sources of error, thereby permitting identification of automated cell washers that are malfunctioning and technologists who need retraining.

Operational Policy

All cell washers shall be subjected to this testing annually.

All personnel who routinely perform antiglobulin tests shall participate in this testing annually.

Limitations

Unwanted Positive Reactions:

- Overcentrifugation.
- Microscopic examination of tests.
- Bacterial contamination of specimen.
- Improper sample.
- Antibody to a reagent constituent.
- Positive DAT on donor RBCs.
- Polyagglutination of donor RBCs.

<u>Unwanted Negative Reactions:</u>

- Failure to wash RBCs adequately.

- Interrupted testing.

- Use of wrong reagent.

- Loss of activity of AHG reagents.

- Failure to add AHG to the test system.

- Too heavy or too light a cell suspension.

- Omission of RBCs or patient's serum or plasma.

Sample Requirements	Anti-D: ACD- or EDTA-anticoagulated plasma, titer 32-64, from an alloim-munized patient (eg, prenatal patient); 4-5 mL. Dispense into 0.2-mL aliquots and store below –20 C.
	Group O, R_1r RBCs from ACD-anticoagulated whole blood. Dilute to a 50% concentration with Alsever's solution.
	Normal plasma, lacking unexpected antibodies and nonreactive in antiglobulin tests with above RBCs.
Equipment/ Materials	Pipettors with disposable tips to deliver 50-100 µL (VWR, Batavia, IL).
	Graduated pipettes and measuring cylinders.
	Laboratory film: Parafilm (VWR, Batavia, IL).
	IgG-coated RBCs.
	AHG: anti-IgG; need not be heavy-chain specific.
Quality Control	Confirm all negative reactions with IgG-coated RBCs (see Step 11 below).

Procedure for RBC Preparation

Use the following steps to prepare the IgG-coated RBCs:

Step	Action
1.	Titrate anti-D against 2% R_1r RBCs in duplicate by Procedure X-D using normal plasma as diluent for anti-D dilutions. Determine the highest anti-D dilution that reliably yields a 1+ reaction. **Note:** To prepare a 2% RBC suspension, mix 0.1 mL 50% RBCs with 2.4 mL Alsever's solution.
2.	Using 100 µL of undiluted anti-D and normal plasma, prepare a bulk anti-D dilution that will yield a 1+ reaction; mix well. **Note:** If titer from Step 1 is 32, use 3.1 mL plasma; if titer is 64, use 6.3 mL plasma, etc.
3.	In a 13 or 16 × 100-mm test tube, mix 0.1 mL of 50% R_1r RBCs with 2.4 mL of the bulk dilution of anti-D.
4.	Similarly, mix 50 µL 50% R_1r RBCs with 1.2 mL of normal plasma.
5.	Cover the tubes with Parafilm and incubate at 37 C for 1 hour; gently invert the tubes periodically during this time.
6.	Mix well and dispense 0.1 mL of RBCs in anti-D into each of 9 appropriately labeled 10 or 12 × 75-mm test tubes.
7.	Similarly, dispense 0.1 mL of RBCs in normal plasma into each of 3 appropriately labeled 10 or 12 × 75-mm test tubes.
8.	Wash each tube three to four times with saline and completely decant the final wash supernate.
9.	To dry cell buttons, add 2 drops of anti-IgG: • Mix and centrifuge. • Dislodge the cell buttons gently. • Examine macroscopically for agglutination. • Grade and record the results.
10.	Add 1 drop of IgG-coated RBCs to all tubes with negative antiglobulin results: • Mix gently. • Centrifuge. • Examine macroscopically for agglutination. • Grade and record the results.

11.	Analyze the reactions of the IgG-coated RBCs as follows:	
	If agglutination or lysis is...	**Then...**
	present	test is complete: • Proceed as described below.
	absent	test is invalid: • Repeat steps 2-12. • Consider cell washer problem or inactive AHG.
12.	Assign score values (using grading system shown in Table I-F-1) to each reaction score obtained in Step 10.	
13.	Add the scores for all 9 tests with anti-D and divide the sum by 9.	

14.	Analyze the data as follows:		
	If in tubes with anti-D...	**And in tubes with normal plasma...**	**Then...**
	all react, and average score is 5-8	all are nonreactive	anti-D dilution is correct: • Administer competency test.
	all react, but scores are not 5-8	all are nonreactive	anti-D dilution is incorrect: • Adjust dilution and repeat steps 1-14.
	some react, and scores are 5-8	all are nonreactive	repeat steps 2-14: • Consider cell washer problem.

Procedure for Administering the Test

Use the following steps to administer the competency test:

Step	Action
1.	For each technologist or automated cell washer to be evaluated, prepare in bulk at least 2 mL of a 2% suspension of anti-D-coated R_1r RBCs using the dilution factors established above. Prepare this suspension in a single tube or glass vessel (eg, conical flask), depending on the volume required.

2.	Similarly, prepare at least 0.8 mL of a 2% suspension of uncoated R_1r RBCs for each individual study to be performed.
3.	Cover the tubes/flask with Parafilm and incubate at 37 C for 1 hour. Gently mix the suspensions periodically during this time.
4.	Mix each suspension well and dispense 0.1 mL of coated RBCs into each of 9 code-labeled 10 or 12 × 75-mm test tubes.
5.	Similarly, dispense 0.1 mL of uncoated RBCs into each of 3 code-labeled 10 or 12 × 75-mm test tubes. **Note:** Keep a record of the tube numbers containing coated and uncoated RBCs. When several technologists are being evaluated, vary the numbers for the tubes containing coated and uncoated RBCs.
6.	Hand the tubes to the technologist(s) participating in the proficiency testing for washing and testing with AHG.
7.	Provide the technologist with a results sheet on which to document observations; this sheet should contain space to record the technologist's name and the identity of the automated cell washer used.

Procedure for Performing the Test

Use the following steps to perform the competency test:

Step	Action
1.	Wash each tube four times with normal saline and completely decant the final wash supernate.
2.	To dry cell buttons, add 2 drops of anti-IgG: • Mix and centrifuge. • Dislodge the cell buttons gently. • Examine macroscopically for agglutination. • Grade and record the results.
3.	Add 1 drop of IgG-coated RBCs to all tubes with negative antiglobulin results: • Mix gently. • Centrifuge. • Examine macroscopically for agglutination. • Grade and record the results.

4.	Analyze the reactions of the IgG-coated RBCs as follows:	
	If agglutination is...	**Then...**
	present	test is complete.
	absent	test is invalid: • Repeat Steps 1-4. • Consider cell washer problem or inactive AHG.
5.	Return worksheet to person administering the test.	

Procedure for Evaluating the Test Results

Use the following steps to evaluate the competency test results for each participant:

Step	Action	
1.	Confirm that the sum of the scores for the 3 tubes containing R_1r RBCs and normal serum (uncoated RBCs) is 0.	
2.	Confirm that all 9 tubes containing R_1r RBCs and dilute anti-D (coated RBCs) were reactive.	
3.	Confirm that all reactive tests were uniformly reactive (scores = ±2).	
4.	Proceed as follows:	
	If above requirements are...	**Then...**
	met	total the scores of the graded reactions and divide by 9.
	not met	have the technologist repeat the test: • Retrain the technologist if problems persist.
5.	Compare the average score for reactive tubes with the mean of the average scores of all participants.	
6.	Evaluate individual performance as follows:	
	If average score is...	**Then...**
	within ±2 of the mean	test has been passed.
	greater than ±2 of mean	have the technologist repeat the test: • Retrain the technologist if problems persist.

Reference Voak D, Downie DM, Moore BP, et al. Replicate tests for the detection and correction of errors in antiglobulin (AHG) tests: Optimum conditions and quality control. Haematologia 1988;21:3-16.

Effective Date

Approved by:	Printed Name	Signature	Date
Laboratory Management			
Medical Director			
Quality Officer			

Section II. Antibody Detection

This section is devoted to test tube methods for detecting antibodies to RBC antigens. With the exception of Procedures II-C and II-F, the antiglobulin methods described may be used instead of Procedure I-C for antibody detection in pretransfusion and prenatal testing or for crossmatching. In addition, the methods are intended for use in antibody identification studies (see Section VIII). They may be adapted and used for testing RBCs with antibodies to human RBC polymorphisms. Alternative procedures using capillary tubes, gel, and solid phase or microplates are given in Section VI.

Suggested Reading

Code of federal regulations. Title 21 CFR Parts 606 and 660. Washington, DC: US Government Printing Office, 2008 (revised annually).

Price TH, ed. Standards for blood banks and transfusion services. 25th ed. Bethesda, MD: AABB, 2008 (or current edition).

Roback J, Combs MR, Grossman B, Hillyer C, eds. Technical manual. 16th ed. Bethesda, MD: AABB, 2008 (or current edition).

II-A. Testing by Albumin Addition/Layering

Purpose

To provide instructions for using albumin as an enhancement medium for:

- Detecting or identifying unexpected antibodies in serum or plasma.

Background Information

IgG antibodies to RBC antigens may coat RBCs in vitro but not agglutinate them. The coated RBCs may be agglutinated by the addition of bovine albumin, which raises the dielectric constant of the reaction milieu and decreases the zeta-potential (negative electric charge) that exists between RBCs in suspension. This reduction in electric charge reduces intercellular distances, making it possible for IgG molecules to span adjacent RBCs. Macromolecules, such as albumin, may also disrupt and disperse water molecules that are bound to RBC membranes, thus increasing the agglutinable properties of RBCs by reducing the steric hindrance caused by bound water.

Contrary to popular belief, albumin as normally used in the United States (see following procedure) does not potentiate the second stage of antigen-antibody reactions. Rather, any enhancement observed is likely due to increased antibody uptake resulting from use of low-ionic-strength albumin solutions. In contrast, this technique, performed routinely in the United Kingdom, has the capacity to detect IgG antibodies by direct agglutination, including IgG antibodies to Rh, Kell, and Duffy antigens that normally are detected only by antiglobulin procedures.

Operational Policy

Microscopic examination is specifically recommended at Step 5.

This procedure should not be the sole method used for pretransfusion/prenatal testing.

An autologous control is not required when performing antibody detection tests but should be performed the first time antibody identification studies are performed using this method.

Limitations

Unwanted Positive Reactions:

- Antibody to a reagent constituent.
- Contaminated reagents or samples.
- Improperly stored albumin.
- Incorrectly prepared serum-albumin.
- Overcentrifugation of tests.
- Use of wrong reagent or sample.

Unwanted Negative Reactions:

- Omission of serum/plasma, albumin, or reagent RBCs.
- Too heavy or too light a cell suspension.
- Use of wrong reagent or sample.

Sample Requirements

Clotted blood as a source of serum.

Autologous RBCs from clotted or anticoagulated blood: wash three times and dilute to a 2% suspension with saline (to serve as an autocontrol in antibody identification studies; not required for antibody detection).

If used for pretransfusion testing, samples should be those required in Procedure I-A.

Equipment/ Materials

RBCs: 2% suspensions of phenotyped homologous group O RBC samples, plus the autologous RBCs.

Serum-albumin: 30% BSA, 20 mL; group AB serum known to lack unexpected antibodies; 10 mL. Store refrigerated.

Microscope: ×10 magnification (eg, VWR, Batavia, IL).

Test tubes: 6 × 50-mm glass culture tubes (eg, VWR, Batavia, IL).

Quality Control

See quality control protocol for Procedure I-B if using this technique solely to screen samples for unexpected antibodies.

In antibody identification studies, the observed reactions should be consistent with those obtained in antibody detection tests (eg, if anti-E is identified, the R_2R_2 sample used for antibody detection should have been the reactive sample).

Procedure   Use the following steps to perform the procedure:

Step	Action
1.	For each RBC sample to be tested, mix 1 drop of test serum with 1 drop of RBCs in a 6 × 50-mm test tube.
2.	Incubate at 37 C for 90 minutes.
3.	Gently layer serum-albumin over the RBCs by allowing 1 drop to trickle down the inside of the test tube.
4.	Incubate at 37 C for 15-30 minutes.
5.	Using a glass Pasteur pipette, smear RBC button onto a glass slide and examine the RBCs microscopically. **Note:** The end of the Pasteur pipette used to smear RBCs onto the glass slide must be level and not jagged, otherwise it will not be possible to remove RBCs without disturbing agglutinates. For the same reason, the internal bore of the pipette should not be too narrow, yet the outer dimensions must be compatible with the internal measurements of the test tubes.
6.	Interpret the reactions as follows:

If agglutination or lysis is…	Then…
present	reactions are positive.
absent	reactions are negative.

Effective Date

Approved by:	Printed Name	Signature	Date
Laboratory Management			
Medical Director			
Quality Officer			

II-B. Testing by Albumin Antiglobulin

Purpose   To provide instructions for using albumin as a medium for:

- Detecting or identifying unexpected antibodies in serum or plasma.

Background Information   Antibodies to RBC antigens may cause direct agglutination or lysis of RBCs or may coat the RBCs with globulins (eg, IgG, C3). Antibody coating may be accelerated in a low-ionic environment; hence the use of bovine albumin.

This procedure is included so that immunohematology reference laboratories can evaluate samples reported to contain unexpected antibodies in albumin tests, although such tests are now infrequently performed in the United States. Performance of this procedure is believed, mistakenly, to enhance the reactions of Rh and other IgG antibodies. The effect of albumin is to potentiate the second stage of RBC antigen-antibody interactions (agglutination); any enhancement noted with this procedure is likely due to increased antibody uptake associated with use of albumin with an osmolarity lower than that of normal saline. Procedure II-A uses albumin in a manner that does potentiate hemagglutination.

Direct agglutination may be observed following centrifugation of RBC-serum mixtures and is a characteristic effect of IgM antibodies.

RBC lysis may be seen with some antibodies, notably C3-binding anti-A, -B, -Le^a, and -P$_1$.

RBCs incubated with serum/plasma in the presence of bovine albumin at 37 C are washed to remove unbound globulins and tested with AHG. Agglutination by AHG indicates that the RBCs are coated with globulin.

Operational Policy   If used for antibody identification, perform an autocontrol the first time the method is used.

DO NOT READ TESTS MICROSCOPICALLY because unwanted positive reactions may occur.

An autologous control is not required when performing antibody detection tests but should be performed the first time antibody identification studies are performed using this method.

Limitations   Unwanted Positive Reactions:

- Antibody to a reagent constituent.
- Contaminated reagents or samples.
- Improperly stored albumin.
- Overcentrifugation of tests.
- Use of wrong reagent or sample.

Unwanted Negative Reactions:

- Contaminated or inactive reagents.
- Contaminated or inactive sample.
- Failure to add active AHG.
- Failure to wash RBCs free of unbound globulins.
- Incorrectly prepared serum-albumin.
- Interrupted testing.
- Omission of serum/plasma, albumin, or reagent RBCs.
- Too heavy or too light a cell suspension.
- Undercentrifugation of tests.
- Use of wrong reagent or sample.

Sample Requirements   EDTA-anticoagulated whole blood as a source of plasma and red cells. Serum should be used if detection of complement-binding antibodies is required.

Note: If used for pretransfusion testing and the patient has been transfused or pregnant within the preceding 3 months, or if the history is uncertain or unavailable, the sample must be obtained within 3 days of scheduled transfusion.

Equipment/ Materials   AHG: polyspecific or anti-IgG; need not be heavy-chain specific.

22% or 30% BSA.

IgG-coated RBCs.

RBCs: 3%-5% suspensions of phenotyped homologous group O RBC samples, plus the autologous RBCs (to serve as an autocontrol in antibody identification studies; not required for antibody detection or crossmatching).

Quality Control

See quality control protocol for Procedure I-B if using this technique solely to screen samples for unexpected antibodies.

In antibody identification studies, the observed reactions should be consistent with those obtained in antibody detection tests (eg, if anti-E is identified, the R_2R_2 sample used for antibody detection should have been the reactive sample).

In general, observed reactions should be consistent with those obtained by other procedures when used.

Confirm all negative reactions with IgG-coated RBCs.

Procedure

Use the following steps to perform the procedure:

Step	Action
1.	For each RBC sample to be tested, mix 3 drops of test serum, 2 drops of albumin, and 1 drop of RBCs in appropriately labeled 10 or 12 × 75-mm test tubes.
2.	Mix and incubate at 37 C for 30 minutes: • Centrifuge. • Dislodge the cell buttons gently. • Examine macroscopically for agglutination and hemolysis. • Grade and record the results.
3.	Interpret the reactions as follows: <table><tr><td>**If agglutination or lysis is...**</td><td>**Then...**</td></tr><tr><td>present</td><td>reactions are positive.</td></tr><tr><td>absent</td><td>reactions are negative.</td></tr></table>
4.	Wash each tube 3-4 times with normal saline and completely decant the final wash supernate.
5.	To the dry cell buttons, add 2 drops of AHG, polyspecific or anti-IgG: • Mix and centrifuge. • Dislodge the cell buttons gently. • Examine macroscopically for agglutination. • Grade and record the results.

6.	Interpret the reactions as follows:	
	If agglutination or lysis is...	**Then...**
	present	reactions are positive.
	absent	reactions are negative.
	Note: In antibody detection tests, samples yielding positive reactions in either Step 4 or Step 7 should be subjected to antibody identification studies.	
7.	Add 1 drop of IgG-coated RBCs to all tubes with negative antiglobulin results: • Mix and centrifuge. • Dislodge the cell buttons gently. • Examine macroscopically for agglutination. • Grade and record the results.	
8.	Interpret the reactions of the IgG-coated RBCs as follows:	
	If agglutination is...	**Then...**
	present	test is complete.
	absent	test is invalid: • Repeat Steps 1-8. • Consider cell washer problem or inactive AHG.

Reference   Roback J, Combs MR, Grossman B, Hillyer C, eds. Technical manual. 16th ed. Bethesda, MD: AABB, 2008 (or current edition).

Effective Date

Approved by:

	Printed Name	Signature	Date
Laboratory Management			
Medical Director			
Quality Officer			

II-C. Testing by Enzyme Antiglobulin

Purpose

To provide instructions for using enzyme-treated RBCs as an enhancement method for:

- Identifying unexpected antibodies in serum or plasma.

Background Information

Antibodies to RBC antigens may cause direct agglutination or lysis of RBCs, or they may coat the RBCs with globulins (eg, IgG, C3). Such reactions are often enhanced when RBCs are pretreated with proteolytic enzymes. Moreover, some IgG antibodies that normally coat but do not agglutinate RBCs may cause direct agglutination of protease-treated RBCs.

Proteolytic enzymes (eg, ficin) remove glycoproteins from RBCs carrying carbohydrate moieties that include the sialic acid N-acetylneuraminic acid (NeuAc). These NeuAc residues contain a carboxyl group that imparts a negative charge to RBCs. Removal of glycoproteins (and, hence, removal of NeuAc) results in a reduction of cell-surface charge such that IgG molecules can span intercellular distances and cause direct agglutination of RBCs. Water molecules bound to RBC membrane carbohydrates are also removed, thus increasing the agglutinable properties of RBCs by reducing the steric hindrance caused by bound water.

Direct agglutination following centrifugation of RBC-serum mixtures may be seen with protease-treated RBCs and IgG antibodies, notably Rh antibodies.

To detect coating antibodies, enzyme-treated RBCs incubated with serum/plasma at 37 C are washed to remove unbound globulins and tested with AHG. Agglutination by AHG indicates that the RBCs are coated with globulins.

Some sera contain panagglutinins that directly agglutinate enzyme-treated RBCs. These panagglutinins are usually non-C3-binding IgM proteins that dissociate from RBCs during the washing phase before AHG is added. They are not associated with RBC destruction in vivo and are distinct from enzyme-potentiated agglutinins seen in sera containing warm-reactive autoantibodies. It is appropriate to ignore this panagglutinin reactivity if the autologous enzyme-treated RBCs react in the same manner as homologous enzyme-treated RBCs, and subsequently performed antiglobulin tests are nonreactive.

Hemolysis of enzyme-treated RBCs is often an indication of antibody specificities such as anti-Le^a, -Le^b, -Jk^a, -Jk^b, -P$_1$, or -Vel. Some examples of warm- or cold-reactive autoantibodies also hemolyze enzyme-treated RBCs.

Blood group antigens denatured by proteolytic enzymes include Fy^a, Fy^b, M, N, S, s, Xg^a, Ch, Rg, JMH, En^a, Pr, In^a, and In^b. Some examples of anti-U, -Ge, and -Yt^a, as well as antibodies directed towards Knops antigens, may also react weakly or not at all with protease-treated RBCs.

Operational Policy

This procedure should not be used for routine detection of unexpected antibodies in pretransfusion or prenatal testing. It is recommended for antibody identification purposes, especially with sera containing multiple antibody specificities, because some blood group antigens are denatured by such treatment, whereas the reactivity of others is enhanced.

Care should be taken not to overread tests with enzyme-treated RBCs, particularly at the antiglobulin phase. When in suspension, enzyme-treated RBCs may manifest a granular appearance, which should not be confused with weak agglutination. DO NOT READ TESTS MICROSCOP-ICALLY because unwanted positive reactions may occur.

Antiglobulin reagents intended for use in tests with enzyme-treated RBCs must be evaluated for their suitability for use by such techniques.

Routine tests with enzyme-treated RBCs at room temperature or 4 C are not advocated because almost all sera will react due to the presence of enzyme-dependent panagglutinins or enzyme-potentiated cold-reactive agglutinins such as anti-I or -IH.

It is not necessary to perform an enzyme autocontrol routinely when performing antibody identification tests with enzyme-treated RBCs. An auto-control may be indicated if all enzyme test results are positive and the DAT results with untreated RBCs are negative.

Limitations

Unwanted Positive Reactions:

- Antibody to a reagent constituent.

- Contaminated reagents or samples.

- Microscopic examination of tests.

- Overcentrifugation of tests.

- Use of wrong reagent or sample.

Unwanted Negative Reactions:

- Contaminated or inactive reagents.

- Contaminated or inactive sample.

- Failure to add active AHG.

- Failure to wash RBCs free of unbound globulins.

- Incorrectly prepared or inactive enzyme solution.

- Interrupted testing.

- Omission of serum/plasma and/or enzyme-treated RBCs.

- Too heavy or too light a cell suspension.

- Undercentrifugation of tests.

- Use of wrong reagent or sample.

Sample Requirements

Clotted blood as a source of serum. Plasma may be used for the detection/identification of non-C3-binding antibodies.

When investigating positive results of antibody identification tests encountered during pretransfusion testing, samples should be those required in Procedure I-A.

Equipment/ Materials

Polyspecific AHG when using serum to detect complement-binding antibodies, or anti-IgG when using plasma.

Enzyme-treated RBCs: 3%-5% suspensions of phenotyped group O RBC samples plus the autologous RBCs (if desired) treated with proteolytic enzyme (eg, papain or ficin). See Section III.

IgG-coated RBCs.

Quality Control

Observed reactions should be consistent with the specificity of the antibody(ies) identified (eg, IgG Rh antibodies should give enhanced reactions with enzyme-treated RBCs; anti-Fy^a should be nonreactive by this procedure).

If enzyme viability is in question, a known weakly reactive antibody enhanced by enzyme-treated RBCs (eg, Rh) and an antibody directed against an antigen destroyed by enzymes (eg, anti-Fy^a) should be tested against enzyme-treated and untreated RBCs.

Confirm all negative reactions with IgG-coated RBCs.

Procedure   Use the following steps to perform the procedure:

Step	Action
1.	For each enzyme-treated RBC sample to be tested, mix 2 or 3 drops of test serum with 1 drop of RBCs in appropriately labeled 10 or 12 × 75-mm test tubes.
2.	Mix and incubate at 37 C for 30-60 minutes: • DO NOT CENTRIFUGE. • Dislodge the cell buttons gently. • Examine the RBCs macroscopically. • Grade and record the results.
3.	Interpret the reactions as follows:

If agglutination or lysis is...	Then...
present	reactions are positive.
absent	reactions are negative.

Step	Action
4.	Wash each tube three to four times with normal saline and completely decant the final wash supernate.
5.	To the dry cell buttons, add 2 drops of AHG: • Mix and centrifuge. • Dislodge the cell buttons gently. • Examine macroscopically for agglutination. • Grade and record the results.
6.	Interpret the reactions as follows:

If agglutination is...	Then...
present	reactions are positive.
absent	reactions are negative.

Step	Action
7.	Add 1 drop of IgG-coated RBCs to all tubes with negative antiglobulin results: • Mix and centrifuge. • Dislodge the cell buttons gently. • Examine macroscopically for agglutination. • Grade and record the results.
8.	Interpret the reactions of the IgG-coated RBCs as follows:

If agglutination is...	Then...
present	test is complete.
absent	test is invalid: • Repeat Steps 1-8. • Consider cell washer problem or inactive AHG.

References

Roback J, Combs MR, Grossman B, Hillyer C, eds. Technical manual. 16th ed. Bethesda, MD: AABB, 2008 (or current edition).

Rolih S, Albietz C, eds. Enzymes, inhibitions, and adsorptions. Washington, DC: AABB, 1981.

Effective Date

Approved by:	Printed Name	Signature	Date
Laboratory Management			
Medical Director			
Quality Officer			

II-D. Testing by LIP Antiglobulin

Purpose   To provide instructions for using the low-ionic Polybrene (Sigma-Aldrich, St Louis, MO) procedure (LIP procedure) as an enhancement method for:

- Detecting and identifying unexpected antibodies in serum or plasma.

Background Information   Cationic polymers such as Polybrene cause aggregation of normal RBCs that can be dispersed with sodium citrate. However, sodium citrate does not disperse Polybrene-induced aggregation of antibody-coated RBCs. In the LIP procedure, RBCs are first incubated with serum under low-ionic conditions to facilitate antibody uptake. Polybrene induces aggregation of RBCs; if antibody has coated the RBCs, immunoglobulin molecules form bridges between adjacent RBCs that persist after sodium citrate is added.

Operational Policy   Do not use polyspecific AHG when testing clotted blood samples because C3 coating will yield unwanted positive tests.

DO NOT READ TESTS MICROSCOPICALLY because unwanted positive reactions may occur.

An autologous control is not required when performing antibody detection tests but should be performed the first time antibody identification studies are performed using this method.

Limitations   Unwanted Positive Reactions:

- Antibody to a reagent constituent.
- Contaminated reagents or samples.
- Improperly stored reagents.
- Incorrectly prepared reagents.
- Microscopic examination of tests.
- Overcentrifugation of tests.
- Use of wrong reagent or sample.

Unwanted Negative Reactions:

- Contaminated or inactive reagents.

- Contaminated or inactive sample.

- Failure to add active AHG.

- Failure to wash RBCs free of unbound globulins.

- Incorrectly prepared reagents.

- Interrupted testing.

- Omission of serum/plasma, LIP solutions, or reagent RBCs.

- Too heavy or too light a cell suspension.

- Use of wrong reagents.

Sample Requirements	Clotted or EDTA-anticoagulated blood as a source of serum/plasma. DO NOT USE SAMPLES ANTICOAGULATED WITH HEPARIN (Polybrene is a heparin antagonist).
	Autologous RBCs from clotted or EDTA-anticoagulated blood: wash three times with saline before use.
	Note: An autologous control is not required when performing antibody detection tests but should be performed the first time antibody identification studies are completed using this method.
	If used for pretransfusion testing, samples should be those required in Procedure I-A.
Equipment/ Materials	AHG: Anti-IgG; need not be heavy-chain specific.
	Control anti-D serum: 1:10,000 dilution (in AB serum) of commercially available, modified tube anti-D serum.
	Note: This yields a negative test result with Rh-positive RBCs in LISS-antiglobulin tests (see following procedure).
	Group AB serum.
	IgG-coated RBCs.
	Low-ionic medium (LIM).
	Polybrene working solution.
	Polybrene neutralizing solution.
	RBCs: 3%-5% suspensions of phenotyped homologous group O RBC samples, plus the autologous RBCs (to serve as an autocontrol in antibody identification studies; not required for antibody detection or crossmatching).

Quality Control

See quality control protocol for Procedure I-B when using this technique solely to screen samples for unexpected antibodies.

Perform positive and negative control tests each time this procedure is performed (see note at Step 1 below).

Observed reactions should be consistent with those obtained in antibody detection tests (eg, if anti-E is identified, the R_2R_2 sample used for antibody detection should have been the reactive sample).

In general, observed reactions should be consistent with those obtained by other procedures when used.

Confirm all negative reactions with IgG-coated RBCs.

Procedure

Use the following steps to perform the procedure:

Step	Action
1.	Wash 1 drop of each RBC sample with normal saline in appropriately labeled 10 or 12 × 75-mm test tubes. **Note:** Include 2 tubes containing Rh-positive RBCs for controls.
2.	Prepare 1% RBC suspensions by gently decanting the supernate and shaking the contents of the tubes lightly to resuspend the RBCs. Decant the tubes to leave 1 drop of 1% RBCs.
3.	Add 0.1 mL of test serum and 1 mL of low-ionic medium to appropriate tubes. Mix and incubate at room temperature for 1 minute.
4.	Similarly, set up positive and negative controls with Rh-positive RBCs and dilute anti-D and AB serum, respectively. Mix and incubate at room temperature for 1 minute.
5.	Add 0.1 mL of aggregating solution to each tube and mix.
6.	Centrifuge at 1000 × g for 10 seconds (or equivalent) and decant the supernate. **Note:** DO NOT RESUSPEND THE RBCs.
7.	Add 0.1 mL of neutralizing solution.
8.	Gently shake the tubes (shake rack gently at 45-degree angle for 10 seconds) and observe for persistent agglutination. Grade and record the results. **Note:** Compare tests with negative control samples when examining for persistence of agglutination after the addition of neutralizing reagent.

9.	Interpret the reactions as follows:	
	If agglutination is...	**Then...**
	present	reactions are positive.
	absent	reactions are negative.

10.	Wash the RBCs three to four times with saline and completely decant the final wash supernate.

11.	To the dry cell buttons, add 2 drops of AHG: • Mix and centrifuge. • Dislodge the cell buttons gently. • Examine macroscopically for agglutination. • Grade and record the results.

12.	Interpret the reactions as follows:	
	If agglutination is...	**Then...**
	present	reactions are positive.
	absent	reactions are negative.

Note: Samples yielding positive reactions in either Step 8 or Step 11 should be subjected to antibody identification studies.

13.	Add 1 drop of IgG-coated RBCs to all tubes with negative antiglobulin results: • Mix and centrifuge. • Dislodge the cell buttons gently. • Examine macroscopically for agglutination. • Grade and record the results.

14.	Interpret the reactions of the IgG-coated RBCs as follows:	
	If agglutination is...	**Then...**
	present	test is complete.
	absent	test is invalid: • Repeat Steps 1-14. • Consider cell washer problem or inactive AHG.

Reference Lalezari P, Jiang AF. The manual Polybrene test: A simple and rapid procedure for detection of red cell antibodies. Transfusion 1980;20:206-11.

**Effective
Date**

Approved by:	Printed Name	Signature	Date
Laboratory Management			
Medical Director			
Quality Officer			

II-E. Testing by LISS Wash Antiglobulin

Purpose

To provide instructions for using a low-ionic-strength saline (LISS) wash solution:

- For detecting or identifying unexpected antibodies in serum or plasma.

- As an alternative to the LISS additive procedure (I-B) in Section I.

Background Information

Antibodies to RBC antigens may cause direct agglutination or complement-mediated lysis of RBCs or may coat RBCs with IgG and/or C3.

Direct agglutination and/or lysis may be observed following centrifugation of RBC/serum mixtures.

Antibody coating may be accelerated in a low-ionic environment; hence the use of LISS.

RBCs incubated with serum/plasma in the presence of LISS at 37 C are washed to remove unbound globulins and tested with AHG. Agglutination by AHG indicates that the RBCs are coated with globulins.

Note: Detection of C3-coating antibodies is not required when performing routine pretransfusion and prenatal testing.

Operational Policy

If used for antibody identification, perform an autocontrol the first time the method is used.

DO NOT READ TESTS MICROSCOPICALLY because unwanted positive reactions may occur.

An autologous control is not required when performing antibody detection tests but should be performed the first time antibody identification studies are performed using this method.

Limitations

Unwanted Positive Reactions:

- Antibody to a reagent constituent.

- Contaminated reagents or samples.

- Improperly stored reagents.

- Incorrectly prepared reagents.

- Microscopic examination of tests.

- Overcentrifugation of tests.

- Use of wrong reagent or sample.

Unwanted Negative Reactions:

- Contaminated or inactive reagents.

- Contaminated or inactive sample.

- Failure to add AHG to the test system.

- Failure to add equal volumes of serum and LISS-suspended RBCs.

- Failure to wash RBCs adequately.

- Interrupted testing.

- Loss of activity of AHG reagents.

- Omission of RBCs or patient's serum or plasma.

- Too heavy or too light a cell suspension.

- Undercentrifugation of tests.

- Use of wrong reagent or sample.

Sample Requirements

EDTA-anticoagulated whole blood as a source of plasma and red cells. Serum should be used if detection of complement-binding antibodies is required.

Note: If used for pretransfusion testing and the patient has been transfused or pregnant within the preceding 3 months, or if the history is uncertain or unavailable, the sample must be obtained within 3 days of scheduled transfusion.

Equipment/ Materials

AHG: polyspecific or anti-IgG.

Filter or tissue paper.

RBCs: 3%-5% suspensions of phenotyped group O RBCs.

IgG-coated RBCs.

LISS wash solution.

Quality Control

See quality control protocol for Procedure I-B if using this technique solely to screen samples for unexpected antibodies.

In antibody identification studies, the observed reactions should be consistent with those obtained in antibody detection tests (eg, if anti-E is identified, the R_2R_2 sample used for antibody detection should have been the reactive sample).

In general, observed reactions should be consistent with those obtained by other procedures when used.

Confirm all negative reactions with IgG-coated RBCs.

Procedure   Use the following steps to perform the procedure:

Step	Action
1.	Wash 1 drop of each RBC sample to be tested with LISS in appropriately labeled 10 or 12 × 75-mm test tubes. Completely decant the supernate and blot the ends of inverted tubes with filter or tissue paper.
2.	Add 2 drops of LISS and 2 drops of test serum to each RBC sample. **Note:** Use uniform-bore Pasteur pipettes to dispense serum and LISS-suspended RBCs to ensure addition of equal volumes of serum/plasma and reagent RBCs.
3.	Mix and incubate at 37 C for 15 minutes: • Centrifuge. • Dislodge the cell buttons gently. • Examine macroscopically for agglutination and hemolysis. • Grade and record the results.
4.	Interpret the reactions as follows:

If agglutination or lysis is...	Then...
present	reactions are positive.
absent	reactions are negative.

Step	Action
5.	Wash each tube three to four times with normal saline and completely decant the final wash supernate.
6.	To the dry cell buttons, add 2 drops of AHG: • Mix and centrifuge. • Dislodge the cell buttons gently. • Examine macroscopically for agglutination. • Grade and record the results.
7.	Interpret the reactions as follows:

If agglutination is...	Then...
present	reactions are positive.
absent	reactions are negative.

Note: In antibody detection tests, samples yielding positive reactions in Steps 4 and/or 7 should be subjected to antibody identification studies.

8.	Add 1 drop of IgG-coated RBCs to all tubes with negative antiglobulin results: • Mix and centrifuge. • Dislodge the cell buttons gently. • Examine macroscopically for agglutination. • Grade and record the results.	
9.	Interpret the reactions of the IgG-coated RBCs as follows:	
	If agglutination is…	**Then…**
	present	test is complete.
	absent	test is invalid: • Repeat Steps 1-9. • Consider cell washer problem or inactive AHG.

Reference   Löw B, Messeter L. Antiglobulin tests in low-ionic strength salt solutions for rapid antibody screening and crossmatching. Vox Sang 1974;26:53-61.

Effective Date

Approved by:	Printed Name	Signature	Date
Laboratory Management			
Medical Director			
Quality Officer			

II-F. Testing by LISS-Ficin Antiglobulin

Purpose

To provide instructions for using enzyme-treated RBCs and LISS as an enhancement method for:

- Identifying unexpected antibodies in serum or plasma—especially Kidd-system antibodies—that do not give clear-cut reactions by LISS or ficin tests alone.

Background Information

It is likely that enhancement of Kidd antibodies results from the combined effect of increased antibody-uptake induced by LISS and the increased complement-binding properties and agglutinability of protease-treated RBCs (see appropriate procedures elsewhere in this Section).

Antibodies to RBC antigens may cause direct agglutination or lysis of RBCs or may coat the RBCs with globulins (eg, IgG, C3). Such reactions are often enhanced when RBCs are pretreated with proteolytic enzymes. Moreover, some IgG antibodies that normally coat but do not agglutinate RBCs may cause direct agglutination of protease-treated RBCs.

Proteolytic enzymes (eg, ficin) remove glycoproteins from RBCs carrying carbohydrate moieties that include the sialic acid *N*-acetylneuraminic acid (NeuAc). These NeuAc residues contain a carboxyl group that imparts a negative charge to RBCs. Removal of glycoproteins (and, hence, removal of NeuAc) results in a reduction of cell surface charge such that IgG molecules can span intercellular distances and cause direct agglutination of RBCs. Water molecules bound to RBC membrane carbohydrates are also removed, thus increasing the agglutinable properties of RBCs by reducing the steric hindrance caused by bound water.

Direct agglutination following centrifugation of RBC/serum mixtures may be seen with protease-treated RBCs and IgG antibodies, notably Rh antibodies. Other antibodies, notably C3-binding anti-A, -B, -Le[a], and -P$_1$, may cause direct lysis of protease-treated RBCs.

To detect coating antibodies, enzyme-treated RBCs incubated with serum/plasma at 37 C are washed to remove unbound globulins and tested with AHG. Agglutination by AHG indicates that the RBCs are coated with globulins.

Some sera contain panagglutinins that directly agglutinate enzyme-treated RBCs. These panagglutinins are usually non-C3-binding IgM proteins that dissociate from RBCs during the washing phase before AHG is added. They are not associated with RBC destruction in vivo and are distinct from enzyme-potentiated agglutinins seen in sera containing warm-reactive autoantibodies. It is appropriate to ignore this panagglutinin reactivity if the autologous enzyme-treated RBCs react in the same manner as homologous enzyme-treated RBCs, and subsequently performed antiglobulin tests are nonreactive.

Hemolysis of enzyme-treated RBCs is often an indication of antibody specificities such as anti-Le^a, -Le^b, -Jk^a, -Jk^b, -P$_1$, or -Vel. Some examples of warm- or cold-reactive autoantibodies also hemolyze enzyme-treated RBCs.

Blood group antigens denatured by proteolytic enzymes include Fy^a, Fy^b, M, N, S, s, Xg^a, Ch, Rg, JMH, En^a, Pr, In^a, and In^b. Some examples of anti-U, -Ge, and -Yt^a, as well as antibodies directed towards Knops antigens, may also react weakly or not at all with protease-treated RBCs.

Operational Policy

This procedure should not be used for routine detection of unexpected antibodies in pretransfusion or prenatal testing. It is recommended for antibody identification purposes only.

Reactivity of enzyme-dependent panagglutinins and cold-reactive auto-antibodies is enhanced by this procedure; their presence can obscure the reactivity of alloantibodies. In cases where Kidd antibodies are suspected, prior adsorption of the serum with ficin-treated Jk(a–) or Jk(b–) RBCs (as appropriate) will facilitate alloantibody recognition.

Care should be taken not to overread tests with enzyme-treated RBCs. When in suspension, enzyme-treated RBCs may manifest a granular appearance, which should not be confused with weak agglutination.

DO NOT READ TESTS MICROSCOPICALLY because unwanted positive reactions may occur.

Routine tests with enzyme-treated RBCs at room temperature or 4 C are not advocated because almost all sera will react due to the presence of enzyme-dependent panagglutinins or enzyme-potentiated cold-reactive agglutinins such as anti-I or -HI.

An autologous control is not required when performing antibody detection tests but should be performed the first time antibody identification studies are performed using this method.

Limitations

Unwanted Positive Reactions:

- Antibody to a reagent constituent.

- Contaminated reagents or samples.

- Improperly stored reagents.

- Incorrectly prepared reagents.

- Microscopic examination of tests.

- Overcentrifugation of tests.

- Use of wrong reagent or sample.

- Overtreatment of RBCs with enzyme.

Unwanted Negative Reactions:

- Contaminated or inactive reagents.

- Contaminated or inactive sample.

- Failure to add AHG to the test system.

- Failure to add equal volumes of serum and LISS-suspended RBCs.

- Failure to wash RBCs adequately.

- Inactive enzyme solution or undertreatment of RBCs with enzyme.

- Interrupted testing.

- Loss of activity of AHG reagents.

- Omission of RBCs or patient's serum or plasma.

- Too heavy or too light a cell suspension.

- Undercentrifugation of tests.

- Use of wrong reagent or sample.

Sample Requirements

Clotted blood as a source of serum. Because the procedure is used to enhance C3-binding Kidd antibodies, the serum should be freshly collected.

Autologous RBCs from clotted or anticoagulated blood: treat with a proteolytic enzyme in parallel with reagent RBCs.

Note: An autocontrol should be tested the first time this procedure is used.

When investigating positive results of antibody identification tests encountered during pretransfusion testing, samples should be those required in Procedure I-A.

Equipment/ Materials

AHG: polyspecific or anti-IgG.

Enzyme-treated RBCs: 3%-5% suspensions of phenotyped group O RBC samples, plus the autologous RBCs (if desired) treated with ficin (see Section III).

Filter or tissue paper.

LISS wash solution.

Quality Control

Reactions should be equal to or stronger than those obtained with LISS alone (Procedure II-E) or by ficin/papain alone (Procedure II-C).

Consider testing an anti-Fy^a and an Rh antibody vs enzyme-treated and untreated RBCs if enzyme viability is in question.

Follow the manufacturer's directions for appropriate quality control when using commercially prepared enzyme solutions.

Confirm all negative reactions with IgG-coated RBCs.

Procedure   Use the following steps to perform the procedure:

Step	Action
1.	Wash 1 drop of each ficin-treated RBC sample with LISS in appropriately labeled 10 or 12 × 75-mm test tubes. Completely decant the supernate and blot the ends of inverted tubes with filter or tissue paper.
2.	To each enzyme-treated RBC sample to be tested, add 2 drops of LISS and 2 drops of test serum. **Note:** Use uniform-bore Pasteur pipettes to dispense serum and LISS-suspended RBCs to ensure addition of equal volumes of serum/plasma and reagent RBCs.
3.	Mix and incubate at 37 C for 30-60 minutes: • Centrifuge. • Dislodge the cell buttons gently. • Examine macroscopically for agglutination and hemolysis. • Grade and record the results.
4.	Interpret the reactions as follows: | If agglutination or lysis is...	Then...
present	reactions are positive.
absent	reactions are negative.	
5.	Wash each tube three to four times with normal saline and completely decant the final wash supernate.
6.	To the dry cell buttons, add 2 drops of polyspecific AHG: • Mix and centrifuge. • Dislodge the cell buttons gently. • Examine macroscopically for agglutination. • Grade and record the results.
7.	Interpret the reactions as follows: | If agglutination is...	Then...
present	reactions are positive.
absent	reactions are negative.	

8.	Add 1 drop of IgG-coated RBCs to all tubes with negative antiglobulin results: • Mix and centrifuge. • Dislodge the cell buttons gently. • Examine macroscopically for agglutination. • Grade and record the results.
9.	Interpret the reactions of the IgG-coated RBCs as follows:

If agglutination is…	Then…
present	test is complete.
absent	test is invalid: • Repeat Steps 1-6. • Consider cell washer problem or inactive AHG.

Reference   Nance S, Gonzalez B, Postoway N, et al. Clinical significance of a primarily complement-dependent anti-Jk^a in a patient who received Jk(a+) red cells (abstract). Transfusion 1985;25:482.

Effective Date

Approved by:	Printed Name	Signature	Date
Laboratory Management			
Medical Director			
Quality Officer			

II-G. Testing by Polyethylene Glycol Antiglobulin

Purpose

To provide instructions for using polyethylene glycol (PEG) as an enhancement medium for:

- Detecting or identifying unexpected antibodies in serum or plasma.

Note: The following procedure is also recommended as an alternative to LISS for routine antibody detection/identification. In addition, it may be used as a supplement to other procedures when weak reactions are encountered.

Background Information

The mechanism by which PEG enhances antigen-antibody interactions is not fully understood. It may pull water molecules away from the RBC membrane. Its effect is to allow for improved antibody sensitization and agglutination.

Serum/plasma proteins can precipitate when PEG is added, giving the test mixture a cloudy appearance.

Anti-IgG is the AHG reagent of choice when using PEG. It is recommended over polyspecific AHG to avoid unwanted positive reactions due to complement-binding cold auto- or alloantibodies.

The addition of PEG to serum or plasma from patients with an IgG monoclonal gammopathy may result in IgG deposition on RBCs. This may lead to the inability to validate negative antiglobulin test results with IgG-coated RBCs. Failure to validate such negative results may also arise from deposition of fibrinogen-IgG complexes onto RBCs when using plasma samples. In such circumstances, additional washes (eg, six to eight washes instead of three to four) may be necessary to validate negative results. If extra washes do not alleviate the problem, an alternative method should be chosen for antibody detection/identification.

PEG is known to enhance autoantibody reactivity. All RBCs will be reactive, including the autocontrol.

Operational Policy

Do not centrifuge after 37 C incubation. RBCs will not resuspend easily.

Microscopic examination is not recommended when using PEG because of increased binding of autoantibodies.

An autologous control is not required when performing antibody detection tests but should be performed the first time antibody identification studies are performed using this method.

Limitations   Underwanted Positive Reactions:

- Antibody to a reagent constituent.

- Contaminated reagents or samples.

- Microscopic examination of tests.

- Overcentrifugation of tests.

- Use of wrong reagent or sample.

Unwanted Negative Reactions:

- Contaminated or inactive reagents.

- Contaminated or inactive sample.

- Failure to add active AHG.

- Failure to wash RBCs free of unbound globulins.

- Fibrinogen-IgG deposition on RBCs when using plasma.

- Interrupted testing.

- Omission of serum/plasma, PEG, or reagent RBCs.

- Too heavy or too light a cell suspension.

- Undercentrifugation of tests.

- Use of wrong reagent or sample.

Sample Requirements   EDTA-anticoagulated whole blood as a source of plasma and red cells.

Note: If used for pretransfusion testing and the patient has been transfused or pregnant within the preceding 3 months, or if the history is uncertain or unavailable, the sample must be obtained within 3 days of scheduled transfusion.

Equipment/ Materials   RBCs: 3%-5% suspensions of phenotyped homologous group O RBC samples, plus the autologous RBCs (to serve as an autocontrol in antibody identification studies; not required for antibody detection or crossmatching).

AHG: anti-IgG.

IgG-coated RBCs.

PEG: 20% wt/vol.

Quality Control

See quality control protocol for Procedure I-B if using this technique solely to screen samples for unexpected antibodies.

Observed reactions should be consistent with those obtained in antibody detection tests (eg, if anti-E is identified, the R_2R_2 sample used for antibody detection should have been the reactive sample).

In general, observed reactions should be consistent with those obtained by other procedures when used.

Confirm all negative reactions with IgG-coated RBCs.

Procedure

Step	Action
1.	For each RBC sample to be tested, mix 2 drops of test serum, 4 drops of PEG, and 1 drop of RBCs in appropriately labeled 10 or 12 × 75-mm test tubes.
2.	Incubate at 37 C for 15-30 minutes.
3.	DO NOT CENTRIFUGE. Wash each tube three to four times with normal saline and completely decant the final wash supernate.
4.	To the dry cell buttons, add 2 drops of AHG: • Mix and centrifuge. • Dislodge the cell buttons gently. • Examine macroscopically for agglutination. • Grade and record the results.
5.	Interpret the reactions as follows:

If agglutination or lysis is…	Then…
present	reactions are positive.
absent	reactions are negative.

Note: In antibody detection tests, samples yielding positive reactions in Step 5 should be subjected to antibody identification studies.

6.	Interpret the reactions as follows:

If agglutination or lysis is…	Then…
present	reactions are positive.
absent	reactions are negative.

Note: In antibody detection tests, samples yielding positive reactions in Step 5 should be subjected to antibody identification studies.

7.	Add 1 drop of IgG-coated RBCs to all tubes with negative antiglobulin results: • Mix gently. • Centrifuge. • Examine macroscopically for agglutination. • Grade and record the results.	
8.	Interpret the reactions of the IgG-coated RBCs as follows:	
	If agglutination is…	**Then…**
	present	test is complete.
	absent	test is invalid: • Repeat Steps 1-8. • Consider cell washer problem or inactive AHG.

Reference

Nance S, Garratty G. Polyethylene glycol: A new potentiator of red blood cell antigen-antibody reactions. Am J Pathol 1987;87:633-5.

Roback J, Combs MR, Grossman B, Hillyer C, eds. Technical manual. 16th ed. Bethesda, MD: AABB, 2008 (or current edition).

Effective Date

Approved by:	Printed Name	Signature	Date
Laboratory Management			
Medical Director			
Quality Officer			

Judd's Methods in Immunohematology
Testing for Cold-Reactive Antibodies by Direct Agglutination
Page 1 of 3

II-H. Testing for Cold-Reactive Antibodies by Direct Agglutination

Purpose

To provide instructions for identification of cold-reactive antibodies:

- IgM alloantibodies (eg, anti-M, -Le^a, -P$_1$).
- IgM autoantibodies (eg, anti-I).

Background Information

IgM antibodies to RBC antigens cause direct agglutination of RBCs. Usually such antibodies are optimally reactive at cold temperatures. Direct agglutination and/or lysis may be observed following centrifugation of RBC/serum mixtures. Agglutination is enhanced if serum/cell mixtures are incubated at or below room temperature before centrifugation.

Given that many cold-reactive autoantibodies possess anti-I, -IH, and -i specificity, it may be helpful to include cord or adult I-negative RBCs in the test.

Operational Policy

Do not allow 4 C tests to warm during centrifugation. If a cold room in which a centrifuge may be placed is not available, return the centrifuged tubes to the refrigerator for 5 minutes before reading.

An autologous control should be performed the first time antibody identification studies are performed using this method.

Limitations

Unwanted Positive Reactions:

- Antibody to a reagent constituent.
- Contaminated reagents or samples.
- Microscopic examination of tests.
- Overcentrifugation of tests.
- Use of wrong reagent or sample.

Unwanted Negative Reactions:

- Omission of plasma, albumin, or reagent RBCs.
- Too heavy or too light a cell suspension.
- Use of wrong reagent or sample.

Sample

Clotted or anticoagulated blood as a source of serum or plasma.

Autologous RBCs from clotted or anticoagulated blood: wash three times with saline before use.

Equipment/ Materials

RBCs: 3%-5% suspensions of phenotyped group O RBCs, including I-negative RBCs; RBCs of the same ABO type as the autologous RBCs (if other than group O) and A_1 status if group A or AB; plus the autologous RBCs (to serve as an autocontrol in antibody identification studies).

Quality Control

Observed reactions should be consistent with those obtained in antibody detection tests (eg, if anti-Le^a is identified, the Le(a+) sample used for antibody detection should have been the reactive sample).

In general, observed reactions should be consistent with those obtained by other procedures when used (eg, reactions with IgM antibodies should be stronger than those obtained in Procedure II-A).

Procedure

Use the following steps to perform antibody detection of cold-reactive allo- and autoantibodies:

Step	Action
1.	For each RBC sample to be tested, mix 2-3 drops of test serum with 1 drop of RBCs in appropriately labeled 10 or 12 × 75-mm test tubes.
2.	Mix and incubate at RT for 15-30 minutes: • Centrifuge. • Dislodge the cell buttons gently. • Examine macroscopically for agglutination and hemolysis. • Grade and record the results.
3.	Interpret the reactions as follows:<table><tr><td>**If agglutination or lysis is…**</td><td>**Then…**</td></tr><tr><td>present</td><td>reactions are positive.</td></tr><tr><td>absent</td><td>reactions are negative.</td></tr></table>
4.	If positive and negative tests are observed, determine the antibody specificity. No further testing is necessary if a blood group specificity may be assigned to the reactions. If not, proceed to Step 5.

5.	Mix and incubate at 4 C for 30-60 minutes:
	• Centrifuge.
	Note: Do not allow 4 C tests to warm during centrifugation. If a cold room in which a centrifuge may be placed is not available, return the centrifuged tubes to the refrigerator for 5 minutes before reading.
	• Dislodge the cell buttons gently.
	• Examine macroscopically for agglutination and hemolysis.
	• Grade and record the results.

6.	Interpret the reactions as follows:	
	If agglutination or lysis is...	**Then...**
	present	reactions are positive.
	absent	reactions are negative.

7.	Determine the antibody specificity and/or perform additional studies as necessary.

Reference   Roback J, Combs MR, Grossman B, Hillyer C, eds. Technical manual. 16th ed. Bethesda, MD: AABB, 2008 (or current edition).

Effective Date

Approved by:

	Printed Name	Signature	Date
Laboratory Management			
Medical Director			
Quality Officer			

II-I. Testing by Saline Indirect Antiglobulin

Purpose

To provide instructions for:

- Detecting or identifying unexpected warm-reactive allo- and autoanti-bodies in serum or plasma without the use of enhancement reagents.

Background Information

Antibodies to RBC antigens may cause direct agglutination or lysis of RBCs or may coat the RBCs with globulins (eg, IgG, C3).

Direct agglutination may be observed following centrifugation of RBC-serum mixtures and is a characteristic effect of IgM antibodies.

RBC lysis may be seen in serum tests with some antibodies, notably C3-binding anti-A, -B, -Le^a, and -P$_1$.

To detect coating antibodies, RBCs incubated with serum/plasma at 37 C are washed to remove unbound globulins and tested with AHG. Agglutination by AHG indicates that the RBCs are coated with globulins.

Operational Policy

Do not allow 4 C tests to warm during centrifugation. If a cold room in which a centrifuge may be placed is not available, return the centrifuged tubes to the refrigerator for 5 minutes before reading.

Refrigerator temperature is suitable for routine 4 C studies.

In instances where both auto- and alloagglutinins are present, elucidation of alloagglutinin specificity may be facilitated by incubation at 12-16 C.

An autologous control is not required when performing antibody detection tests but should be performed the first time antibody identification studies are performed using this method.

Limitations

Unwanted Positive Reactions:

- Antibody to a reagent constituent.
- Contaminated reagents or samples.
- Microscopic examination of tests.
- Overcentrifugation of tests.
- Use of wrong reagent or sample.

Unwanted Negative Reactions:

- Omission of serum/plasma, albumin, or reagent RBCs.

- Too heavy or too light a cell suspension.

- Use of wrong reagent or sample.

Sample Requirements

EDTA-anticoagulated whole blood as a source of plasma and red cells. Serum should be used if detection of complement-binding antibodies is required.

Note: If used for pretransfusion testing and the patient has been transfused or pregnant within the preceding 3 months, or if the history is uncertain or unavailable, the sample must be obtained within 3 days of scheduled transfusion.

Equipment/ Materials

AHG: polyspecific or anti-IgG; need not be heavy-chain specific.

IgG-coated RBCs.

RBCs: 3%-5% suspensions of phenotyped homologous group O RBC samples, plus the autologous RBCs (to serve as an autocontrol in antibody identification studies; not required for antibody detection or crossmatching).

Quality Control

See quality control protocol for Procedure I-B if using this technique solely to screen samples for unexpected antibodies.

In antibody identification studies, the observed reactions should be consistent with those obtained in antibody detection tests (eg, if anti-E is identified, the R_2R_2 sample used for antibody detection should have been the reactive sample).

In general, observed reactions should be consistent with those obtained by other procedures when used.

Confirm all negative reactions with IgG-coated RBCs.

Procedure

Use the following steps to perform the procedure:

Step	Action
1.	For each RBC sample to be tested, mix 3 drops of test serum and 1 drop of RBCs in appropriately labeled 10 or 12 × 75-mm test tubes.

2.	Mix and incubate at 37 C for 30-60 minutes: • Centrifuge. • Dislodge the cell buttons gently. • Examine macroscopically for agglutination and hemolysis • Grade and record the results.
3.	Interpret the reactions as follows: **If agglutination or lysis is...** / **Then...** present / reactions are positive. absent / reactions are negative.
4.	Wash each tube three to four times with normal saline and completely decant the final wash supernate.
5.	To the dry cell buttons, add 2 drops of AHG: • Mix and centrifuge. • Dislodge the cell buttons gently. • Examine macroscopically for agglutination. • Grade and record the results.
6.	Interpret the reactions as follows: **If agglutination or lysis is...** / **Then...** present / reactions are positive. absent / reactions are negative. **Note:** In antibody detection tests, samples yielding positive reactions in either Step 3 or Step 6 should be subjected to antibody identification studies.
7.	Add 1 drop of IgG-coated RBCs to all tubes with negative antiglobulin results: • Mix and centrifuge. • Dislodge the cell buttons gently. • Examine macroscopically for agglutination. • Grade and record the results.
8.	Interpret the reactions of the IgG-coated RBCs as follows: **If agglutination is...** / **Then...** present / test is complete. absent / test is invalid: • Repeat Steps 1-8. • Consider cell washer problem or inactive AHG.

Reference   Roback J, Combs MR, Grossman B, Hillyer C, eds. Technical manual. 16th ed. Bethesda, MD: AABB, 2008 (or current edition).

Effective Date

Approved by:	Printed Name	Signature	Date
Laboratory Management			
Medical Director			
Quality Officer			

Section III. Enzyme Techniques

The treatment of RBCs with proteolytic enzymes is invaluable in blood group serology. The serologic reactivity of some antibodies may be enhanced, whereas that of others is abolished. This results from the susceptibility of RBC membrane proteins to different proteolytic enzymes.

Serologic enhancement is due, at least in part, to cleavage of glycoproteins that carry *N*-acetylneuraminic acid, a sialic acid with a negatively charged carboxyl group that contributes considerably to the RBC surface charge. Because like charges repel, normal RBCs are kept apart at a distance too great for IgG immunoglobulin molecules to span. It is the second stage (cross-linking) of the antigen-antibody reaction that is primarily influenced through the use of proteases. Removal of sialic acid-bearing glycoproteins reduces RBC surface charge and conceivably permits RBCs to come close enough together to enable coating antibodies to form intercellular bridges. Other factors that contribute to enhancement of hemagglutination include the removal of RBC membrane-bound water, the clustering of antigen sites, and the alteration of RBC surface conformation. In addition, the first stage of the reaction (coating) may be influenced by the removal of structures that otherwise sterically hinder attachment of antibody to antigen.

Enhancement of serologic reactivity is a consequence of altered physical factors in the reaction. However in antibody identification, the loss of serologic reactivity following protease treatment is often a clear indication of antibody specificity. Because most of the membrane components carrying blood group antigens are well characterized, the protease sensitivity of the different antigens is often indicative of the component on which they are carried. Similarly, the ability to hemolyze protease-treated RBCs is a characteristic of certain complement-binding antibodies Thus, reaction patterns with enzyme-treated RBCs provide important clues to antibody identification. In addition, proteases are used 1) to enhance the adsorptive capacity of RBCs; 2) in conjunction with a sulphydryl compound to remove RBC-bound autoantibodies; 3) to convert RBC-bound human complement fragments C3b and C4b into C3d and C4d, respectively; and 4) to cleave specific blood-group-active RBC membrane structures.

Suggested Reading

Ellisor SS. Action and application of enzymes in immunohematology. In: Bell CA, ed. Seminar on antigen-antibody reactions revisited. Arlington, VA: AABB, 1982:133-74.

Pollack W, Hager HJ, Reckel R, Toren DA. A study of the forces involved in the second stage of hemagglutination. Transfusion 1965;5:158-83.

Reid ME, Lomas-Francis C. Blood group antigen factsbook. 2nd ed. San Diego, CA: Academic Press, 2004.

Reid ME, Lomas-Francis C. Blood group antigens and antibodies: A clinical and technical guide. New York: Star Bright Books, 2007.

Steane EA. Red blood cell agglutination: a current perspective. In: Bell CA, ed. Seminar on antigen-antibody reactions revisited. Arlington, VA: AABB, 1982:67-98.

Voak D, Cawley JC, Emmines JP, Barker CR. The role of enzymes and albumin in hemagglutination reactions: A serological and ultrastructural study with ferritin labeled anti-D. Vox Sang 1974;27:156-70.

III-A. Detecting Antibodies with the Bromelain One-Stage Method

Purpose

To provide instructions for using bromelain in a one-stage enzyme technique:

- Antibody detection, especially Rh antibodies.

Background Information

Incubation of serum and RBCs in the presence of a proteolytic enzyme such as bromelain results in the enhancement of agglutination and/or hemolysis with some blood group antibodies (eg, Rh and Jk antibodies).

This is a one-stage technique that requires no pretreatment of test RBCs.

Operational Policy

Because some antigens are denatured by treating RBCs with proteolytic enzymes, this method should not be used as the sole method for detecting antibodies in patients or blood donors. Use only in conjunction with an IAT with untreated RBCs.

DO NOT READ TESTS MICROSCOPICALLY because unwanted positive reactions may occur.

Do not refreeze thawed enzyme solutions.

Limitations

Unwanted Positive Reactions:

- Serum/plasma contains a broad-specificity antibody directed at all bromelain-treated RBCs.

Unwanted Negative Reactions:

- Enzyme is inactive.
- Incorrect technique is used.
- Enzyme preparation buffer is the wrong pH.
- A test component has been omitted.

Sample Requirements

Clotted or EDTA-anticoagulated blood as a source of serum or plasma.

**Equipment/
Materials**

Bromelain: 2% wt/vol.

Glass Pasteur pipettes (eg, VWR, Batavia, IL).

RBCs: 3%-5% saline suspensions of phenotyped group O, R_1R_1 and R_2R_2 RBCs.

Normal serum/plasma known to lack unexpected antibodies: 10-12 examples.

Weak Rh antibody: eg, anti-c; titer ≤ 16.

6×50-mm glass culture tubes (eg, VWR, Batavia, IL).

**Quality
Control**

For quality control of stock enzyme solution:

- Test normal sera by this procedure, using group O reagent RBCs. Decrease enzyme concentration by 0.2% if unwanted positive reactions occur.

- Prepare dilutions of anti-c (titer ≥ 16) and test against R_1r RBCs by this method and by the saline antiglobulin technique described in Procedure II-I. Comparable titration values should be obtained.

At each time of use, demonstrate that the method detects weakly reactive antibody, (eg, dilute anti-c described above).

Procedure

Use the following steps to perform the procedure:

Step	Action
1.	For each serum sample to be tested, mix 1 drop of serum, 1 drop of RBCs, and 1 drop of bromelain in a 6×50-mm test tube.
2.	Incubate at 37 C for 1 hour.
3.	Using a glass Pasteur pipette, smear RBC button onto a glass slide and examine the RBCs microscopically. **Note:** The end of the Pasteur pipette used to smear RBCs onto the glass slide must be level and not jagged; otherwise it will not be possible to remove RBCs without disturbing agglutinates. For the same reason, the internal bore of the pipette should not be too narrow, yet the outer dimensions must be compatible with the internal measurements of the test tubes.
4.	Interpret the reaction as follows: <table><tr><th>If agglutination or lysis is...</th><th>Then...</th></tr><tr><td>present</td><td>reactions are positive.</td></tr><tr><td>absent</td><td>reactions are negative.</td></tr></table>

5.	Interpret the reactions with weak Rh antibody as follows:		
	If the treated RBCs are…	**And the normal sera are…**	**Then the enzyme…**
	reactive	nonreactive	was used correctly.
	reactive	reactive	concentration may be too high, or panaglutinins are present in normal sera.
	nonreactive	reactive or nonreactive	is unsuitable for use: • Repeat enzyme preparation. • Consider alternative sources of bromelain.

References

Ellisor SS. Enzymes used in immunohematology. In: Rolih S, Albeitz C, eds. Enzymes, inhibitions, and adsorptions. Washington DC: AABB, 1981:1-37.

Marsh WL. Recent advances in laboratory serological techniques. Prog Med Lab Technol 1962;1:1-11.

Effective Date

Approved by:	**Printed Name**	**Signature**	**Date**
Laboratory Management			
Medical Director			
Quality Officer			

III-B. Treating RBCs with α-Chymotrypsin

Purpose

To provide instructions for α-chymotrypsin treatment of RBCs:

- Studies on MNS-related antibodies.
- Identification of antibodies to antigens of high prevalence.

Background Information

Treatment with α-chymotrypsin cleaves proteins at specific amino acids, namely the carboxyl terminus of the amino acids leucine, phenylalanine, tryptophan, and tyrosine. On the RBC, several blood-group-carrying proteins are susceptible to α-chymotrypsin treatment, notably glycophorin B (GPB), the Duffy glycoprotein, and decay accelerating factor (DAF), among others (See Table IX-2). In contrast, glycophorin A (GPA) is not affected by such treatment. This method is suitable for studies on MNS-related blood group antigens and for investigation of antibodies to antigens of high prevalence.

Operational Policy

Naturally occurring antibodies to enzyme-treated RBCs may interfere with the results of antibody identification studies using this procedure. The presence of such antibodies can be determined by performing an enzyme autocontrol. Interference by such antibodies can be eliminated by either adsorbing the antibody with enzyme-treated autologous RBCs or purifying the antibody by adsorption-elution.

DO NOT READ TESTS MICROSCOPICALLY because unwanted positive reactions may occur.

Do not refreeze thawed enzyme solutions.

Limitations

Unwanted Positive Reactions:

- Serum/plasma contains a broad specificity antibody directed at all α-chymotrypsin-treated RBCs.

Unwanted Negative Reactions:

- Enzyme is inactive.
- Incorrect technique is used.
- Enzyme preparation buffer is the wrong pH.
- A test component has been omitted.

Sample Requirements

Antibody under investigation and 0.25 mL reactive packed test RBCs, washed three times with saline before use.

**Equipment/
Materials**

α-chymotrypsin: 5 mg/mL.

Control M+N–S+s– RBCs: wash 0.25 mL packed RBCs three times with saline.

100 mM PBS at pH 8.0.

Vicia graminea lectin: see Section XIV.

Pipettors with disposable tips to deliver 0.25 mL to 1 mL (eg, VWR, Batavia, IL)

**Quality
Control**

Test untreated and α-chymotrypsin-treated M+N–S+s– RBCs with *V. graminea.*

Untreated RBCs will react strongly with *V. graminea*; treated RBCs should be nonreactive with *V. graminea.*

Procedure

Use the following steps to perform the procedure:

Step	Action
1.	Mix 0.25 mL RBCs with 1 mL of α-chymotrypsin.
2.	Incubate at 37 C for 30 minutes.
3.	Wash RBCs three times with saline.
4.	Dilute α-chymotrypsin-treated RBCs to a 3%-5% suspension with Alsever's solution. Store at 4 C.
5.	Test the treated and untreated RBCs with *V. graminea.*
6.	Interpret the reactions with *V. graminea* as follows:

If the treated RBCs are…	And the untreated RBCs are…	Then the enzyme treatment…
nonreactive	reactive	is complete.
nonreactive	nonreactive	results are unknown: • Consider inactive *V. graminea.*

	If the treated RBCs are...	And the untreated RBCs are...	Then the enzyme treatment...
	reactive	reactive	is incomplete: • Consider inactive enzyme.
	reactive	nonreactive	results are unknown: • Test was improperly performed.
7.	Provided the control tests above react as expected, test the antibody under investigation (by Procedure II-H if agglutinating or II-I if coating) against untreated and chymotrypsin-treated RBCs.		
8.	Evaluate the results of the treated and untreated RBCs as follows:		

If the untreated RBCs are...	And the treated RBCs are...	Then the antibody defines a...
reactive	nonreactive	chymotrypsin-sensitive structure.
reactive	reactive	chymotrypsin-resistant structure.

References

Daniels G. Effects of enzymes on and chemical modifications of high-frequency red cell antigens. Immunohematology 1992;8:53-57.

Judson PA, Anstee DJ. Comparative effect of trypsin and α-chymotrypsin on blood group antigens. Med Lab Sci 1977;34:1-6.

Reid ME, Lomas-Francis C. Blood group antigen factsbook 2nd ed. San Diego, CA: Academic Press, 2004.

Effective Date

Approved by:

	Printed Name	Signature	Date
Laboratory Management			
Medical Director			
Quality Officer			

III-C. Detecting Antibodies with the Ficin One-Stage Method

Purpose

To provide instructions for using ficin in a one-stage enzyme technique:

- Antibody detection, especially Rh antibodies.

Background Information

Incubation of serum and RBCs in the presence of a proteolytic enzyme such as ficin results in enhancement of agglutination and/or hemolysis with some blood group antibodies (eg, Rh and Jk antibodies).

This is a one-stage technique that requires no pretreatment of test RBCs.

Operational Policy

DO NOT READ TESTS MICROSCOPICALLY because unwanted positive reactions may occur.

Do not refreeze thawed enzyme solutions.

Limitations

Unwanted Positive Reactions:

- Serum/plasma contains a broad-specificity antibody directed at all ficin-treated RBCs.

Unwanted Negative Reactions:

- Enzyme is inactive.
- Incorrect technique is used.
- Enzyme preparation buffer is the wrong pH.
- A test component has been omitted.

Sample Requirements

Clotted or EDTA-anticoagulated blood as a source of serum/plasma and autologous RBCs.

Equipment/ Materials

Ficin: 1% wt/vol.

Glass Pasteur pipettes.

Normal serum known to lack unexpected antibodies: 10-12 examples.

6 × 50-mm glass culture tubes (eg, VWR, Batavia, IL).

Weak Rh antibody: eg, anti-c; titer ≤16.

Quality Control

For quality control of stock enzyme solution:

- Test normal sera by this procedure, using group O reagent RBCs. Decrease enzyme concentration by 0.1% if unwanted positive reactions occur.

- Prepare dilutions of anti-c (titer ≥16) and test against R_1r RBCs by this method and by the saline antiglobulin technique described in Procedure II-H. Comparable titration values should be obtained.

At each time of use, demonstrate that the method detects weakly reactive antibody (eg, dilute anti-c as described above).

Procedure

Use the following steps to perform the procedure:

Step	Action
1.	For each RBC sample to be tested, mix 1 drop of test serum, 1 drop of RBCs, and 1 drop of ficin in a 6 × 50-mm test tube.
2.	Incubate at 37 C for 1 hour.
3.	Observe for hemolysis, then smear RBC button onto a glass slide and examine macroscopically over a white illuminated background. Grade and record the results. **Note:** The end of the Pasteur pipette used to smear RBCs onto the glass slide must be level so as not to disturb agglutinates.
4.	Interpret the reactions as follows:

If agglutination or lysis is…	Then…
present	reactions are positive.
absent	reactions are negative.

5.	Interpret the reactions with weak Rh antibody as follows		
	If the treated RBCs are...	**And the normal sera are...**	**Then the enzyme...**
	reactive	nonreactive	is suitable for use.
	reactive	reactive	concentration may be too high or panaglutinins are present in normal sera.
	nonreactive	reactive or nonreactive	is unsuitable for use: • Repeat enzyme preparation. • Consider alternative sources of ficin.

References

Ellisor SS. Enzymes used in immunohematology. In: Rolih S, Albeitz C, eds. Enzymes, inhibitions, and adsorptions. Washington DC: AABB, 1981:1-37.

Marsh WL. Recent advances in laboratory serological techniques. Prog Med Lab Technol 1962;1:1-11.

Effective Date

Approved by:	Printed Name	Signature	Date
Laboratory Management			
Medical Director			
Quality Officer			

III-D. Treating RBCs with Ficin

Purpose

To provide instructions for ficin treatment of RBCs:

- Antibody identification.

Background Information

Treatment of RBCs with proteolytic enzymes such as ficin results in enhancement of agglutination and/or hemolysis with some blood group antibodies (eg, Rh and Jk antibodies, respectively) and loss of reactivity with others (eg, MNS and Fy antibodies).

Ficin cleaves proteins at specific amino acids, namely the carboxyl terminus of the amino acids alanine, aspartic acid, glycine, leucine, lysine, tyrosine, and valine. Ficin cleaves the same blood-group-carrying antigens as papain (see Table IX-2), most notably glycophorins A and B (GPA and GPB), which carry most of the negatively charged sialic acid residues. Consequently, the effect of ficin treatment is both specific, with regard to enzyme susceptibility, and nonspecific, because most of the sialic acid is removed and RBCs can come close enough together to be directly agglutinated by IgG antibodies. Enhancement of reactivity in antiglobulin tests is a consequence of altered physical factors leading to an increase in antibody uptake. This method is suitable for treating RBCs for use in the detection and investigation of unexpected antibodies.

Operational Policy

Naturally occurring antibodies to enzyme-treated RBCs may interfere with the results of antibody identification studies using this procedure. The presence of such antibodies can be determined by performing an enzyme autocontrol. Interference by such antibodies can be eliminated by either adsorbing the antibody with enzyme-treated autologous RBCs or purifying the antibody by adsorption-elution.

DO NOT READ TESTS MICROSCOPICALLY because unwanted positive reactions may occur.

Do not refreeze thawed enzyme solutions.

Limitations

Unwanted Positive Reactions:

- Serum/plasma contains a broad-specificity antibody directed at all ficin-treated RBCs.

Unwanted Negative Reactions:

- Enzyme is inactive.

- Incorrect technique is used.

- Enzyme preparation buffer is the wrong pH.

- A test component has been omitted.

Sample Requirements

RBC samples for treatment: wash 0.25 mL packed RBCs three times with saline before use.

Equipment/ Materials

Ficin: 1% wt/vol.

Normal serum known to lack unexpected antibodies: 10-12 examples.

Anti-Fy^a: titer ≥16.

Control Fy(a+b−) RBCs: wash 0.25 mL packed RBCs three times with saline.

10 mM PBS at pH 7.3.

0.1% Polybrene or *Glycine max* lectin: see Section XIV.

Weak Rh antibody: eg, anti-c; titer ≤16.

Pipettors with disposable tips to deliver 0.1 mL to 0.5 mL (eg, VWR, Batavia, IL).

Quality Control

1) For quality control of stock ficin solution:

   a) Treat Fy(a+b−) RBCs with enzyme for 15 minutes at 37 C as described below. Test anti-Fy^a with enzyme-treated and untreated Fy(a+b−) RBCs, in parallel, as described in Procedure II-C. If Fy(a+b−) RBCs are still reactive, then increase enzyme incubation time by 1 minute and repeat.

   b) Treat group O reagent RBCs with enzyme for the time established in Step 1a above and test against normal sera by Procedure II-C. If ≥2 of 10 sera are reactive, reduce enzyme incubation time by 1 minute intervals until Fy^a antigen is denatured but normal sera do not react with ficin-treated RBCs by procedure II-C.

Quality Control

c) Prepare dilutions of IgG Rh antibody (titer ≤16) and test against enzyme-treated RBCs (using the incubation time established above) and untreated RBCs (use RBCs with single-dose antigen expression) by Procedure II-C. Dilutions of Rh antibody should cause direct agglutination of enzyme-treated (but not untreated RBCs) after 37 C incubation. Enhancement with enzyme-treated RBCs should be observed at the antiglobulin phase.

2) Following preparation of enzyme-treated RBCs:

a) Test with diluted Rh antibody from Step 1c above. Weak Rh antibody should cause direct agglutination of antigen-positive enzyme-treated RBCs.

b) Alternatively, test with 0.1% Polybrene or with *Glycine max* lectin. Enzyme-treated RBCs should not aggregate when suspended in 0.1% Polybrene. Enzyme-treated RBCs should be agglutinated (3+ to 4+) by *Glycine max*.

Procedure

Use the following steps to perform the procedure:

Step	Action
1.	Dilute 1 part of 1% ficin solution with 9 parts of pH 7.3 PBS. **Note:** Dilute ficin solution may be kept at room temperature for 1 hour, after which it should be discarded.
2.	Mix 0.1 mL of each RBC sample with 0.5 mL dilute ficin.
3.	Incubate at 37 C using the time established in Step 1a and/or 1b under Quality Control.
4.	Wash RBCs three times with saline.
5.	Dilute ficin-treated RBCs to a 3%-5% suspension with saline and store for up to 72 hours at 4 C. **Note**: RBCs may also be prepared as a 0.8 or 1% suspension in the card manufacturer's diluent for use in column agglutination tests.
6.	Test by an indirect antiglobulin technique such as Procedure II-C.
7.	Interpret the reactions as follows: | If agglutination is...	Then...
present	reactions are positive.
absent	reactions are negative.	

8.	Interpret the reactions with weak Rh antibody as follows:		
	If the treated RBCs are…	**And the normal sera are…**	**Then the enzyme…**
	reactive	nonreactive	is suitable for use.
	reactive	reactive	concentration may be too high, or panaglutinins are present in normal sera.
	nonreactive	reactive or nonreactive	is unsuitable for use: • Repeat enzyme preparation. • Consider alternative sources of ficin.

References

Ellisor SS. Enzymes used in immunohematology. In: Rolih S, Albeitz C, eds. Enzymes, inhibitions and adsorptions. Washington DC: AABB, 1981:1-37.

Haber G, Rosenfield RE. Ficin treated red cells for hemagglutination studies. In: Anderson PH. Papers in dedication of his 60th birthday. Copenhagen: Munksgaard, 1957:45.

Effective Date

Approved by:	Printed Name	Signature	Date
Laboratory Management			
Medical Director			
Quality Officer			

III-E. Treating RBCs with Neuraminidase (T-Activation)

Purpose
To provide instructions for the sialidase modification of RBCs for:

- Investigation of RBC polyagglutination (T-activation).
- Lectin studies.
- Investigation of MNS-related antigens and antibodies.

Background Information
Neuraminidase cleaves *N*-acetylneuraminic acid (NeuAc), a sialic acid with a negatively charged carboxyl group that contributes considerably to the RBC surface charge. The abundant glycophorins A and B (GPA and GPB) are heavily glycosylated with NeuAc and some MNS antigens are dependent on NeuAc for expression. Removal of NeuAc exposes T receptors, which are galactose residues linked to *N*-acetylgalactosamine (GalNAc). The disaccharide structure Gal(β,1-3)GalNAc is a potent inhibitor of the peanut lectin (*Arachis hypogaea)*, and T-exposed RBCs react strongly with this lectin. All normal adult human sera contain a naturally occurring anti-T that will react with neuraminidase-treated RBCs.

Operational Policy
Because serum/plasma contains anti-T that reacts with all neuraminidase-treated RBCs, use eluates of human antibodies to assess loss of antibody reactivity following treatment of RBCs with neuraminidase.

DO NOT READ TESTS MICROSCOPICALLY because unwanted positive reactions may occur.

Limitations
Unwanted Positive Reactions:

- Anti-T is present in normal serum/plasma.

Unwanted Negative Reactions:

- Enzyme is inactive.
- Incorrect technique is used.
- Enzyme preparation buffer is the wrong pH.
- A test component has been omitted.

Sample Requirements
RBC samples for treatment: wash 0.25 mL packed RBCs three times with saline before use.

Equipment/ Materials

Neuraminidase from *Vibrio cholerae*, 1 IU/mL: EMD Biosciences (San Diego, CA).

pH 7.3 PBS.

Arachis hypogaea (PNA) lectin. (See Section XIV.)

Pipettors with disposable tips to deliver 0.1 mL to 0.25 mL (eg, VWR, Batavia, IL).

Quality Control

Test neuraminidase-treated RBCs and untreated RBCs with a 1:256 dilution of *A. hypogaea* lectin. The treated RBCs should react ≥3+ with dilute *A. hypogaea*. Untreated RBCs should be negative.

Procedure

Use the following steps to perform the procedure:

Step	Action
1.	Dilute 1 part of neuraminidase with 9 parts of pH 7.3 PBS.
2.	Mix 0.1 mL of each RBC sample with 0.l mL of dilute neuraminidase.
3.	Incubate at 37 C for 15 minutes.
4.	Wash RBCs three times with saline.
5.	Dilute neuraminidase-treated RBCs to a 3%-5% suspension with saline. Store in Alsever's solution at 4 C.
6.	Test with a 1:256 dilution of *A. hypogaea* lectin.
7.	Interpret the reactions with *A. hypogaea* lectin as follows:

If agglutination is...	Then...
present, ≥3+	RBCs are T-activated: • Use as desired.
present, <3+	neuraminidase treatment is insufficient: • Repeat treatment, increasing incubation time by 1 minute intervals until 3+ reactivity occurs with *A. hypogaea* lectin.
absent	procedure failed: • Investigate cause.

Reference

Judd WJ, Issitt PD, Pavone BG. The Can serum: Demonstrating further polymorphism of M and N blood group antigens. Transfusion 1979;19-7-11.

**Effective
Date**

Approved by:	Printed Name	Signature	Date
Laboratory Management			
Medical Director			
Quality Officer			

III-F. Detecting Antibodies with the Papain One-Stage Method

Purpose

To provide instructions using papain in a one-stage enzyme technique:

- Antibody detection, especially Rh antibodies.

Background Information

Incubation of serum and RBCs in the presence of a proteolytic enzyme such as papain results in enhancement of agglutination and/or hemolysis with some blood group antibodies (eg, Rh and Jk antibodies).

This is a one-stage technique that requires no pretreatment of test RBCs.

Operational Policy

DO NOT READ TESTS MICROSCOPICALLY because unwanted positive reactions may occur.

Do not refreeze thawed enzyme solutions.

Limitations

Unwanted Positive Reactions:

- Serum/plasma contains a broad-specificity antibody directed at all papain-treated RBCs.

Unwanted Negative Reactions:

- Enzyme is inactive.
- Incorrect technique is used.
- Enzyme preparation buffer is the wrong pH.
- A test component has been omitted.

Sample Requirements

Clotted or EDTA-anticoagulated blood as a source of serum/plasma and autologous RBCs.

Equipment/ Materials

Papain: 1% wt/vol.

Glass Pasteur pipettes (eg, VWR, Batavia, IL)

Normal serum known to lack unexpected antibodies: 10-12 examples.

6 × 50-mm glass culture tubes (eg, VWR, Batavia, IL).

Weak Rh antibody: eg, anti-c; titer ≤16.

Judd's Methods in Immunohematology
Detecting Antibodies with the Papain One-Stage Method
Page 2 of 3

Quality Control

For quality control of stock enzyme solution:

- Test normal sera by this procedure, using group O reagent RBCs. Decrease enzyme concentration by 0.1% if unwanted positive reactions occur.

- Prepare dilutions of anti-c (titer ≥16) and test against R_1r RBCs by this method and by the saline antiglobulin technique described in Procedure II-I. Comparable titration values should be obtained.

- At each time of use, demonstrate that the method detects weakly reactive antibody (eg, dilute anti-c described above).

Procedure

Use the following steps to perform the procedure:

Step	Action
1.	For each RBC sample to be tested, mix 1 drop of test serum, 1 drop of RBCs, and 1 drop of papain in a 6 × 50-mm test tube.
2.	Incubate at 37 C for 1 hour.
3.	Observe for hemolysis, then smear RBC button onto a glass slide and examine macroscopically over a white illuminated background. Grade and record the results. **Note:** The end of the Pasteur pipette used to smear RBCs onto the glass slide must be level so as not to disturb agglutinates.
4.	Interpret the reactions as follows:

If agglutination or lysis is...	Then...
present	reactions are positive.
absent	reactions are negative.

Step	Action
5.	Interpret the reactions with weak Rh antibody as follows:

If the treated RBCs are...	And the normal sera are...	Then the enzyme...
reactive	nonreactive	is suitable for use.
reactive	reactive	concentration may be too high, or panaglutinins are present in normal sera.
nonreactive	reactive or nonreactive	is unsuitable for use: • Repeat enzyme preparation. • Consider alternative sources of papain.

Reference   Nance S, Gonzalez B, Postoway N, et al. Clinical significance of a primarily complement-dependent anti-Jk^a in a patient who received Jk(a+) red cells (abstract). Transfusion 1985;25(Suppl):482.

Effective Date

Approved by:	Printed Name	Signature	Date
Laboratory Management			
Medical Director			
Quality Officer			

III-G. Treating RBCs with Papain

Purpose	To provide instructions for papain treatment of RBCs:
	• Antibody identification.

Background Information

Treatment of RBCs with proteolytic enzymes such as papain results in enhancement of agglutination and/or hemolysis with some blood group antibodies (eg, Rh and Jk antibodies, respectively) and loss of reactivity with others (eg, MNS and Fy antibodies).

Papain cleaves proteins at specific amino acids, namely the carboxyl terminus of the amino acids arginine, lysine, and phenylalanine. Many blood-group-carrying proteins on the RBC are susceptible to papain treatment (see Table IX-2), most notably glycophorins A and B (GPA and GPB), which carry most of the negatively charged sialic acid. Consequently, the effect of papain treatment is both specific, with regard to enzyme susceptibility, and nonspecific, because most of the sialic acid is removed and RBCs can come close enough together to be directly agglutinated by IgG antibodies. Enhancement of reactivity in antiglobulin tests is a consequence of altered physical factors leading to an increase in antibody uptake. This method is suitable for treating RBCs for use in the detection and investigation of unexpected antibodies.

Operational Policy

Naturally occurring antibodies to enzyme-treated RBCs may interfere with the results of antibody identification studies using this procedure. The presence of such antibodies can be determined by performing an enzyme autocontrol. Interference by such antibodies can be eliminated by either adsorbing the antibody with enzyme-treated autologous RBCs or purifying the antibody by adsorption-elution.

DO NOT READ TESTS MICROSCOPICALLY because unwanted positive reactions may occur.

Do not refreeze thawed enzyme solutions.

Limitations

Unwanted Positive Reactions:

- Serum/plasma contains a broad-specificity antibody directed at all papain-treated RBCs.

Unwanted Negative Reactions:

- Enzyme is inactive.

- Incorrect technique is used.

- Enzyme preparation buffer is the wrong pH.

- A test component has been omitted.

Sample Requirements

RBC samples for treatment: wash 0.25 mL packed RBCs three times with saline before use.

Equipment/ Materials

Papain: 1% wt/vol.

Normal serum known to lack unexpected antibodies: 10-12 examples.

Anti-Fy^a: titer ≥16.

Control Fy(a+b−) RBCs: wash 0.25 mL packed RBCs three times with saline.

10 mM PBS at pH 7.3.

0.1% Polybrene or *Glycine max* lectin: see Section XIV.

Weak Rh antibody: eg, anti-c; titer ≤16.

Pipettors with disposable tips to deliver 0.1 mL to 0.25 mL (eg, VWR, Batavia, IL).

Quality Control

1) For quality control of stock papain solution:

   a) Treat Fy(a+b−) RBCs with enzyme for 15 minutes at 37 C as described below. Test anti-Fy^a with enzyme-treated and untreated Fy(a+b−) RBCs in parallel as described in Procedure II-C. If Fy(a+b−) RBCs are still reactive, then increase enzyme incubation time by 1 minute and repeat.

   b) Treat group O reagent RBCs with enzyme for the time established in Step 1a above and test against normal sera by Procedure II-C. If ≥2 of 10 sera are reactive, then reduce enzyme incubation time by 1 minute intervals until Fy^a antigen is denatured but normal sera do not react with papain-treated RBCs by Procedure II-C.

c) Prepare dilutions of IgG Rh antibody (titer ≤16) and test against enzyme-treated RBCs (using the incubation time established in Step 1b above) and untreated RBCs (use RBCs with single-dose antigen expression) by Procedure II-C. Dilutions of Rh antibody should cause direct agglutination of enzyme-treated (but not un-treated) RBCs after 37 C incubation. Enhancement with enzyme-treated RBCs should be observed at the antiglobulin phase.

2) Following preparation of enzyme-treated RBCs:

a) Test with dilute Rh antibody from Step 1c above. Weak Rh anti-body should cause direct agglutination of antigen-positive enzyme-treated RBCs.

b) Alternatively, test with 0.1% Polybrene or with *Glycine max* lectin. Enzyme-treated RBCs should not aggregate when suspended in 0.1% Polybrene. Enzyme-treated RBCs should be agglutinated (3+ to 4+) by *Glycine max.*

Procedure   Use the following steps to perform the procedure:

Step	Action
1.	Dilute 1 part of 1% papain solution with 19 parts of pH 7.3 PBS. **Note:** Dilute papain solution may be kept at room temperature for 1 hour, after which it should be discarded.
2.	Mix 0.1 mL of each RBC sample with 0.5 mL dilute ficin.
3.	Incubate at 37 C using the time established in Step 1a and/or 1b under Quality Control.
4.	Wash RBCs three times with saline.
5.	Dilute ficin-treated RBCs to a 3%-5% suspension with saline and store for up to 72 hours at 4 C. **Note:** RBCs may also be prepared as a 0.8 or 1% suspension in the card manufacturer's diluent for use in column agglutination tests.
6.	Test by an indirect antiglobulin technique such as Procedure II-C.
7.	Interpret the reactions as follows: 	If agglutination or lysis is...	Then...	 	present	reactions are positive.	 	absent	reactions are negative.	

8.	Interpret the reactions with weak Rh antibody as follows:		
	If the treated RBCs are…	**And the normal sera are…**	**Then the enzyme…**
	reactive	nonreactive	is suitable for use.
	reactive	reactive	concentration may be too high, or panaglutinins are present in normal sera.
	nonreactive	reactive or nonreactive	is unsuitable for use: • Repeat enzyme preparation. • Consider alternative sources of papain.

Reference   Ellisor SS. Enzymes used in immunohematology. In: Rolih S, Albeitz C, eds. Enzymes, inhibitions, and adsorptions. Washington DC: AABB, 1981:1-37.

Effective Date

Approved by:	Printed Name	Signature	Date
Laboratory Management			
Medical Director			
Quality Officer			

III-H. Treating RBCs with Pronase

Purpose
To provide instructions for pronase treatment of RBCs:

- Antibody identification.

Background Information
Treatment of RBCs with proteolytic enzymes such as pronase results in enhancement of agglutination and/or hemolysis with some blood group antibodies (eg, Rh and Jk antibodies, respectively) and loss of reactivity with others (eg, MNS and Fy antibodies).

Pronase cleaves proteins at the carboxyl terminus of any hydrophobic amino acid (eg, arginine, histidine, lysine, aspartic acid, or glutamic acid). Many blood-group-carrying proteins on the RBC are susceptible to pronase treatment (see Table X-1), most notably glycophorins A and B (GPA and GPB), which carry most of the negatively charged sialic acid. Consequently, the effect of pronase treatment is both specific, with regard to enzyme susceptibility, and nonspecific, because most of the sialic acid is removed and RBCs can come close enough together to be directly agglutinated by IgG antibodies. Enhancement of reactivity in antiglobulin tests is a consequence of altered physical factors leading to an increase in antibody uptake. This method is suitable for treating RBCs for use in the detection and investigation of unexpected antibodies.

Operational Policy
Naturally occurring antibodies to enzyme-treated RBCs may interfere with the results of antibody identification studies using this procedure. The presence of such antibodies can be determined by performing an enzyme autocontrol. Interference by such antibodies can be eliminated by either adsorbing the antibody with enzyme-treated autologous RBCs or purifying the antibody by adsorption-elution.

DO NOT READ TESTS MICROSCOPICALLY because unwanted positive reactions may occur.

Do not refreeze thawed enzyme solutions.

Limitations Unwanted Positive Reactions:

- Serum/plasma contains a broad-specificity antibody directed at all pronase-treated RBCs.

Unwanted Negative Reactions:

- Enzyme is inactive.

- Incorrect technique is used.

- Enzyme preparation buffer is the wrong pH.

- A test component has been omitted.

Sample Requirements RBC samples for treatment: wash 0.25 mL packed RBCs three times with saline before use.

Equipment/ Materials Pronase: 2.5 mg/mL.

Normal serum known to lack unexpected antibodies: 10-12 examples.

Anti-Fy^a: titer ≥16.

Control Fy(a+b–) RBCs: wash 0.25 mL packed RBCs three times with saline.

10 mM PBS at pH 8.0.

0.1% Polybrene or *Glycine max* lectin: see Section XIV.

Weak Rh antibody: eg, anti-c; titer ≤16.

Pipettors with disposable tips to deliver 0.25 mL to 1 mL (eg, VWR, Batavia, IL).

Quality Control

1) For quality control of pronase solution:

   a) Treat Fy(a+b–) RBCs with enzyme for 30 minutes at 37 C as described below. Test anti-Fy^a with enzyme-treated and untreated Fy(a+b–) RBCs in parallel as described in Procedure II-C. If Fy(a+b–) RBCs are still reactive, then increase enzyme incubation time by 1 minute and repeat.

   b) Treat group O reagent RBCs with enzyme for the time established in Step 1a above and test against normal sera by Procedure II-C. If ≥2 of 10 sera are reactive, reduce enzyme incubation time by 1 minute intervals until Fy^a antigen is denatured but normal sera do not react with papain-treated RBCs by Procedure II-C.

c) Prepare dilutions of IgG Rh antibody (titer ≤16) and test against enzyme-treated RBCs (using the incubation time established in Step 1b above) and untreated RBCs (use RBCs with single-dose antigen expression) by Procedure II-C. Dilutions of Rh antibody should cause direct agglutination of enzyme-treated (but not untreated) RBCs after 37 C incubation. Enhancement with enzyme-treated RBCs should be observed at the antiglobulin phase.

2) Following preparation of enzyme-treated RBCs:

a) Test with dilute Rh antibody from Step 1c above. Weak Rh antibody should cause direct agglutination of antigen-positive enzyme-treated RBCs.

b) Alternatively, test with 0.1% Polybrene or with *Glycine max* lectin. Enzyme-treated RBCs should not aggregate when suspended in 0.1% Polybrene. Enzyme-treated RBCs should be agglutinated (3+ to 4+) by *Glycine max.*

Procedure   Use the following steps to perform the procedure:

Step	Action
1.	Mix 0.25 mL of each RBC sample with 1 mL of pronase.
2.	Incubate at 37 C using the time established in Step 1a and/or 1b under Quality Control.
3.	Wash RBCs three times with saline.
4.	Dilute pronase-treated RBCs to a 3%-5% suspension with saline and store for up to 72 hours at 4 C. **Note**: RBCs may also be prepared as a 0.8 or 1% suspension in the card manufacturer's diluent for use in column agglutination tests.
5.	Test by an indirect antiglobulin technique such as Procedure II-C.
6.	Interpret the reactions as follows:

If agglutination or lysis is...	Then...
present	reactions are positive.
absent	reactions are negative.

7.	Interpret the reactions with weak Rh antibody as follows:		
	If the treated RBCs are…	**And the normal sera are…**	**Then the enzyme…**
	reactive	nonreactive	is suitable for use.
	reactive	reactive	concentration may be too high, or panaglutinins are present in normal sera.
	nonreactive	reactive or nonreactive	is unsuitable for use: • Repeat enzyme preparation. • Consider alternative sources of papain.

References

Daniels G. Effect of enzymes on and chemical modifications of high-frequency red cell antigens. Immunohematology 1992;8:53-7.

Reid ME, Green CA, Hoffer J, Oyen R. Effect of pronase on high-incidence blood group antigens and the prevalence of antibodies to pronase-treated erythrocytes. Immunohematology 1996;4:139-42.

Effective Date

Approved by:	**Printed Name**	**Signature**	**Date**
Laboratory Management			
Medical Director			
Quality Officer			

III-I. Treating RBCs with Trypsin (Crude Enzyme)

Purpose

To provide instructions for trypsin treatment of RBCs:

- Antibody detection.
- Preparation of C3d/C4d-coated RBCs.

Background Information

Treatment of RBCs with proteolytic enzymes such as trypsin results in enhancement of agglutination and/or hemolysis with some blood group antibodies (eg, Rh and Jk antibodies, respectively) and loss of reactivity with others (eg, some MNS antibodies).

Trypsin cleaves proteins at the carboxyl terminus of arginine and lysine. Many blood-group-carrying proteins on the RBC are susceptible to trypsin treatment (see Table IX-2), most notably glycophorin A (GPA), which carries much of the negatively charged sialic acid. Consequently, the effect of trypsin treatment is both specific, with regard to enzyme susceptibility, and nonspecific, because most of the sialic acid is removed and RBCs can come close enough together to be directly agglutinated by IgG antibodies. Enhancement of reactivity in antiglobulin tests is a consequence of altered physical factors leading to an increase in antibody uptake. Trypsin can also be used to modify complement components when bound to RBCs—eg, treatment of RBC-bound C3b results in breakdown of C3b to C3c and C3d; C3c is released, leaving the RBCs coated with C3d. Trypsin causes similar changes to C4b.

Applications of this procedure include the detection and identification of unexpected antibodies and the preparation of C3d- or C4d-coated RBCs for recognition of anti-Ch/-Rg or evaluating AHG reagents.

Operational Policy

DO NOT READ TESTS MICROSCOPICALLY because unwanted positive reactions may occur.

Limitations   Underlined: Unwanted Positive Reactions:

- Serum/plasma contains a broad-specificity antibody directed at all trypsin-treated RBCs.

Unwanted Negative Reactions:

- Enzyme is inactive.

- Incorrect technique is used.

- Enzyme preparation buffer is the wrong pH.

- A test component has been omitted.

Sample Requirements   RBC samples for treatment: wash 0.25 mL packed RBCs three times with saline before use.

Note: If RBCs are to be used to aid in the identification of an unknown antibody, then treat autologous RBCs in parallel to exclude enzyme-specific autoantibodies.

Equipment/ Materials   Trypsin: 1% wt/vol.

Anti-M: titer ≥8, or commercially available.

Control M+N– RBCs: wash 0.25 mL packed RBCs three times with saline.

Normal serum known to lack unexpected antibodies: 10-12 examples.

100 mM PBS at pH 7.7.

0.1% Polybrene or *Glycine max* lectin: see Section XIV.

Weak Rh antibody: eg, anti-c; titer ≤16.

Pipettors with disposable tips to deliver 0.1 mL to 0.25 mL (eg, VWR, Batavia, IL).

Quality Control   1) For quality control of stock trypsin solution:

a) Treat M+N– RBCs with enzyme for 30 minutes at 37 C as described below. Test anti-M with enzyme-treated and untreated M+N– RBCs in parallel by Procedure II-H (at room temperature only) or as described in the reagent manufacturer's instructions. If M+N– RBCs are still reactive, then increase enzyme incubation time by 5 minutes and repeat.

b) Treat group O reagent RBCs with enzyme for the time established in Step 1a above and test against normal sera by Procedure II-C. If ≥2 of 10 sera are reactive, then reduce enzyme incubation time by 1 minute intervals until M antigen is denatured but normal sera do not react with trypsin-treated RBCs by Procedure II-C.

c) Prepare dilutions of IgG Rh antibody (titer ≤16) and test against enzyme-treated RBCs (using the incubation time established above) and untreated RBCs (use RBCs with single-dose antigen expression) by Procedure II-C. Dilutions of Rh antibody should cause direct agglutination of enzyme-treated (but not untreated) RBCs after 37 C incubation. Enhancement with enzyme-treated RBCs should be observed at the antiglobulin phase.

2) Following preparation of enzyme-treated RBCs:

a) Test with dilute Rh antibody from Step 1c above. Weak Rh antibody should cause direct agglutination of antigen-positive enzyme-treated RBCs.

b) Alternatively, test with 0.1% Polybrene or with *Glycine max* lectin. Enzyme-treated RBCs should not aggregate when suspended in 0.1% Polybrene. Enzyme-treated RBCs should be agglutinated (2+ to 3+) by *Glycine max.*

Procedure   Use the following steps to perform the procedure:

Step	Action
1.	Dilute 1 part of trypsin with 9 parts of pH 7.7 PBS.
2.	Mix 0.1 mL of RBCs with 0.1 mL of dilute trypsin.
3.	Incubate at 37 C using the time established in Step 1a and/or 1b under Quality Control.
4.	Wash RBCs three times with saline.
5.	Dilute trypsin-treated RBCs to a 3%-5% suspension with saline. Store for up to 72 hours at 4 C. **Note**: RBCs may also be prepared as a 0.8 or 1% suspension in the card manufacturer's diluent for use in column agglutination tests.
6.	Test by an indirect antiglobulin technique such as Procedure II-C.

7.	Interpret the reactions as follows:	
	If agglutination or lysis is...	**Then...**
	present	reactions are positive.
	absent	reactions are negative.

8.	Interpret the reactions with weak Rh antibody as follows:		
	If the treated RBCs are...	**And the normal sera are...**	**Then the enzyme...**
	reactive	nonreactive	is suitable for use.
	reactive	reactive	concentration may be too high, or panaglutinins are present in normal sera.
	nonreactive	reactive or nonreactive	is unsuitable for use: • Repeat enzyme preparation. • Consider alternative sources of trypsin.

References

Daniels G. Effect of enzymes on and chemical modifications of high-frequency red cell antigens. Immunohematology 1992;8:53-7.

Morton JA, Pickles M. Use of trypsin in the detection of incomplete Rh antibodies. Nature 1947;159:779.

Effective Date

Approved by:

	Printed Name	Signature	Date
Laboratory Management			
Medical Director			
Quality Officer			

III-J. Treating RBCs with Trypsin (Purified Enzyme)

Purpose

To provide instructions for trypsin treatment of RBCs:

- Studies on MNS-related antibodies.

- Identification of antibodies to high-incidence antigens.

Background Information

Treatment of RBCs with proteolytic enzymes such as trypsin results in enhancement of agglutination and/or hemolysis with some blood group antibodies (eg, Rh and Jk antibodies, respectively) and loss of reactivity with others (eg, some MNS antibodies).

Trypsin cleaves proteins at the carboxyl terminus of arginine and lysine. Many blood-group-carrying proteins on the RBC are susceptible to trypsin treatment (see Table IX-2), most notably glycophorin A (GPA), which carries much of the negatively charged sialic acid. Consequently, the effect of trypsin treatment is both specific, with regard to enzyme susceptibility, and nonspecific, because most of the sialic acid is removed and RBCs can come close enough together to be directly agglutinated by IgG antibodies. Enhancement of reactivity in antiglobulin tests is a consequence of altered physical factors leading to an increase in antibody uptake.

Under controlled conditions, trypsin cleaves GPA but not glycophorin B (GPB) on intact RBCs. The first 26 N-terminal amino acids of N-active GPA and normal GPB (from S+ and/or s+ individuals) are identical; ie, both are N-active structures. 'N' (N-quotes) is used when referring to the N antigen carried on GPB.

At the appropriate dilution, *Vicia graminea* lectin (anti-N_{VG}) reacts preferentially with RBCs from *MN* and *NN* individuals. M+N– RBCs can be made to react strongly with anti-N_{VG} by treating them with trypsin, which removes sterically hindering GPA and makes 'N' on GPB accessible to the lectin. The primary application of this procedure is for the detection of 'N' on abnormal GPB and hybrid sialoglycoproteins.

Operational Policy

Naturally occurring antibodies to enzyme-treated RBCs may interfere with the results of antibody identification studies using this procedure. The presence of such antibodies can be determined by performing an enzyme autocontrol. Interference by such antibodies can be eliminated by either adsorbing the antibody with enzyme-treated autologous RBCs or purifying the antibody by adsorption-elution.

DO NOT READ TESTS MICROSCOPICALLY because unwanted positive reactions may occur.

Do not refreeze thawed enzyme solutions.

Limitations

Unwanted Positive Reactions:

- Serum/plasma contains a broad-specificity antibody directed at all trypsin-treated RBCs.

Unwanted Negative Reactions:

- Enzyme is inactive.

- Incorrect technique is used.

- Enzyme preparation buffer is the wrong pH.

- A test component has been omitted.

Sample Requirements

Antibody under investigation and 0.25 mL reactive packed test RBCs, washed three times with saline before use.

Equipment/ Materials

Trypsin: 180,000 BAEE units/mL.

100 mM PBS at pH 7.7.

Vicia graminea lectin: see Section XIV.

M+N–S+s+ and M–N+S–s– RBCs: wash 0.25 mL packed RBCs three times with saline.

Pipettors with disposable tips to deliver 0.1 mL to 0.25 mL (eg, VWR, Batavia, IL).

**Quality
Control**

Test untreated and trypsin-treated M+N–S+s+U+ and M–N+S–s–U– RBCs with *V. graminea*:

- Trypsin-treated M+N–S+s+U+ RBCs should react (≥2+) with *V. graminea*; the untreated RBCs should be nonreactive.

- Trypsin-treated M–N+S–s–U– RBCs should be nonreactive with *V. graminea*; the untreated RBCs should be strongly (3+ to 4+) reactive.

Procedure

Use the following steps to perform the procedure:

Step	Action
1.	Mix 0.1 mL of RBCs with 0.1 mL of trypsin.
2.	Incubate at 37 C for 30 minutes.
3.	Wash RBCs three times with saline.
4.	Dilute trypsin-treated RBCs to a 3%-5% suspension with saline. Store for up to 72 hours at 4 C. **Note**: RBCs may also be prepared as a 0.8 or 1% suspension in the card manufacturer's diluent for use in column agglutination tests.
5.	Test the control samples with *V. graminea* lectin.
6.	Interpret the reactions with *V. graminea* as follows:

If the treated M+N–S+s+U+ RBCs are...	And the treated M–N+S–s–U– RBCs are...	Then the enzyme treatment is....
nonreactive	reactive	is complete: • Reactions with unknown antibody are valid.
nonreactive	nonreactive	results are unknown: • Consider inactive *V. graminea*.
reactive	reactive	is incomplete.
reactive	nonreactive	results are unknown: • Test was improperly performed.

Step	Action
7.	Provided the control tests above react as expected, test the antibody under investigation, by procedure II-H if agglutinating or II-I if coating) against untreated and trypsin-treated RBCs.

8.	Evaluate the results of the treated and untreated RBCs as follows:		
	If the untreated RBCs are...	**And the treated RBCs are...**	**Then the antibody defines a....**
	reactive	nonreactive	trypsin-sensitive structure.
	reactive	reactive	trypsin-resistant structure.

References

Daniels G. Effect of enzymes on and chemical modifications of high-frequency red cell antigens. Immunohematology 1992;8:53-7.

Morton JA, Pickles M. Use of trypsin in the detection of incomplete Rh antibodies. Nature 1947;159:779.

Pavone BG, Billman R, Bryant J, et al. An auto-anti-En[a] inhibitable by MN sialoglycoprotein. Transfusion 1981;21:25-31.

Effective Date

Approved by:	Printed Name	Signature	Date
Laboratory Management			
Medical Director			
Quality Officer			

Section IV. Elution Techniques

Elution, as applied in immunohematology, entails the removal of antibody from coated RBCs, the primary objective being to recover bound antibody for study by routine serologic techniques. The results of such studies are an important part of the laboratory diagnosis of immune-mediated RBC destruction caused by autoantibodies to intrinsic RBC antigens, alloantibodies made in response to recent transfusions, and drug-induced phenomena. In combination with an in-vitro adsorption technique, elution procedures are used to purify blood group antibodies, to detect weakly expressed antigens, to concentrate antibody-containing solutions, or to resolve multiple antibody specificities present in a single serum. In other instances, elution is undertaken to remove coating antibody, rendering RBCs negative by the direct antiglobulin test and thereby allowing the RBCs to be tested with antisera reactive by the indirect antiglobulin test.

For effective elution, the binding forces between RBC antigens and coating antibody molecules must be reversed or neutralized. This can be accomplished by heat, alterations to pH or salt concentration, sonication, use of detergents or organic solvents, or combinations of two or more of these.

There are several procedures described in this section for recovering RBC-bound antibody for use in serologic testing. Selection of any given procedure for routine use is often a matter of personal preference, governed by availability of the necessary reagents and equipment. In the authors' experience, heat elution or sonication techniques are best reserved for elution of primarily cold-reactive (IgM) antibodies. For optimal recovery of warm-reactive allo- or autoantibodies, few procedures compare, in terms of serologic effectiveness, with elution by ether or xylene. However, because of safety concerns, many workers use commercially prepared kits based on a cold acid elution technique. Nonetheless, elution procedures that entail use of organic solvents have been included for the sake of completeness.

Suggested Reading

Issitt PD, Anstee DJ. Applied blood group serology. 4th ed. Durham, NC: Montgomery Scientific Publications, 1998.

Judd WJ. Antibody elution from red cells. In: Bell CA, ed. Seminar on antigen-antibody reactions revisited. Arlington, VA: AABB, 1982:175-221.

Judd WJ. Elution—dissociation of antibody from red blood cells: Theoretical and practical considerations. Transfus Med Rev, 1999;13:297-310.

South SF, Rea AE, Tregellas WM. An evaluation of 11 red cell elution procedures. Transfusion 1986;26:167-70.

IV-A. Washing Before Eluting

Purpose   To provide instructions for washing antibody-coated RBCs before antibody elution.

Background Information   To ensure that antibody recovered in eluates is RBC-membrane-derived and does not represent "free" unbound antibody, RBC samples for elution must be adequately washed before performing the elution procedure. Either normal or buffered saline, or LISS, may be used to wash RBCs before elution. Using ice-cold saline or LISS may help prevent dissociation of low-affinity antibodies during the washing process. This method is suitable for the preparation of most eluates, although some variations may be desirable, as indicated in the specific procedures described elsewhere in this Section.

Operational Policy   When washing RBCs coated in vitro with antibody, transfer the washed RBCs into a clean test tube before elution. Antibody may bind to glass during the coating phase and dissociate during the elution process, thereby contaminating the eluate.

Limitations   Unwanted Positive Eluates:

- Incomplete washing.

Unwanted Negative Eluates:

- Antibody dissociation during washing.

Sample Requirements   Any RBC sample may be subjected to elution. However, it is most convenient to use RBCs from an anticoagulated sample (eg, EDTA). For diagnostic testing, a volume of 1-2 mL usually will suffice.

Equipment/ Materials   AHG: anti-IgG; need not be heavy-chain specific.

IgG-coated RBCs.

Wash solution (saline, pH 7.3 PBS or LISS wash solution). May be used cold, from the refrigerator.

Vacuum aspiration equipment: for efficient removal of wash supernates (optional).

Quality Control   A quality control method for the washing process is included in the proce-dure.

Procedure   Use the following steps to perform the procedure:

Step	Action
1.	Wash the RBCs six times in the chosen wash solution, saving approximately 2 mL of the final wash supernate for testing as described below and later in parallel testing with the eluate.
2.	Mix 1 drop of anti-IgG with 1 drop of supernate in a 10 or 12 × 75-mm test tube.
3.	Incubate at room temperature for 5 minutes.
4.	Add 1 drop of IgG-coated RBCs: • Mix gently. • Centrifuge. • Examine macroscopically for agglutination. • Grade and record results.
5.	Interpret the results and proceed as follows:

If agglutination is…	Then…
present	washing is complete: • Prepare eluate.
absent	washing is inadequate: • Wash the RBCs twice more and repeat from Step 2.

Effective Date

Approved by:	Printed Name	Signature	Date
Laboratory Management			
Medical Director			
Quality Officer			

IV-B. Eluting Antibodies with Chloroform

Purpose   To provide instructions for eluting IgG auto- and alloantibodies from RBCs using chloroform:

- In the investigation of immune hemolysis due to autoantibodies, allo-antibodies or drugs.

- In conjunction with an adsorption technique:

  o   To confirm the presence or absence of an antigen on RBCs.

  o   To concentrate an antibody.

  o   To isolate an antibody in pure form from a serum containing multi-ple alloantibodies.

Background Information   Organic solvents probably influence antigen-antibody dissociation by sev-eral mechanisms, including:

Alteration of the tertiary structure of antibody molecules.

Disruption of the RBC membrane bilipid layer.

Reversal of the forces of attraction between antigen and antibody.

The first two mechanisms result in loss of structural complementarity be-tween antigen and antibody.

Operational Policy   Inhalation of chloroform in large doses may cause hypotension, cardiac and respiratory depression, and death. Also, chloroform is carcinogenic in laboratory animals. Consequently, the following safety precautions should be followed:

Store bulk quantities of organic solvents in an explosion-proof refrigerator or cabinet. Small amounts (eg, 4 oz) may be kept at room temperature in a stoppered container.

Discard organic solvents when the container is one-quarter full. Some or-ganic solvents become acidic during storage, probably as the result of pe-roxide formation. This may account for apparent nonspecific activity of eluates when the solvent used has been taken from an almost empty con-tainer.

Use organic solvents in a well-ventilated area away from heat, flame, and electrical outlets; a properly constructed chemical hood is preferred.

Store waste chloroform underwater in a large, dark glass bottle and keep under a chemical hood. Dispose according to state and federal guidelines.

Limitations

Unwanted Positive Reactions:

- Incomplete washing of RBCs.

- Matuhasi-Ogata phenomenon.

- Incomplete removal of organic solvent

Unwanted Negative Reactions:

- Incomplete removal of organic solvent.

- Incorrect technique.

Sample Requirements

RBCs for elution studies, washed as described in Procedure IV-A.

Equipment/ Materials

6% BSA.

Chloroform: $CHCl_3$ (reagent grade).

Cork stoppers: size #2 (eg, VWR, Batavia, IL).

Note: Cork stoppers should be used when agitating eluates prepared with organic solvents. Cork allows the tube to "breathe" during agitation, thereby minimizing gas build-up that may cause the contents to splatter when the stopper is removed.

Glass Pasteur pipettes.

Quality Control

Save the supernate from the final wash (see Procedure IV-A) for parallel testing with the eluate.

In combined adsorption-elution studies, reserve an aliquot of the adsorbing RBC sample (uncoated) for testing with the eluate.

Procedure   Use the following steps to perform the procedure:

Step	Action
1.	Wash the RBCs as described in Procedure IV-A. **Note:** Save the supernate from the final wash for parallel testing with the eluate.
2.	Mix 1 vol of RBCs, 1 vol of 6% BSA, and 2 vol of chloroform in a 13×100-mm test tube.
3.	Stopper the tube and agitate for 15 seconds. Mix by inversion for 1 minute.
4.	Remove stopper and place tube at 56 C for 5 minutes. Stir periodically with applicator sticks.
5.	Centrifuge to remove particulate matter and harvest the eluate (upper layer).
6.	Test the eluate and the final wash supernate against the desired RBCs by one of the IAT methods described in Section II. **Note:** Dilute protein solutions (eg, eluates) are unstable and should be tested directly following preparation. If storage is necessary, the protein concentration should be adjusted to around 6 g/dL with bovine albumin. Eluates thus treated retain their antibody activity for several months when frozen.
7.	Interpret the results and proceed as follows:

If eluate is...	And final wash supernate is...	Then...
reactive	nonreactive	eluate reactions are valid: • Interpret results.
nonreactive	nonreactive	no antibody was eluted: • Consider passive ABO or drug-dependent antibody.
reactive	reactive	eluate reactions are invalid: • Repeat Steps 1- 7; extra washes of the RBCs before elution may be necessary.

Reference   Branch DR, Hian ALS, Petz LD. A new elution procedure using a nonflammable organic solvent (abstract). Transfusion 1980;20:635.

**Effective
Date**

Approved by:	Printed Name	Signature	Date
Laboratory Management			
Medical Director			
Quality Officer			

IV-C. Eluting Antibodies with Chloroform/Trichloroethylene

Purpose

To provide instructions for eluting IgG auto- and alloantibodies from RBCs using a mixture of chloroform and trichloroethylene:

- In the investigation of immune hemolysis due to autoantibodies, allo-antibodies, or drugs.

- In conjunction with an adsorption technique:

  o To confirm the presence or absence of an antigen on RBCs.

  o To concentrate an antibody.

  o To isolate an antibody in pure form from a serum containing multiple alloantibodies.

Background Information

Organic solvents probably influence antigen-antibody dissociation by several mechanisms, including:

- Alteration of the tertiary structure of antibody molecules.

- Disruption of the RBC membrane bilipid layer.

- Reversal of the forces of attraction between antigen and antibody.

The first two mechanisms result in loss of structural complementarity between antigen and antibody.

Operational Policy

Inhalation of chloroform in large doses may cause hypotension, cardiac and respiratory depression, and death, whereas moderate exposure to trichloroethylene can cause symptoms similar to alcohol inebriation and narcosis at high concentrations. Also, chloroform is carcinogenic in laboratory animals. Consequently, the following safety precautions should be followed:

- Store bulk quantities of organic solvents in an explosion-proof refrigerator or cabinet. Small amounts (eg, 4 oz) may be kept at room temperature in a stoppered container.

- Discard organic solvents when the container is one-quarter full. Some organic solvents become acidic during storage, probably as the result of peroxide formation. This may account for apparent nonspecific activity of eluates when the solvent used has been taken from an almost empty container.

- Use organic solvents in a well-ventilated area away from heat, flame, and electrical outlets; a properly constructed chemical hood is preferred.

- Store waste chloroform underwater in a large dark glass bottle and keep under a chemical hood. Dispose according to state and federal guidelines.

Limitations

Unwanted Positive Reactions:

- Incomplete washing of RBCs.

- Matuhasi-Ogata phenomenon.

- Incomplete removal of organic solvent.

Unwanted Negative Reactions:

- Incomplete removal of organic solvent.

- Incorrect technique.

Sample Requirements

RBCs for elution studies, washed as described in Procedure IV-A.

Equipment/ Materials

Chloroform: $CHCl_3$ (reagent grade).

Trichloroethylene: C_2HCl_3 (reagent grade).

Cork stoppers: size #2 (eg, VWR, Batavia, IL).

Note: Cork stoppers should be used when agitating eluates prepared with organic solvents. Cork allows the tube to "breathe" during agitation, thereby minimizing gas build-up that may cause the contents to splatter when the stopper is removed.

Glass Pasteur pipettes.

Quality Control

Save the supernate from the final wash (see Procedure IV-A) for parallel testing with the eluate.

In combined adsorption-elution studies, reserve an aliquot of the adsorbing RBC sample (uncoated) for testing with the eluate.

Procedure   Use the following steps to perform the procedure:

Step	Action
1.	Wash the RBCs as described in Procedure IV-A. **Note:** Save the supernate from the final wash for parallel testing with the eluate.
2.	Mix 1 vol of RBCs, 1 vol of saline, 1 vol of chloroform, and 1 vol of trichloroethylene in a 13 × 100-mm test tube.
3.	Stopper the tube and agitate for 15 seconds. Mix by inversion for 1 minute.
4.	Remove stopper and place tube at 37 C for 10 minutes. Stir periodically with applicator sticks.
5.	Centrifuge to remove particulate matter and harvest the eluate (upper layer).
6.	Test the eluate and the final wash supernate against the desired RBCs by one of the IAT methods described in Section II. **Note:** Dilute protein solutions (eg, eluates) are unstable and should be tested directly following preparation. If storage is necessary, the protein concentration should be adjusted to around 6 g/dL with bovine albumin. Eluates thus treated retain their antibody activity for several months when frozen.
7.	Interpret the results and proceed as follows:

If eluate is...	And final wash supernate is...	Then...
reactive	nonreactive	eluate reactions are valid: • Interpret results.
nonreactive	nonreactive	no antibody was eluted: • Consider passive ABO or drug-dependent antibody.
reactive	reactive	eluate reactions are invalid: • Repeat Steps 1-7; extra washes of the RBCs before elution may be necessary.

Reference   Massuet L, Martin C, Ribera A, et al. Antibody elution from red blood cells by chloroform and trichloroethylene. Transfusion 1982;22:359-61.

**Effective
Date**

Approved by:	Printed Name	Signature	Date
Laboratory Management			
Medical Director			
Quality Officer			

IV-D. Eluting Antibodies with Citric Acid

Purpose

To provide instructions for eluting IgG auto- and alloantibodies from RBCs using citric acid:

- In the investigation of immune hemolysis caused by autoantibodies, alloantibodies, or drugs.

- In conjunction with an adsorption technique:

  o To confirm the presence or absence of an antigen on RBCs.

  o To concentrate an antibody.

  o To isolate an antibody in pure form from a serum containing multiple alloantibodies.

To provide instructions for dissociating IgG from RBCs without compromising the integrity of RBC membrane antigens:

- To render DAT-positive RBCs DAT-negative, thereby permitting phenotyping with antisera that require use of the IAT (eg, anti-S, anti-Fy^a).

- Treatment of IgG-coated RBCs for autologous adsorption.

Background Information

Acids probably influence elution of antibody from coated RBCs by lowering the pH of antigen and antibody proteins such that they both become protonated. The antigens and antibodies lose their ability to attract one another through electrostatic bonding and may be forced apart by repulsion of like charges. The tertiary structure of proteins may be affected; hydrogen (H^+) ions are attracted to hydroxyl (OH^-) groups on aspartic and glutamic acids, resulting in molecular unfolding with consequential loss of structural complementarity between antigen and antibody.

Operational Policy

Do not test RBCs treated with citric acid for Kell antigens; these antigens are denatured by this procedure.

Limitations

Unwanted Positive Reactions:

- Incomplete washing of RBCs.

- Matuhasi-Ogata phenomenon.

- Failure to remove particulate matter before testing the eluate.

Unwanted Negative Reactions:

- Failure to adjust the pH of the eluate correctly.

- Incorrect technique.

Sample Requirements

RBCs for elution studies, washed as described in Procedure IV-A.

Equipment/ Materials

Citric acid eluting solution.

Neutralizing solution.

Litmus paper (range = pH 6-8).

Cork stoppers: size #2 (eg, VWR, Batavia, IL).

Quality Control

Save the supernate from the final wash (see Procedure IV-A) for parallel testing with the eluate.

In combined adsorption-elution studies, reserve an aliquot of the adsorbing RBC sample (uncoated) for testing with the eluate.

Procedure

Use the following steps to perform the procedure:

Step	Action
1.	Chill all reagents to 4 C before use.
2.	Wash the RBCs as described in Procedure IV-A. **Note:** Save the supernate from the final wash for parallel testing with the eluate, if required.
3.	Place 1 vol of packed RBCs in a 13 × 100-mm test tube.
4.	Add 1 vol of eluting solution and note the time.
5.	Stopper the tube and mix by inversion for exactly 90 seconds.
6.	Remove stopper and promptly centrifuge the tube at 1000 × g for 45 seconds (or equivalent).

7.	Transfer supernate to a clean test tube and add 5-6 drops of neutralizing solution.
8.	When performing adsorption or phenotyping studies, wash RBCs four times and test vs anti-IgG.
9.	Interpret the reactions and proceed as follows:

If the DAT is...	Then...
negative	• Confirm with IgG-coated RBCs. • Wash the total sample of treated RBCs and use for phenotyping or adsorption.
positive	procedure may be repeated once more.

10.	When performing elution studies, check pH of supernate and adjust if necessary to pH 7.0 by adding more neutralizing solution.
11.	Centrifuge to remove precipitate that forms after neutralization and harvest the supernate.
12.	Test the eluate and the final wash supernate against the desired RBCs by one of the IAT methods described in Section II. **Note:** Dilute protein solutions (eg, eluates) are unstable and should be tested directly following preparation. If storage is necessary, the protein concentration should be adjusted to around 6 g/dL with bovine albumin. Eluates thus treated retain their antibody activity for several months when frozen.
13.	Interpret the results and proceed as follows:

If eluate is...	And final wash supernate is...	Then...
reactive	nonreactive	eluate reactions are valid: • Interpret results.
nonreactive	nonreactive	no antibody was eluted: • Consider passive ABO or drug-dependent antibody.
reactive	teactive	eluate reactions are invalid: • Repeat Steps 1-7 and 10-13; extra washes of the RBCs before elution may be necessary.

Reference

Burich MA, AuBuchon JP, Anderson HJ. Antibody elution using citric acid (letter). Transfusion 1986;26:116-7.

Effective Date

Approved by

	Printed Name	Signature	Date
Laboratory Management			
Medical Director			
Quality Officer			

IV-E. Eluting Antibodies with Cold Acid

Purpose

To provide instructions for eluting IgG auto- and alloantibodies from RBCs using a cold acid solution:

- In the investigation of immune hemolysis caused by autoantibodies, alloantibodies, or drugs.

- In conjunction with an adsorption technique:

  o To confirm the presence or absence of an antigen on RBCs.

  o To concentrate an antibody.

  o To isolate an antibody in pure form from a serum containing multiple alloantibodies.

To provide for dissociating IgG from RBCs without compromising the integrity of RBC membrane antigens:

- To render DAT-positive RBCs DAT-negative, thereby permitting phenotyping with antisera that require use of the IAT (eg, anti-S, anti-Fy^a).

- Treatment of IgG-coated RBCs for autologous adsorption.

Background Information

Acids probably influence elution of antibody from coated RBCs by lowering the pH of antigen and antibody proteins such that they both become protonated. The antigens and antibodies lose their ability to attract one another through electrostatic bonding and may be forced apart by repulsion of like charges. The tertiary structure of proteins may be affected; hydrogen (H$^+$) ions are attracted to hydroxyl (OH$^-$) groups on aspartic and glutamic acids, resulting in molecular unfolding with consequential loss of structural complementarity between antigen and antibody.

The low pH of the glycine buffer enhances antibody dissociation from RBCs; addition of phosphate buffer restores neutrality to the acidic eluate.

Operational Policy

Do not test RBCs treated with citric acid for Kell antigens; these antigens are denatured by this procedure.

Persisting acidity may result in hemolysis of reagent RBCs. The addition of bovine albumin (1 part to 4 parts of eluate) may reduce such hemolysis. The addition of albumin also increases the stability of the eluted antibody, permitting frozen storage if needed.

Limitations

Unwanted Positive Reactions:

- Incomplete washing of RBCs.
- Matuhasi-Ogata phenomenon.
- Failure to remove particulate matter before testing the eluate.

Unwanted Negative Reactions:

- Failure to adjust the pH of the eluate correctly.
- Incorrect technique.

Sample Requirements

RBCs for elution studies, washed as described in Procedure IV-A.

Equipment/ Materials

Glycine: 0.1 M (pH 3.0; store refrigerated).

Phosphate buffer: 0.8 M (pH 8.2; store refrigerated).

Normal saline (store refrigerated).

Litmus paper (range = pH 6-8).

Cork stoppers: size #2 (eg, VWR, Batavia, IL).

Ice bath.

Quality Control

Save the supernate from the final wash (see Procedure IV-A) for parallel testing with the eluate.

In combined adsorption-elution studies, reserve an aliquot of the adsorbing RBC sample (uncoated) for testing with the eluate.

Procedure

Use the following steps to perform the procedure:

Step	Action
1.	Chill all reagents to 4 C before use.
2.	Wash the RBCs as described in Procedure IV-A. **Note:** Save the supernate from the final wash for parallel testing with the eluate, if required.
3.	Place 1 vol of packed RBCs in a 13 × 100-mm test tube.
4.	Add 1 vol of chilled saline and 2 vol of glycine solution.
5.	Stopper the tube and place in an ice bath for 1 minute.

6.	Remove stopper and promptly centrifuge the tube at $1000 \times g$ for 45 seconds (or equivalent).
7.	Transfer supernate to a clean test tube and add 5-6 drops of phosphate buffer.
8.	When performing adsorption or phenotyping studies, wash RBCs four times and test vs anti-IgG.

9.	Interpret the reactions and proceed as follows:

If the DAT is...	Then...
negative	• Confirm with IgG-coated RBCs. • Wash the total sample of treated RBCs and use for phenotyping or adsorption.
positive	procedure may be repeated once more.

10.	When performing elution studies, check pH of supernate and adjust if necessary to pH 7.0 by adding more phosphate buffer.
11.	Centrifuge to remove precipitate that forms after neutralization and harvest the supernate.
12.	Test the eluate and the final wash supernate against the desired RBCs by one of the IAT methods described in Section II. **Note:** Dilute protein solutions (eg, eluates) are unstable and should be tested directly following preparation. If storage is necessary, the protein concentration should be adjusted to around 6 g/dL with bovine albumin. Eluates thus treated retain their antibody activity for several months when frozen.
13.	Interpret the results and proceed as follows:

If eluate is...	And final wash supernate is...	Then...
reactive	nonreactive	eluate reactions are valid: • Interpret results.
nonreactive	nonreactive	no antibody was eluted: • Consider passive ABO or drug-dependent antibody.
reactive	reactive	eluate reactions are invalid: • Repeat Steps 1-13; extra washes of the RBCs before elution may be necessary.

Reference   Rekvig OP, Hannestad K. Acid elution of blood group antibodies from intact erythrocytes. Vox Sang 1977;33:280-5.

Effective Date

Approved by

	Printed Name	Signature	Date
Laboratory Management			
Medical Director			
Quality Officer			

IV-F. Eluting Antibodies from Stroma

Purpose

To provide instructions for preparing hemoglobin-free eluates from RBC stroma using a cold acid solution:

- In the investigation of immune hemolysis caused by autoantibodies, alloantibodies, or drugs.

- In conjunction with an adsorption technique:

  o To confirm the presence or absence of an antigen on RBCs.

  o To concentrate an antibody.

  o To isolate an antibody in pure form from a serum containing multiple alloantibodies.

Background Information

Acids probably influence elution of antibody from coated RBCs by lowering the pH of antigen and antibody proteins such that they both become protonated. The antigens and antibodies lose their ability to attract one another through electrostatic bonding and may be forced apart by repulsion of like charges. The tertiary structure of proteins may be affected; hydrogen (H^+) ions are attracted to hydroxyl (OH^-) groups on aspartic and glutamic acids, resulting in molecular unfolding with consequential loss of structural complementarity between antigen and antibody.

The low pH of the glycine buffer enhances antibody dissociation from RBCs; addition of phosphate buffer restores neutrality to the acidic eluate.

Operational Policy

Use this procedure when hemoglobin-free eluates are required (eg, in the preparation of typing reagents suitable for all ABO types using a combined adsorption-elution technique.

Persisting acidity may result in hemolysis of reagent RBCs. The addition of bovine albumin (1 part to 4 parts of eluate) may reduce such hemolysis. The addition of albumin also increases the stability of the eluted antibody, permitting frozen storage if needed.

Note: Digitonin is an irritant and may cause death if swallowed or adsorbed through the skin.

If inhaled, remove to fresh air. If breathing is difficult, give oxygen.

In case of contact, immediately flush eyes or skin with large amounts of water for at least 15 minutes; remove contaminated clothing.

Wash contaminated clothing before reuse.

Limitations

Unwanted Positive Reactions:

- Incomplete washing of RBCs.
- Matuhasi-Ogata phenomenon.
- Failure to remove particulate matter before testing the eluate.

Unwanted Negative Reactions:

- Failure to adjust the pH of the eluate correctly.
- Incorrect technique.

Sample Requirements

RBCs for elution studies, washed as described in Procedure IV-A.

Equipment/ Materials

Digitonin: 0.5% wt/vol.

Glycine: 0.1 M (pH 3.0).

Phosphate buffer: 0.8 M (pH 8.2).

Normal saline (store refrigerated).

Litmus paper (range = pH 6-8).

Cork stoppers: size #6 (eg, VWR, Batavia, IL).

Pipettors with disposable tips to deliver 0.5 mL to 1 mL (eg, VWR, Batavia, IL).

10-mL graduated pipettes (eg, VWR, Batavia, IL).

Quality Control

Save the supernate from the final wash (see Procedure IV-A) for parallel testing with the eluate.

In combined adsorption-elution studies, reserve an aliquot of the adsorbing RBC sample (uncoated) for testing with the eluate.

Procedure   Use the following steps to perform the procedure:

Step	Action
1.	Warm reagents to 37 C before use and mix well.
2.	Wash the RBCs as described in Procedure IV-A. **Note:** Save the supernate from the final wash (see Procedure IV-A) for parallel testing with the eluate.
3.	Mix 1 mL of RBCs and 9 mL of saline in a 16 × 100-mm test tube.
4.	Add 0.5 mL of digitonin. Stopper the tube and mix by inversion until lysis is complete (at least 1 minute).
5.	Remove stopper and centrifuge the tube to deposit the stroma. Discard the supernate.
6.	Wash the stroma until it appears white (at least 5 washes). Centrifuge at $1000 \times g$ for 2 minutes (or equivalent) per wash.
7.	Discard the supernate wash solution and add 2 mL of glycine.
8.	Stopper the tube and mix by inversion for at least 1 minute.
9.	Remove stopper and centrifuge the tube to remove particulate matter.
10.	Transfer the eluate into a clean test tube and add 0.2 mL of phosphate buffer.
11.	Mix and centrifuge again to remove any precipitate and harvest the supernate.
12.	Check pH of supernate and adjust if necessary to pH 7.0 by adding more phosphate buffer.
13.	Test the eluate and the final wash supernate against the desired RBCs by one of the IAT methods described in Section II. **Note:** Dilute protein solutions (eg, eluates) are unstable and should be tested directly following preparation. If storage is necessary, the protein concentration should be adjusted to around 6 g/dL with bovine albumin. Eluates thus treated retain their antibody activity for several months when frozen.

14.	Interpret the results and proceed as follows:		
	If eluate is...	**And final wash supernate is...**	**Then...**
	reactive	nonreactive	eluate reactions are valid: • Interpret results.
	nonreactive	nonreactive	no antibody was eluted: • Consider passive ABO or drug-dependent antibody.
	reactive	reactive	eluate reactions are invalid: • Repeat Steps 1-14; extra washes of the RBC/stroma before elution may be necessary.

References

Araszkiewicz P, Huff SR, Szymanski IO. Modification of acid stromal elution for complete recovery of bound antibodies. Transfusion 1983;23:72-4.

Jenkins DE, Moore WH. A rapid procedure for the preparation of high-potency auto- and alloantibody eluates. Transfusion 1977;17:110-7.

Effective Date

Approved by

Laboratory Management

Medical Director

Quality Officer

Printed Name	Signature	Date

IV-G. Eluting Antibodies with Ether

Purpose

To provide instructions for eluting IgG auto- and alloantibodies from RBCs using ether:

- In the investigation of immune hemolysis caused by autoantibodies, alloantibodies, or drugs.

- In conjunction with an adsorption technique:

  o To confirm the presence or absence of an antigen on RBCs.

  o To concentrate an antibody.

  o To isolate an antibody in pure form from a serum containing multiple alloantibodies.

Background Information

Organic solvents probably influence antigen-antibody dissociation by several mechanisms, including:

- Alteration of the tertiary structure of antibody molecules.

- Disruption of the RBC membrane bilipid layer.

- Reversal of the forces of attraction between antigen and antibody.

The first two mechanisms result in loss of structural complementarity between antigen and antibody.

Operational Policy

Ether is an explosion hazard, a mild skin irritant, and a narcotic in high concentrations. Consequently, the following safety precautions should be followed:

- Store bulk quantities of organic solvents in an explosion-proof refrigerator or cabinet. Small amounts (eg, 4 oz) may be kept at room temperature in a stoppered container.

- Discard organic solvents when the container is one-quarter full. Some organic solvents become acidic during storage, probably as the result of peroxide formation. This may account for apparent nonspecific activity of eluates when the solvent used has been taken from an almost empty container.

- Use organic solvents in a well-ventilated area away from heat, flame, and electrical outlets; a properly constructed chemical hood is preferred.

Limitations   Unwanted Positive Reactions:

- Incomplete washing of RBCs.

- Matuhasi-Ogata phenomenon.

- Incomplete removal of organic solvent.

Unwanted Negative Reactions:

- Incomplete removal of organic solvent.

- Incorrect technique.

Sample   RBCs for elution studies, washed as described in Procedure IV-A.
Requirements

Equipment/   Diethyl ether: $C_4H_{10}O$ (anesthesia/reagent grade).
Materials
Cork stoppers: size #2 (eg, VWR, Batavia, IL).

Note: Cork stoppers should be used when agitating eluates prepared with organic solvents. Cork allows the tube to "breathe" during agitation, thereby minimizing gas build-up that may cause the contents to splatter when the stopper is removed.

Glass Pasteur pipettes.

Quality   Save the supernate from the final wash (see Procedure IV-A) for parallel
Control   testing with the eluate.

In combined adsorption-elution studies, reserve an aliquot of the adsorbing RBC sample (uncoated) for testing with the eluate.

Procedure   Use the following steps to perform the procedure:

Step	Action
1.	Wash the RBCs as described in Procedure IV-A. **Note:** Save the supernate from the final wash for parallel testing with the eluate.
2.	Mix equal volumes of RBCs and ether in a 13 × 100-mm test tube.
3.	Stopper the tube and agitate vigorously for 1-2 minutes.

4.	Remove stopper and place tube at 37 for 15 minutes. Stir periodically with applicator sticks.
5.	Centrifuge to remove particulate matter. Remove upper layer of ether and discard.
6.	With a glass Pasteur pipette, carefully transfer hemoglobin-stained eluate beneath stromal layer into a clean tube.
7.	Place at 37 C and periodically bubble air through eluate, using a Pasteur pipette, to facilitate removal of residual ether.
8.	When the eluate no longer smells of ether, centrifuge to remove particulate matter and harvest the supernate.
9.	Test the eluate and the final wash supernate against the desired RBCs by one of the IAT methods described in Section II. **Note:** Dilute protein solutions (eg, eluates) are unstable and should be tested directly following preparation. If storage is necessary, the protein concentration should be adjusted to around 6 g/dL with bovine albumin. Eluates thus treated retain their antibody activity for several months when frozen.
10.	Interpret the results and proceed as follows:

If eluate is...	And final wash supernate is...	Then...
reactive	nonreactive	eluate reactions are valid: • Interpret results.
nonreactive	nonreactive	no antibody was eluted: • Consider passive ABO or drug-dependent antibody.
reactive	reactive	eluate reactions are invalid: • Repeat Steps 1-10; extra washes of the RBCs before elution may be necessary.

References   Rubin H. Antibody elution from red blood cells. J Clin Path 1963;16:70-3.

Vos G. The evaluation of specific anti-G (CD) eluates obtained by a double adsorption and elution procedure. Vox Sang 1960;5:472-8.

Effective Date

Approved by	Printed Name	Signature	Date
Laboratory Management			
Medical Director			
Quality Officer			

IV-H. Eluting Antibodies by Freezing-Thawing (Lui Method)

Purpose   To provide instructions for eluting ABO antibodies:

- Investigation of ABO HDFN.

- Detection of weak A and B antigens on RBCs (combined adsorption-elution procedure with polyclonal antibodies).

- Detection of passive anti-A and/or anti-B in recipients of non-ABO-type-specific, plasma-containing components or marrow.

Background Information   As RBCs freeze, extracellular ice crystals form that attract pure water from their surroundings, resulting in an increase in the osmolarity of the extracellular fluid that then attracts intracellular water molecules. The RBCs shrink, then hemolyze. RBC membranes are disrupted, with resultant loss of structural complementarity between antigen and antibody.

Operational Policy   Rarely do elution studies provide useful additional information when investigating ABO HDFN. The diagnosis of ABO HDFN can be made from clinical observations and by demonstrating ABO incompatibility between maternal plasma and the infant's RBCs.

Polyclonal anti-A and/or anti-B should be used in combined adsorption-elution procedures because unwanted negative results may be encountered with monoclonal antibodies. See Procedure XIII-K for selecting high-titer anti-A and anti-B.

Limitations   Unwanted Positive Reactions:

- Incomplete washing of RBCs.

- Matuhasi-Ogata phenomenon.

- Failure to remove particulate matter before testing the eluate.

Unwanted Negative Reactions:

- Incorrect technique.

Sample Requirements   RBCs for elution studies, washed as described in Procedure IV-A.

Equipment/ Materials

Cork stoppers: size #2 (eg, VWR, Batavia, IL).

Freezer at –20 C or below.

Water faucet with running warm water.

Pipettors with disposable tips to deliver 0.5 mL (eg, VWR, Batavia, IL).

Quality Control

Save the supernate from the final wash (see Procedure IV-A) for parallel testing with the eluate.

In combined adsorption-elution studies, reserve an aliquot of the adsorbing RBC sample (uncoated) for testing with the eluate.

Procedure

Use the following steps to perform the procedure:

Step	Action
1.	Wash the RBCs as described in Procedure IV-A. **Note:** Save the supernate from the final wash for parallel testing with the eluate.
2.	Mix 0.5 mL RBCs with 3 drops isotonic saline in a 13 × 100-mm glass test tube.
3.	Stopper the tube and rotate to coat glass surface with RBCs.
4.	Place at –20 C for 10 minutes. **Note:** RBCs may be kept frozen overnight.
5.	Thaw the RBCs rapidly under warm running tap water.
6.	Remove stopper and centrifuge the tube to remove particulate matter; then harvest the supernate.
7.	Test the eluate and the final wash supernate against the desired RBCs by direct agglutination and/or one of the IAT methods described in Section II.

8.	Interpret the results and proceed as follows:		
	If eluate is...	**And final wash supernate is...**	**Then...**
	reactive	nonreactive	eluate reactions are valid: • Interpret results.
	nonreactive	nonreactive	no antibody was eluted.
	reactive	reactive	eluate reactions are invalid: • Repeat Steps 1-8; extra washes of the RBCs before elution may be necessary.

Reference

Feng CS, Kirkley KC, Eicher CA, de Jongh DS. The Lui elution technique: A simple and efficient procedure for eluting ABO antibodies. Transfusion 1985;25:433-4.

Effective Date

	Printed Name	Signature	Date
Approved by			
Laboratory Management			
Medical Director			
Quality Officer			

IV-I. Eluting Antibodies by Freezing-Thawing (Wiener Method)

Purpose

To provide instructions for antibody elution using an organic solvent in conjunction with a freeze-thaw procedure:

- Investigation of ABO HDFN.

- Detection of weak A and B antigens on RBCs (combined adsorption-elution procedure with polyclonal antibodies).

- Detection of passive anti-A and/or anti-B in recipients of non-ABO-type-specific, plasma-containing components or marrow.

Background Information

This procedure uses an organic solvent and the action of freezing and thawing to dissociate antigen-antibody complexes. Organic solvents probably influence antigen-antibody dissociation by several mechanisms, including 1) alteration of the tertiary structure of antibody molecules, 2) disruption of the RBC membrane bilipid layer, and 3) reversal of the forces of attraction between antigen and antibody. The first two mechanisms result in loss of structural complementarity between antigen and antibody. As RBCs freeze, extracellular ice crystals form that attract pure water from their surroundings, resulting in an increase in the osmolarity of the extracellular fluid that then attracts intracellular water molecules. The RBCs shrink, then hemolyze. RBC membranes are disrupted, with resultant loss of structural complementarity between antigen and antibody.

Operational Policy

The following safety precautions should be followed:

- Store bulk quantities of organic solvents in an explosion-proof refrigerator or cabinet. Small amounts (eg, 4 oz) may be kept at room temperature in a stoppered container.

- Discard organic solvents when the container is one-quarter full. Some organic solvents become acidic during storage, probably as the result of peroxide formation. This may account for apparent nonspecific activity of eluates when the solvent used has been taken from an almost empty container.

- Use organic solvents in a well-ventilated area away from heat, flame, and electrical outlets; a properly constructed chemical hood is preferred.

- Store waste ethanol in a large, dark glass bottle and keep under a chemical hood. Dispose according to state and federal guidelines.

Rarely do elution studies provide useful additional information when investigating ABO HDFN. The diagnosis of ABO HDFN can be made from clinical observations and by demonstrating ABO incompatibility between maternal plasma and the infant's RBCs.

Polyclonal anti-A and/or anti-B should be used in combined adsorption-elution procedures because unwanted negative results may be encountered with monoclonal antibodies. See Procedure XIII-K for selecting high-titer anti-A and anti-B.

Limitations

Unwanted Positive Reactions:

- Incomplete washing of RBCs.

- Matuhasi-Ogata phenomenon.

- Failure to remove particulate matter before testing the eluate.

Unwanted Negative Reactions:

- Incorrect technique.

Sample Requirements

RBCs for elution studies, washed as described in Procedure IV-A.

Equipment/ Materials

Cork stoppers: size #2 (eg, VWR, Batavia, IL).

Note: Cork stoppers should be used when agitating eluates prepared with organic solvents. Cork allows the tube to "breathe" during agitation, thereby minimizing gas build-up that may cause the contents to splatter when the stopper is removed.

Glass Pasteur pipettes.

Freezer at –20 C and –70 C.

Water faucet with running warm water.

6% BSA.

50% Ethanol: C_2H_5OH, 1 part; distilled water, 1 part.

Pipettors with disposable tips to deliver 0.5 mL to 1 mL (eg, VWR, Batavia, IL).

10-mL graduated pipettes (eg, VWR, Batavia, IL).

Note: Cool ethanol mixture to –6 C in the freezing compartment of an explosion-proof refrigerator before use.

Quality Control

Save the supernate from the final wash (see Procedure IV-A) for parallel testing with the eluate.

In combined adsorption-elution studies, reserve an aliquot of the adsorbing RBC sample (uncoated) for testing with the eluate.

Procedure

Use the following steps to perform the procedure:

Step	Action
1.	Wash the RBCs as described in Procedure IV-A. **Note:** Save the supernate from the final wash for parallel testing with the eluate.
2.	Transfer 1 mL washed RBCs into a stoppered 16 × 100-mm test tube and place at −70 C for 10 minutes.
3.	Thaw the RBCs rapidly under warm running tap water.
4.	Add 10 mL of cold ethanol. Stopper the tube with a cork, mix well by inversion and place the tube at −20 C for 1 hour.
5.	Centrifuge to remove particulate matter and discard the supernate.
6.	Break up the RBC stroma with applicator sticks and wash once with distilled water. Centrifuge to remove particulate matter and completely discard the supernate.
7.	Add 1 mL of 6% albumin and mix well, using applicator sticks to break up the stroma.
8.	Incubate at 37 C for 1 hour.
9.	Centrifuge to remove particulate matter and harvest the supernate.
10.	Test the eluate and the final wash supernate against the desired RBCs by direct agglutination and/or one of the IAT methods described in Section II.

11.	Interpret the results and proceed as follows:		
	If eluate is…	**And final wash supernate is…**	**Then…**
	reactive	nonreactive	eluate reactions are valid: • Interpret results.
	nonreactive	nonreactive	no antibody was eluted.
	reactive	reactive	eluate reactions are invalid: • Repeat Steps 1-11; extra washes of the RBCs before elution may be necessary.

Reference   Wiener W. Eluting red-cell antibodies: A procedure and its application. Br J Haematol 1957;3:276.

Effective Date

Approved by

	Printed Name	Signature	Date
Laboratory Management			
Medical Director			
Quality Officer			

IV-J. Eluting Antibodies by Heat

Purpose

To provide instructions for elution using heat:

- Investigation of ABO HDFN.

- Detection of weak A and B antigens on RBCs (combined adsorption-elution procedure with polyclonal antibodies).

Background Information

The exothermic reaction for the formation of antibody-antigen complexes can be represented by the following equation:

$$Ag + Ab \leftrightarrows [AgAb] + calories$$

Thus, an increase in temperature results in displacement of the equation to the left or dissociation of [AgAb].

Operational Policy

Rarely do elution studies provide useful additional information when investigating ABO HDFN. The diagnosis of ABO HDFN can be made from clinical observations and by demonstrating ABO incompatibility between maternal plasma and the infant's RBCs.

Polyclonal anti-A and/or anti-B should be used in combined adsorption-elution procedures because unwanted negative results may be encountered with monoclonal antibodies. See Procedure XIII-K for selecting high-titer anti-A and anti-B.

Limitations

Unwanted Positive Reactions:

- Incomplete washing of RBCs.

- Matuhasi-Ogata phenomenon.

Unwanted Negative Reactions:

- Incorrect technique.

Sample Requirements

RBCs for elution studies, washed as described in Procedure IV-A.

Equipment/ Materials	6% BSA.
	Applicator sticks.
	Water bath at 56 C.

Quality Control	Save the supernate from the final wash (see Procedure IV-A) for parallel testing with the eluate.
	In combined adsorption-elution studies, reserve an aliquot of the adsorbing RBC sample (uncoated) for testing with the eluate.

Procedure Use the following steps to perform the procedure:

Step	Action
1.	Wash the RBCs as described in Procedure IV-A. **Note:** For optimal recovery of cold-reactive antibodies, RBCs should be washed in ice-cold saline to prevent dissociation of bound antibody before elution. **Note:** Save the supernate from the final wash for parallel testing with the eluate.
2.	Mix equal volumes of 6% BSA and RBCs.
3.	Incubate at 56 C for 10 minutes, stirring periodically with applicator sticks.
4.	Centrifuge to remove particulate matter and harvest the supernate using a heated centrifuge, if available.
5.	Test the eluate and the final wash supernate against the desired RBCs by direct agglutination and/or one of the IAT methods described in Section II.
6.	Interpret the results and proceed as follows: <table><tr><th>If eluate is...</th><th>And final wash supernate is...</th><th>Then...</th></tr><tr><td>reactive</td><td>nonreactive</td><td>eluate reactions are valid: • Interpret results.</td></tr><tr><td>nonreactive</td><td>nonreactive</td><td>no antibody was eluted.</td></tr><tr><td>reactive</td><td>reactive</td><td>eluate reactions are invalid: • Repeat Steps 1-10; extra washes of the RBCs before elution may be necessary.</td></tr></table>

Reference   Landsteiner K, Miller CP. Serological studies on the blood of primates. II. The blood groups in anthropoid apes. J Exp Med 1925;42:853-62.

**Effective
Date**

Approved by	Printed Name	Signature	Date
Laboratory Management			
Medical Director			
Quality Officer			

IV-K. Eluting Antibodies with Methylene Chloride

Purpose

To provide instructions for eluting IgG auto- and alloantibodies from RBCs using methylene chloride:

- In the investigation of immune hemolysis caused by autoantibodies, alloantibodies, or drugs

- In conjunction with an adsorption technique:

  o To confirm the presence or absence of an antigen on RBCs.

  o To concentrate an antibody.

  o To isolate an antibody in pure form from a serum containing multiple alloantibodies.

Background Information

Organic solvents probably influence antigen-antibody dissociation by several mechanisms, including:

- Alteration of the tertiary structure of antibody molecules.

- Disruption of the RBC membrane bilipid layer.

- Reversal of the forces of attraction between antigen and antibody.

The first two mechanisms result in loss of structural complementarity between antigen and antibody.

Operational Policy

Methylene chloride is a narcotic in high concentrations. Consequently, the following safety precautions should be followed:

- Store bulk quantities of organic solvents in an explosion-proof refrigerator or cabinet. Small amounts (eg, 4 oz) may be kept at room temperature in a stoppered container.

- Discard organic solvents when the container is one-quarter full. Some organic solvents become acidic during storage, probably as the result of peroxide formation. This may account for apparent nonspecific activity of eluates when the solvent used has been taken from an almost empty container.

- Use organic solvents in a well-ventilated area away from heat, flame, and electrical outlets; a properly constructed chemical hood is preferred.

- Allow organic solvents to evaporate in a large, dark glass vessel and keep under a chemical hood. Dispose according to state and federal guidelines.

Limitations

Unwanted Positive Reactions:

- Incomplete washing of RBCs.
- Matuhasi-Ogata phenomenon.
- Incomplete removal of organic solvent.

Unwanted Negative Reactions:

- Incomplete removal of organic solvent.
- Incorrect technique.

Sample Requirements

RBCs for elution studies, washed as described in Procedure IV-A.

Equipment/ Materials

22% or 30% BSA.

Methylene chloride (dichloromethane): CH_2Cl_2.

Cork stoppers: size #2 (eg, VWR, Batavia, IL).

Note: Cork stoppers should be used when agitating eluates prepared with organic solvents. Cork allows the tube to "breathe" during agitation, thereby minimizing gas build-up that may cause the contents to splatter when the stopper is removed.

Glass Pasteur pipettes.

Quality Control

Save the supernate from the final wash (see Procedure IV-A) for parallel testing with the eluate.

In combined adsorption-elution studies, reserve an aliquot of the adsorbing RBC sample (uncoated) for testing with the eluate.

Procedure

Use the following steps to perform the procedure:

Step	Action
1.	Wash the RBCs as described in Procedure IV-A. **Note:** Save the supernate from the final wash for parallel testing with the eluate.
2.	Mix 1 mL of RBCs, 1 mL of saline, and 2 mL of methylene chloride.

3.	Stopper the tube and mix by gentle agitation for 1 minute.
4.	Remove stopper and centrifuge the tube at 1000 × g (or equivalent) for 10 minutes.
5.	Remove lower layer of methylene chloride with a Pasteur pipette and discard.
6.	Place tube at 56 C for 10 minutes and stir periodically with applicator sticks.
7.	Centrifuge at 1000 × g for 10 minutes (or equivalent) and harvest the supernate.
8.	Test the eluate and the final wash supernate against the desired RBCs by direct agglutination and/or one of the IAT methods described in Section II.
9.	Interpret the results and proceed as follows:

If eluate is...	And final wash supernate is...	Then...
reactive	nonreactive	eluate reactions are valid: • Interpret results.
nonreactive	nonreactive	no antibody was eluted: • Consider passive ABO or drug-dependent antibody.
reactive	reactive	eluate reactions are invalid: • Repeat Steps 1-8; extra washes of the RBCs before elution may be necessary.

Reference   Ellisor SS, Papenfus L, Sugasawara E, Azzi R. Dichloromethane (DCM) elution procedure (abstract). Transfusion 1982;22:409.

**Effective
Date**

Approved by	Printed Name	Signature	Date
Laboratory Management			
Medical Director			
Quality Officer			

IV-L. Eluting Antibodies with Microwaves

Purpose

To provide a method for antibody elution using microwaves:

- Investigation of ABO HDFN.

- Detection of weak A and B antigens on RBCs (combined adsorption-elution procedure with polyclonal antibodies).

Background Information

The exothermic reaction for the formation of antibody-antigen complexes can be represented by the following equation:

$$Ag + Ab \leftrightarrows [AgAb] + calories$$

Thus, an increase in temperature results in displacement of the equation to the left or dissociation of [AgAb].

Operational Policy

To ensure a constant final output temperature, accuracy of RBC suspensions and cooling before elution are essential.

Rarely do elution studies provide useful additional information when investigating ABO HDFN. The diagnosis of ABO HDFN can be made from clinical observations and by demonstrating ABO incompatibility between maternal plasma and the infant's RBCs.

Polyclonal anti-A and/or anti-B should be used in combined adsorption-elution procedures because unwanted negative results may be encountered with monoclonal antibodies. See Procedure XIII-K for selecting high-titer anti-A and anti-B.

Limitations

Unwanted Positive Reactions:

- Incomplete washing of RBCs.

- Matuhasi-Ogata phenomenon.

Unwanted Negative Reactions:

- Incorrect technique.

Sample Requirements

RBCs for elution studies, washed as described in Procedure IV-A.

Equipment/ Materials

Graduated conical centrifuge tubes: 10-mL to 15-mL capacity (eg, VWR, Batavia, IL).

12 × 75-mm polypropylene tubes (BD, Franklin Lakes, NJ).

Microwave oven using 2450 mHz microwaves (any conventional microwave oven). Calibrate for use as follows:

- Place a plastic test tube rack in the oven and mark its location. Always replace the rack at that location.

- Prepare an accurate 50% suspension of RBCs with saline. Dispense 2-mL aliquots into 12 × 75-mm polypropylene tubes. Place tubes in melting ice for 5 minutes.

- Use a constant power setting and vary the time to test different tube locations within the rack. Remove the tubes to measure the final output temperature.

Note: Samples must be microwaved individually.

- Mark those tube locations and note the time setting at which the final output temperature is between 56 C and 62 C. Use these locations when performing microwave elutions.

Quality Control

Save the supernate from the final wash (see Procedure IV-A) for parallel testing with the eluate.

In combined adsorption-elution studies, reserve an aliquot of the adsorbing RBC sample (uncoated) for testing with the eluate.

Procedure

Use the following steps to perform the procedure:

Step	Action
1.	Wash the RBCs as described in Procedure IV-A. **Note:** Save the supernate from the final wash for parallel testing with the eluate.
2.	Place 1 mL RBCs in a 10-mL to 15-mL graduated conical centrifuge tube. Fill the tube with saline and centrifuge at 1000 × g (or equivalent) for 10 minutes.
3.	Remove supernate and add sufficient saline to yield a 50% RBC suspension.
4.	Transfer 2 mL of 50% RBCs into a 12 × 75-mm polypropylene tube and place in melting ice for 5 minutes.
5.	Place the polypropylene tube in the predetermined rack position and expose to microwaves using the established time and power settings.

6.	Centrifuge to remove particulate matter and harvest the supernate.
7.	Test the eluate and the final wash supernate against the desired RBCs by direct agglutination and/or one of the IAT methods described in Section II.
8.	Interpret the results and proceed as follows:

If eluate is...	And final wash supernate is...	Then...
reactive	nonreactive	eluate reactions are valid: • Interpret results.
nonreactive	nonreactive	no antibody was eluted.
reactive	reactive	eluate reactions are invalid: • Repeat Steps 1-8; extra washes of the RBCs before elution may be necessary.

Reference

Meier TJ, Wilkinson SL, Utz G. Elution of antibody from sensitized red blood cells using a conventional microwave oven (abstract). Transfusion 1983;23:411.

Effective Date

Approved by

Laboratory Management

Medical Director

Quality Officer

	Printed Name	Signature	Date

IV-M. Eluting Antibodies from Placental Tissue

Purpose

To provide a method for recovering antibody from placental tissue.

- Preparation of large volumes of antibody for phenotyping.

Background Information

The placenta is an abundant source of immunoglobulins. When obtained from an alloimmunized pregnancy, the placenta can be used to prepare large volumes of hemoglobin-free, specific antibody for phenotyping purposes.

Acids probably influence elution of antibody from coated RBCs by lowering the pH of antigen and antibody proteins such that they both become protonated. The antigens and antibodies lose their ability to attract one another through electrostatic bonding and may be forced apart by repulsion of like charges. The tertiary structure of proteins may be affected; hydrogen (H^+) ions are attracted to hydroxyl (OH^-) groups on aspartic and glutamic acids, resulting in molecular unfolding with consequential loss of structural complementarity between antigen and antibody.

Operational Policy

Persisting acidity may result in hemolysis of reagent RBCs; the addition of bovine albumin (1 part to 4 parts of eluate) may reduce such hemolysis. The addition of albumin also increases the stability of the eluted antibody, permitting frozen storage if needed.

Note: Digitonin is an irritant and may cause death if swallowed or adsorbed through the skin.

If inhaled, remove to fresh air. If breathing is difficult, give oxygen.

In case of contact, immediately flush eyes or skin with large amounts of water for at least 15 minutes; remove contaminated clothing.

Wash contaminated clothing before reuse.

Limitations

Unwanted Positive Reactions:

- Failure to remove particulate matter before testing the eluate.

Unwanted Negative Reactions:

- Failure to adjust the pH of the eluate correctly.
- Incorrect technique.

Sample Requirements

Placenta from an alloimmunized pregnancy. Placental tissue should be fresh and unfixed but may be covered with saline for transportation to the laboratory. Dissect into cubes (approximately 2 cm^2).

Equipment/ Materials

30% BSA.

Digitonin: 0.5% wt/vol.

Glycine: 0.1 M (pH 3.0).

Phosphate buffer: 0.8 M (pH 8.2).

Normal saline (store refrigerated).

Litmus paper (range = pH 6-8).

Waring blender (eg, VWR, Batavia, IL).

100-mL and 1-L measuring cylinders and 1-L flasks (eb, VWR, Batavia, IL).

RC-3C regrigerated centrifuge (eg, Thermo Fisher Scientific, Waltham, MA).

Quality Control

Check specificity and titer of eluted antibody. Titer should be ≥8 for reagent use.

Procedure

Use the following steps to perform the procedure:

Step	Action
1.	Warm reagents to 37 C before use and mix well.
2.	Centrifuge placenta and harvest supernate. **Note:** This is a source of serum that can be evaluated for antibody activity.
3.	Place residual tissue in the blender and add 100 mL of digitonin and 200 mL of saline. Homogenize tissue to a fine emulsion.
4.	Centrifuge to pack the residue (10 minutes at 1000 × g, or equivalent). Discard the supernate.
5.	Wash residual material four times with saline. Ensure adequate mixing with saline during each wash.
6.	Add 400 mL of glycine and mix in the blender for 1 minute.
7.	Allow to stand at room temperature for 10 minutes and mix again.

8.	Centrifuge at $1000 \times g$ for 10 minutes (or equivalent) and harvest supernate.
9.	Add 1 mL of 0.8 M phosphate buffer per 10 mL of eluate and mix well. Check pH, adjusting to pH 7.0 ± 0.5 with 1 N NaOH or 1 N HCl as necessary.
10.	Centrifuge at $1000 \times g$ for 10 minutes (or equivalent) and harvest the supernate.
11.	Add 2 mL of 30% BSA per 10 mL of eluate.
12.	Test for specificity and potency (titer) by saline IAT using 30 minutes incubation and anti-IgG. See Section VIII and Procedures II-I and X-D.
13.	Proceed as follows:

14.	**If...**	**Then...**
	titer ≥8 and specificity is confirmed	dispense into convenient aliquots and store below –20 C for future testing.
	unable to confirm specificity, or titer <8	eluate is unsuitable for confirmatory phenotyping but may be suitable for screening purposes.

Reference   Moulds JJ, Mallory D, Zodin V. Placental eluates: An economical source of antibodies (abstract). Transfusion 1978;18:388.

Effective Date

Approved by

	Printed Name	Signature	Date
Laboratory Management			
Medical Director			
Quality Officer			

IV-N. Eluting Antibodies Using Ultrasound

Purpose   To provide instructions for elution using ultrasound:

- Investigation of ABO HDFN.

- Detection of weak A and B antigens on RBCs (combined adsorption-elution procedure with polyclonal antibodies).

- Detection of passive anti-A and/or anti-B in recipients of non-ABO-type-specific, plasma-containing components or marrow.

Background Information   High-frequency sound waves cause rapid alternation in pressure within fluids such that minute gas bubbles are formed. As these bubbles grow to a critical size, they implode, causing shock waves that exert considerable shearing forces. Antibody molecules are shaken off the RBCs.

Operational Policy   Rarely do elution studies provide useful additional information when investigating ABO HDFN. The diagnosis of ABO HDFN can be made from clinical observations and by demonstrating ABO incompatibility between maternal plasma and the infant's RBCs.

Polyclonal anti-A and/or anti-B should be used in combined adsorption-elution procedures because unwanted negative results may be encountered with monoclonal antibodies. See Procedure XIII-K for selecting high-titer anti-A and anti-B.

Limitations   Unwanted Positive Reactions:

- Incomplete washing of RBCs.

- Matuhasi-Ogata phenomenon.

Unwanted Negative Reactions:

- Incorrect technique.

Sample Requirements   RBCs for elution studies, washed as described in Procedure IV-A.

Equipment/ Materials	6% BSA.
	Applicator sticks.
	Ultrasound cleaning bath (eg, VWR, Batavia, IL).
	Pipettors with disposable tips to deliver 1 mL (eg, VWR, Batavia, IL).

Quality Control	Save the supernate from the final wash (see Procedure IV-A) for parallel testing with the eluate.
	In combined adsorption-elution studies, reserve an aliquot of the adsorbing RBC sample (uncoated) for testing with the eluate.

Procedure   Use the following steps to perform the procedure:

Step	Action
1.	Wash the RBCs as described in Procedure IV-A. **Note:** Save the supernate from the final wash for parallel testing with the eluate.
2.	Mix 1 mL of 6% BSA and 1 mL of RBCs.
3.	Place the tube in the center of the ultrasound bath, resting the tube on the bottom of the bath. Keep the tube in this position and sonicate for approximately 1 minute. Mix contents of the tube with applicator sticks during this time.
4.	Centrifuge to remove particulate matter and harvest the supernate.
5.	Test the eluate and the final wash supernate against the desired RBCs by direct agglutination and/or one of the IAT methods described in Section II.
6.	Interpret the results and proceed as follows: <table><tr><th>If eluate is…</th><th>And final wash supernate is…</th><th>Then…</th></tr><tr><td>reactive</td><td>nonreactive</td><td>eluate reactions are valid: • Interpret results.</td></tr><tr><td>nonreactive</td><td>nonreactive</td><td>no antibody was eluted.</td></tr><tr><td>reactive</td><td>reactive</td><td>eluate reactions are invalid: • Repeat Steps 1-6; extra washes of the RBCs before elution may be necessary.</td></tr></table>

References   Bird GWG, Wingham J. A new procedure for elution of erythrocyte-bound antibody. Acta Haematol 1972;47:344-7.

Jimerfield CA. A rapid and simple procedure for preparing red cell eluates using ultrasound. Am J Med Technol 1977;43:187-9.

**Effective
Date**

Approved by	Printed Name	Signature	Date
Laboratory Management			
Medical Director			
Quality Officer			

IV-O. Eluting Antibodies with Xylene/<u>D</u>-Limonene

Purpose

To provide instructions for eluting IgG auto- and alloantibodies from RBCs using xylene or <u>D</u>-Limonene:

- In the investigation of immune hemolysis caused by autoantibodies, alloantibodies, or drugs.

- In conjunction with an adsorption technique:

  o To confirm the presence or absence of an antigen on RBCs.

  o To concentrate an antibody.

  o To isolate an antibody in pure form from a serum containing multiple alloantibodies.

Background Information

Organic solvents probably influence antigen-antibody dissociation by several mechanisms, including:

- Alteration of the tertiary structure of antibody molecules.

- Disruption of the RBC membrane bilipid layer.

- Reversal of the forces of attraction between antigen and antibody.

The first two mechanisms result in loss of structural complementarity between antigen and antibody.

Operational Policy

Xylene is carcinogenic, flammable (but less so than ether), and narcotic in high concentration. <u>D</u>-Limonene is a skin irritant but is otherwise less toxic than xylene. Consequently, the following safety precautions should be followed:

- Store bulk quantities of organic solvents in an explosion-proof refrigerator or cabinet. Small amounts (eg, 4 oz) may be kept at room temperature in a stoppered container.

- Discard organic solvents when the container is one-quarter full. Some organic solvents become acidic during storage, probably as the result of peroxide formation. This may account for apparent nonspecific activity of eluates when the solvent used has been taken from an almost empty container.

- Use organic solvents in a well-ventilated area away from heat, flame, and electrical outlets; a properly constructed chemical hood is preferred.

- Allow organic solvents to evaporate in a large, dark glass vessel and keep under a chemical hood. Dispose according to state and federal guidelines.

Limitations

<u>Unwanted Positive Reactions:</u>

- Incomplete washing of RBCs.

- Matuhasi-Ogata phenomenon.

- Incomplete removal of organic solvent.

<u>Unwanted Negative Reactions:</u>

- Incomplete removal of organic solvent.

- Incorrect technique.

Sample Requirements

RBCs for elution studies, washed as described in Procedure IV-A.

Equipment/ Materials

22% or 30% BSA.

<u>D</u>-Limonene or xylene: $C_{10}H_{16}$ or $C_6H_4(CH_3)_2$ (reagent grade).

Cork stoppers: size #2 (eg, VWR, Batavia, IL).

Note: Cork stoppers should be used when agitating eluates prepared with organic solvents. Cork allows the tube to "breathe" during agitation, thereby minimizing gas build-up that may cause the contents to splatter when the stopper is removed.

Glass Pasteur pipettes.

Procedure

Use the following steps to perform the procedure:

Step	Action
1.	Wash the RBCs as described in Procedure IV-A. **Note:** Save the supernate from the final wash for parallel testing with the eluate.
2.	Mix equal volumes of RBCs and xylene or <u>D</u>-Limonene.

3.	Stopper tube and agitate 1-2 minutes.
4.	Incubate at 56 C for 10 minutes and stir periodically with applicator sticks.
5.	Centrifuge at 1000 × *g* for 10 minutes (or equivalent). Remove upper layer of xylene (or D-Limonene) and stroma by vacuum aspiration and harvest the eluate.
6.	To minimize hemolysis due to residual organic solvent, add 1 drop of BSA to 2 drops of eluate before testing with RBCs.

7.	Interpret the results and proceed as follows:		
	If eluate is...	**And final wash supernate is...**	**Then...**
	reactive	nonreactive	eluate reactions are valid: • Interpret results.
	nonreactive	nonreactive	no antibody was eluted: • Consider passive ABO or drug-dependent antibody.
	reactive	reactive	eluate reactions are invalid: • Repeat Steps 1-7; extra washes of the RBCs before elution may be necessary.

References

Bueno R, Garratty G, Postoway N. Elution of antibody from red blood cells using xylene, a superior procedure. Transfusion 1981;21:157-62.

Chan-Shu SA, Blair O. A new procedure of antibody elution from red blood cells. Transfusion 1979;19:182-5.

Deisting B, Douglas D, Ellisor S. D-Limonene: A xylene substitute for elution procedures (abstract). Transfusion 1986;26:549.

Garratty G, O'Neill P. Overcoming lysis of test RBCs following xylene elution (letter). Transfusion 1986;26:487.

**Effective
Date**

	Printed Name	Signature	Date
Approved by			
Laboratory Management			
Medical Director			
Quality Officer			

IV-P. Dissociating of IgG with EDTA-Glycine-HCl

Purpose   To provide instructions for dissociating IgG from RBCs without compromising the integrity of RBC membrane antigens:

- To render DAT-positive RBCs DAT-negative, thereby permitting phenotyping with antisera that require use of the IAT (eg, anti-S, anti-Fy[a]).

- Treatment of IgG-coated RBCs for autologous adsorption.

Background Information   Acids probably influence elution of antibody from coated RBCs by lowering the pH of antigen and antibody proteins such that they both become protonated. The antigens and antibodies lose their ability to attract one another through electrostatic bonding and may be forced apart by repulsion of like charges. The tertiary structure of proteins may be affected; hydrogen (H^+) ions are attracted to hydroxyl (OH^-) groups on aspartic and glutamic acids, resulting in molecular unfolding, with consequential loss of structural complementarity between antigen and antibody.

Operational Policy   Do not test RBCs treated with acid for Kell antigens; these antigens are denatured by this procedure.

Limitations   Failure to Dissociate IgG:

- Incorrect technique.

- Use of wrong reagent.

Note: Approximately 80% of IgG-coated RBC samples can be rendered DAT-negative by this technique.

Sample Requirements   IgG-coated RBCs, washed three times in saline, 0.1 mL.

Equipment/ Materials Na_2EDTA: 10% wt/vol.

Glycine: 0.1 M (pH 1.5).

TRIS base: 1 M.

Pipettors with disposable tips to deliver 0.1 mL to 1 mL (eg, VWR, Batavia, IL).

Judd's Methods in Immunohematology
Dissociating of IgG with EDTA-Glycine-HCl
Page 2 of 3

Quality Control

When phenotyping with antiglobulin-reactive antisera:

- Treat an aliquot of RBCs known to carry a single dose of the antigen(s) under investigation in parallel with the test sample.

- Perform an IAT-control using treated RBCs and 6% BSA.

Procedure

Use the following steps to perform the procedure:

Step	Action
1.	Mix 0.8 mL of glycine-HCl and 0.2 mL of EDTA in a 16 × 100-mm test tube.
2.	Immediately add 0.1 mL of washed packed RBCs and mix well.
3.	Incubate at room temperature for no longer than 2 minutes.
4.	Immediately add 0.2 mL TRIS base.
5.	Wash the RBCs three times with saline.
6.	To 1 drop of 3%-5% washed RBCs in saline, add 2 drops of anti-IgG: • Mix and centrifuge. • Dislodge the cell buttons gently. • Examine macroscopically for agglutination. • Grade and record results.

Step	If the DAT is...	Then...
7.	negative	confirm with IgG-coated RBCs.
	positive	procedure may be repeated once more.

Reference

Louie J, Jiang A, Zaroulis C. Preparation of intact antibody-free red blood cells in autoimmune hemolytic anemia (abstract). Transfusion 1986;26: 550.

**Effective
Date**

Approved by	Printed Name	Signature	Date
Laboratory Management			
Medical Director			
Quality Officer			

IV-Q. Dissociating of IgG with Chloroquine Diphosphate

Purpose   To provide instructions for dissociating IgG from RBCs without compromising the integrity of RBC membrane antigens:

- To render DAT-positive RBCs DAT-negative, thereby permitting phenotyping with antisera that require use of the IAT (eg, anti-S, anti-Fy^a).

Background Information   Chloroquine diphosphate causes elution of bound antibody without disrupting RBC membrane antigens. The most likely mechanism involves neutralization of charged groups on amino acids that govern the tertiary structure of antibody molecules (ie, R groups that are involved with intermolecular bonds).

Operational Policy   Do not extend incubation beyond 2 hours at room temperature (RT) or 30 minutes at 37 C because antigen denaturation may occur.

Do not use chloroquine-treated RBCs in direct agglutination tests, especially Rh phenotyping, because unwanted negative reactions can occur.

Limitations   Failure to Dissociate IgG:

- Incorrect technique.
- Use of wrong reagent.

Note: Some 80% of IgG-coated RBC samples can be rendered DAT-negative by this technique. In other instances, elution of IgG may be facilitated by incubation at 37 C; however, RBCs should be tested with anti-IgG at 5-minute intervals, and the total incubation at 37 C should not exceed 30 minutes.

Sample Requirements   IgG-coated RBCs, washed three times in saline; 0.2 mL.

Equipment/ Materials   Chloroquine diphosphate (20% wt/vol).

AHG: anti-IgG.

IgG-coated RBCs.

Pipettors with disposable tips to deliver 0.2 mL to 1 mL (eg, VWR, Batavia, IL).

Quality Control

In parallel with the test sample, treat an aliquot of RBCs known to carry a single dose of the antigen(s) under investigation.

When phenotyping with antiglobulin-reactive antisera, perform an IAT-control using treated RBCs and 6% BSA.

RT Procedure

Use the following steps to perform the procedure at RT:

Step	Action
1.	Wash the RBCs four times with saline.
2.	Mix 0.2 mL of washed RBCs and 0.8 mL of chloroquine diphosphate.
3.	Incubate at RT for 30 minutes.
4.	Remove a small aliquot of RBCs and wash four times with saline.
5.	To 1 drop of 3%-5% washed RBCs in saline, add 2 drops of anti-IgG: • Mix and centrifuge. • Dislodge the cell buttons gently. • Examine macroscopically for agglutination. • Grade and record the results.
6.	Interpret the reactions and proceed as follows: | If the DAT is…	Then…
---	---
negative	• Confirm with IgG-coated RBCs. • Wash the total sample of treated RBCs and type with antisera for use by the IAT.
positive	repeat Step 3 at 30-minute intervals for up to 2 hours.	

37 C Procedure

Use the following steps to perform the procedure at 37 C:

Step	Action
1.	Wash the RBCs four times with saline.
2.	Mix 0.2 mL of washed RBCs and 0.8 mL of chloroquine diphosphate.
3.	Incubate at 37 C for 5 minutes.
4.	Remove a small aliquot of RBCs and wash four times with saline.

5.	To 1 drop of 3%-5% washed RBCs in saline, add 2 drops of anti-IgG: • Mix and centrifuge. • Dislodge the cell buttons gently. • Examine macroscopically for agglutination. • Grade and record the results.	
6.	Interpret the reactions and proceed as follows:	
	If the DAT is…	**Then…**
	negative	• Confirm with IgG-coated RBCs. • Wash the total sample of treated RBCs and type with antisera for use by the IAT.
	positive	repeat Step 3 at 5-minute intervals for up to 30 minutes.

Reference

Edwards JM, Moulds JJ, Judd WJ. Chloroquine diphosphate dissociation of antigen-antibody complexes: A new technique for phenotyping red cells with a positive direct antiglobulin test. Transfusion 1982;22:59-61.

Effective Date

Approved by:

	Printed Name	Signature	Date
Laboratory Management			
Medical Director			
Quality Officer			

Section V. Cell Separation Methods

RBC separation methods used in immunohematology generally entail either 1) differential agglutination coupled with sedimentation or slow centrifugation, or 2) differential centrifugation at high speed. The former is particularly suited to the investigation of RBC mosaicism caused by rare genetic disorders, such as chimerism and dispermy, or induced artificially by hematopoietic stem cell transplantation. RBCs are separated on the basis of differences in the blood group phenotype between the two (rarely more) RBC populations, using agglutinating antisera. A method for separating mixed-cell populations on the basis of differences in ABO group is presented in Section XIII, whereas a method for separation based on other polymorphisms is included in this Section. High-speed centrifugation is applied to the separation of homologous RBCs from autologous RBCs in recently transfused patients. The procedure uses the principle that newly formed autologous RBCs (ie, reticulocytes) have a lower specific gravity than transfused stored RBCs; the less dense cells migrate to the top of an RBC column during centrifugation. The harvested reticulocytes can be subjected to direct antiglobulin testing, phenotyping, or autologous adsorption. For further information, the interested reader is referred to the sources listed below.

Suggested Reading

Garratty G. Predicting the clinical significance of alloantibodies and determining the in vivo survival of transfused red cells. In: Judd WJ, Barnes A, eds. Clinical and serological aspects of transfusion reactions. Arlington VA: AABB, 1982:91-119.

Mougey R. Red cell separation techniques and their applications. In: Myers M, Reynolds A, eds. Micromethods in blood group serology. Arlington, VA: AABB, 1984:19-36.

Race R, Sanger R. Blood groups in man. 6th ed. Oxford, UK: Blackwell Scientific Publications, 1975.

Roback J, Combs MR, Grossman B, Hillyer C, eds. Technical manual. 16th ed. Bethesda, MD: AABB, 2008 (or current edition).

Wallas CH, Tanley PC, Gorrell LP. Recovery of autologous erythrocytes in transfused patients. Transfusion 1980;20:332-6.

V-A. Harvesting Autologous RBCs by Direct Centrifugation

Purpose

To provide instructions for separating autologous RBCs from donor RBCs in recently transfused patients, using high-speed microhematocrit centrifugation. The separated autologous RBCs can be used for:

- Phenotyping.
- Autoadsorption studies.
- Direct antiglobulin testing.

Background Information

Young autologous RBCs (ie, reticulocytes), with a specific gravity lower than that of transfused RBCs, may be separated from the transfused population by simple centrifugation in microhematocrit tubes. The autologous RBCs concentrate at the top of a centrifuged microhematocrit tube. Separation efficacy is comparable to the phthalate ester technique.

Operational Policy

Use Procedure V-D for separating autologous RBCs in patients with sickle cell disease.

Separation is best accomplished when blood samples are obtained 3 days or more after transfusion.

Mix packed RBCs continuously during filling of microhematocrit tubes.

Limitations

Incorrect Results:

- Improper storage of reagents.
- Use of incorrect technique.
- Use of wrong reagent.
- Marrow aplasia.
- Use of aged samples.

Sample Requirements

Whole blood: freshly collected (ie, within the past 24 hours, if possible) and anticoagulated with EDTA/ACD/CPD; 7 mL (more if patient is anemic).

**Equipment/
Materials**

Reagent antisera for phenotyping.

Metal file: to cut microhematocrit tubes.

Microhematocrit equipment (eg, VWR, Batavia, IL).

Microhematocrit centrifuge (eg, VWR, Batavia, IL).

Plain (not heparinized) glass, plastic, or plastic-coated microhematocrit tubes (eg, VWR, Batavia, IL).

Sealant (eg, VWR, Batavia, IL).

**Quality
Control**

For each antisera used, compare the results of phenotyping tests (especially Rh and MN) on separated and unseparated RBCs. Separated RBCs should give clear-cut positive and negative reactions with blood typing reagents, and the unseparated RBCs should show mixed-field agglutination with most reagents.

Procedure

Use the following steps to perform the procedure:

Step	Action
1.	Wash the RBCs three times with saline.
2.	Centrifuge the last wash to pack the RBCs. Remove as much of the residual supernate as is possible without disturbing the buffy-coat. Mix thoroughly.
3.	Save an aliquot of washed RBCs for quality control purposes (see above).
4.	Fill up to 10 microhematocrit tubes with 60 mm of packed RBCs. **Note:** Care should be taken to ensure that the packed RBCs are mixed continuously during the filling of microhematocrit tubes.
5.	Seal the end of the tubes with sealant.
6.	Centrifuge all tubes in a microhematocrit centrifuge for 15 minutes.
7.	Cut the microhematocrit tubes 5 mm below the top of the centrifuged RBC column.
8.	Place the cut microhematocrit tubes into a clean, appropriately labeled 10 × 75-mm or 12 × 75-mm test tube.
9.	Fill the test tube containing the cut microhematocrit tubes with saline.

10.	Centrifuge for 1 minute. Decant the microhematocrit tubes and supernatant saline into a waste container. **Note:** RBCs will be at the bottom of the test tube.
11.	Wash the separated RBCs two to three additional times with saline.
12.	Type the separated RBCs from Step 11 and the unseparated RBCs from Step 3 with desired antisera.
13.	Interpret the reactions as follows:

If some tests with separated RBCs show...	And tests with unseparated RBCs show...	Then...
no or scant agglutination	a mixed-field reaction	cell separation is complete: • Reactions with antisera and separated RBCs are valid.
a mixed-field reaction	a mixed-field reaction	separation failed: • Repeat separation after 3 days have elapsed since last transfusion.

Reference   Reid ME, Toy P. Simplified method for recovery of autologous red blood cells from transfused patients. Am J Clin Path 1983;79:364-6.

Effective Date

Approved by:

	Printed Name	Signature	Date
Laboratory Management			
Medical Director			
Quality Officer			

V-B. Harvesting Autologous RBCs Using Phthalate Esters

Purpose

To provide instructions for separating autologous RBCs from donor RBCs in recently transfused patients, using high-speed microhematocrit centrifugation pththalate esters. The separated RBCs can be used for:

- Phenotyping.

- Autoadsorption studies.

- Direct antiglobulin testing.

Background Information

RBCs released from marrow have a specific gravity (SG) of about 1.078, which changes to around 1.114 as RBCs become older. In recently transfused patients, the RBCs with the lowest SG are likely to be the autologous reticulocytes. They can be separated from transfused RBCs and the patient's older RBCs by centrifugation through water-immiscible solutions of defined SG, such as mixtures of dibutyl and dimethyl phthalates. RBCs with a SG lower than the ester mixture remain above the ester layer. At a certain SG, which varies from patient to patient, only the autologous RBCs remain above the ester layer.

Accuracy is essential when preparing ester mixtures. Preparation by weight is preferred, although volume measurements are satisfactory if performed carefully. Use graduated conical tubes. Add one ester to all tubes first, and allow to settle. Because the esters are viscous, it will be necessary to adjust the volumes of the first ester before adding the second.

Operational Policy

Use Procedure V-D for separating autologous RBCs in patients with sickle cell disease.

Separation is best accomplished when blood samples are obtained 3 days or more after transfusion.

Mix packed RBCs continuously during the filling of microhematocrit tubes.

Limitations

Incorrect Results:

- Improper storage of reagents.

- Use of incorrect technique.

- Use of wrong reagent.

- Marrow aplasia.

- Use of aged samples.

Sample Requirements	Whole blood: freshly collected (ie, within the past 24 hours, if possible) and anticoagulated with EDTA/ACD/CPD, 7 mL (more if patient is anemic).

Equipment/ Materials	Reagent antisera for phenotyping.
	22% or 30% BSA.
	Metal file, to cut microhematocrit tubes.
	Microhematocrit equipment (eg, VWR, Batavia, IL).
	Microhematocrit centrifuge (eg, VWR, Batavia, IL).
	Plain (not heparinized) glass, plastic, or plastic-coated microhematocrit tubes (eg, VWR, Batavia, IL).
	Sealant (eg, VWR, Batavia, IL).
	Phthalate ester mixtures.
	Syringe: 2 mL with 23-gauge needle.

Quality Control	Compare the results of phenotyping tests (especially Rh and MN) on separated and unseparated RBCs. Separated RBCs should give clear-cut positive and negative reactions with blood typing reagents, and the unseparated RBCs should show mixed-field agglutination with most reagents.

Procedure   Use the following steps to perform the procedure:

Step	Action
1.	Wash the RBCs three times with saline.
2.	Centrifuge the last wash to pack the RBCs. Remove as much of the residual supernate as is possible without disturbing the buffy-coat. Mix thoroughly.
3.	Save an aliquot of washed RBCs for quality control purposes (see above).
4.	For each ester mixture, fill a microhematocrit tube with 5 mm of ester and 60 mm of packed RBCs.
5.	Seal the end of the tubes with sealant.
6.	Centrifuge all tubes in a microhematocrit centrifuge for 10 minutes.

7.	Examine the tubes and select the phthalate ester mixture that corresponds to the tube containing approximately 5 mm of RBCs above the ester layer.
8.	Prepare a number of tubes containing packed RBCs and the selected ester mixture. Normally, 10 such tubes will suffice.
9.	Centrifuge the tubes in a microhematocrit centrifuge for 10 minutes.
10.	Cut the microhematocrit tubes at the interface of the ester layer and the upper layer of packed RBCs.
11.	Place the cut microhematocrit tubes containing the 5-mm RBCs into a clean test tube.
12.	Fill the test tube containing the cut microhematocrit tubes with saline.
13.	Centrifuge for 1 minute. Decant the microhematocrit tubes and supernatant saline into a waste container. **Note:** RBCs will be at the bottom of the test tube.
14.	Centrifuge to pack the RBCs, and add 1 mL of BSA. Mix well.
15.	Centrifuge to pack the RBCs, and discard the supernate.
16.	Wash the separated RBCs three times with saline.
17.	Resuspend the RBCs to a 3%-5% suspension for phenotyping. Proceed to the next step or use packed RBCs in micro-autoadsorption tests (see Section XI).
18.	Type the separated RBCs from Step 17 and the unseparated RBCs from Step 3 with desired antisera.
19.	Interpret the reactions as follows:

If some tests with separated RBCs show...	And tests with unseparated RBCs show...	Then...
no or scant agglutination	a mixed-field reaction	cell separation is complete: • Reactions with antisera and separated RBCs are valid.
a mixed-field reaction	a mixed-field reaction	separation failed: • Repeat separation after 3 days have elapsed since last transfusion.

Reference   Wallas CH, Tanley PC, Gorrell LP. Recovery of autologous erythrocytes in transfused patients. Transfusion 1980;20:332-6.

**Effective
Date**

Approved by:	Printed Name	Signature	Date
Laboratory Management			
Medical Director			
Quality Officer			

V-C. Cell Separation Using Percoll-Renografin Procedure

Purpose
To provide instructions for separating autologous RBCs from donor RBCs in recently transfused patients, using a density gradient of Percoll-Renografin and high-speed centrifugation. The separated autologous RBCs can be used for:

- Phenotyping.
- Autoadsorption studies.
- Direct antiglobulin testing.

Background Information
Young autologous RBCs (ie, reticulocytes), with a specific gravity lower than that of transfused RBCs, may be separated from the transfused population by centrifugation through a density gradient. Top layers will contain autologous RBCs; lower bands will contain older or transfused RBCs.

Operational Policy
See Procedure V-D for separating autologous RBCs in patients with sickle cell disease.

Separation is best accomplished when blood samples are obtained 3 days or more after transfusion.

Limitations
Incorrect Results:

- Improper storage of reagents.
- Use of incorrect technique.
- Use of wrong reagent.
- Marrow aplasia.
- Use of aged samples.

Sample Requirements
Whole blood: freshly collected (ie, within the past 24 hours, if possible) and anticoagulated with EDTA/ACD/CPD; 7 mL (more if patient is anemic).

Equipment/ Materials

Reagent antisera for phenotyping.

Alsever's Solution.

α-cellulose (eg, Sigma-Aldrich, St Louis, MO).

Microcrystalline cellulose (eg, Sigma-Aldrich, St Louis, MO).

Percoll (eg, Sigma-Aldrich, St Louis, MO).

Renografin 60 (eg, Bracco Diagnostics, Inc, Princeton, NJ).

0.9% NaCl.

Syringe: 20 mL.

High-speed centrifuge: angle rotor, refrigerated centrifuge, capable of centrifuging 5-mL volumes at $35,000 \times g$ (eg, Allegra 64, Beckman Coulter, Inc, Fullerton, CA).

Quality Control

Compare the results of phenotyping tests (especially Rh and MN) on separated and unseparated RBCs. Separated RBCs should give clear-cut positive and negative reactions with blood typing reagents, and the unseparated RBCs should show mixed-field agglutination with most reagents.

Procedure

Use the following steps to perform the procedure:

Step	Action
1.	Save an aliquot of whole blood for parallel testing with the separated RBCs.
2.	Pack the syringe cylinder with approximately 2-5 cm of microcrystalline cellulose and α-cellulose in a 1:1 ratio by weight.
3.	Centrifuge the leukocyte-reduced blood to pack the RBCs.
4.	Discard the supernatant plasma and mix 1 mL of packed RBCs with 10 mL of Percoll-Renografin. Mix well.
5.	Divide the mixture in half and place into 2 centrifuge tubes.
6.	Centrifuge at $35,000 \times g$ for 5 minutes at 4 C.
7.	Examine the tubes for bands of RBCs. Remove the upper bands (reticulocytes) and place into a clean test tube.
8.	Wash the RBCs four times with saline before use.

9.	Resuspend the RBCs to a 3%-5% suspension for phenotyping. Proceed to the next step or use packed RBCs in micro-autoadsorption tests (see Section XI).
10.	Type the separated RBCs from Step 8 and the unseparated RBCs from Step 1 with desired antisera.
11.	Interpret the reactions as follows:

If some tests with separated RBCs show...	And tests with unseparated RBCs show...	Then...
no or scant agglutination	a mixed-field reaction	cell separation is complete: • Reactions with antisera and separated RBCs are valid.
a mixed-field reaction	a mixed-field reaction	separation failed: • Repeat separation after 3 days have elapsed since last transfusion.

Reference

Branch DR, Hian AI, Carlson F. Erythrocyte age-fractionation using a Percoll-Renografin density gradient: Application to autologous red cell antigen determinations in recently transfused patients. Am J Clin Pathol 1983;80: 453-8.

Effective Date

Approved by:

	Printed Name	Signature	Date
Laboratory Management			
Medical Director			
Quality Officer			

V-D. Harvesting Autologous RBCs in Hemoglobin S or Sickle Cell Disease

Purpose

To provide instructions for separating autologous RBCs from donor RBCs in recently transfused patients with hemoglobin S or sickle cell disease, using hypotonic saline to lyse transfused red cells. The separated RBCs may be used for:

- Phenotyping.
- Autoadsorption studies.
- Direct antiglobulin testing.

Background Information

RBCs from patients with hemoglobin S or sickle cell disease are resistant to lysis by hypotonic saline, in contrast to normal donor RBCs and RBCs from donors with hemoglobin S trait.

Operational Policy

Separation is best accomplished when blood samples are obtained 3 days or more after transfusion.

Limitations

Incorrect Results:

- Improper storage of reagents.
- Use of incorrect technique.
- Use of wrong reagent.
- Marrow aplasia.
- Use of aged samples.

Sample Requirements

Packed RBCs from whole blood: freshly collected (ie, within the past 24 hours, if possible) and anticoagulated with EDTA/ACD/CPD; 7 mL (more if patient is anemic).

Equipment/ Materials

0.3% NaCl.

0.9% NaCl.

Reagent antisera for phenotyping.

**Quality
Control**

Compare the results of phenotyping tests (especially Rh and MN) on separated and unseparated RBCs. Separated RBCs should give clear-cut positive and negative reactions with blood typing reagents, and the unseparated RBCs should show mixed-field agglutination with most reagents.

Procedure

Use the following steps to perform the procedure:

Step	Action
1.	Place 4 to 5 drops of packed RBCs into a 10 or 12 × 75-mm test tube. **Note:** Larger volumes, for use in adsorption studies, can be processed in a 16 × 100-mm test tube.
2.	Wash the RBCs six times with 0.3% NaCl or until gross hemolysis is no longer apparent. Use centrifugation at $1000 \times g$ for 1 minute (or equivalent) per wash.
3.	Wash the RBCs two times with 0.9% NaCl to restore tonicity. Use centrifugation at $200 \times g$ for 2 minutes (or equivalent) per wash to facilitate removal of residual stroma.
4.	Resuspend the RBCs to a 3%-5% suspension for phenotyping. Proceed to the next step or use packed RBCs in micro-autoadsorption tests (see Section XI).
5.	Type the separated RBCs from the previous step and the unseparated RBCs with desired antisera.
6.	Interpret the reactions as follows:

If some tests with separated RBCs show...	And tests with unseparated RBCs show...	Then...
no or scant agglutination	a mixed-field reaction	cell separation is complete: • Reactions with antisera and separated RBCs are valid.
a mixed-field reaction	a mixed-field reaction	separation failed: • Repeat separation after 3 days have elapsed since last transfusion.

Reference

Brown D. A rapid method for harvesting autologous red cells from patients with hemoglobin S disease (abstract). Transfusion 1986;26:572.

**Effective
Date**

Approved by:	Printed Name	Signature	Date
Laboratory Management			
Medical Director			
Quality Officer			

V-E. Separating Mixed-Cell Populations with Antibodies

Purpose

To provide instructions for separating mixed RBC populations with blood group antisera, including antisera reactive by IAT:

- Studies on generic or artificial chimeras.

Background Information

Mixed RBC populations, as may occur in rare genetic disorders such as chimerism or dispermy or as may be seen following transfusion or marrow transplantation, may be separated using antisera that discriminate between the different RBC populations.

Ideally, potent agglutinating reagents (reactive at immediate-spin or room-temperature incubation) should be used, although this technique works in situations requiring use of antiglobulin-reactive antisera. With either type of antisera, weak agglutinates are formed with one RBC population and are separated from the other (non-agglutinated) RBCs by differential sedimentation through a dextrose column.

Limitations

Incorrect Results:

- Improper storage of reagents.

- Use of incorrect technique.

- Use of wrong reagent.

- Marrow aplasia.

- Use of aged samples.

Sample Requirements

Whole blood: freshly collected (ie, within the past 24 hours, if possible) and anticoagulated with EDTA/ACD/CPD; 7 mL (more if patient is anemic).

Note: Volume will depend on the number of tubes required in Step 1 below.

Equipment/ Materials

AB serum.

Note: A single-source sample will suffice.

AHG: anti-IgG (required when using coating antibodies).

Petri dish (eg, VWR, Batavia, IL).

Pipettors with disposable tips to deliver 0.5, 1.0, 2.0, and 20 mL (eg, VWR, Batavia, IL).

pH 7.3 PBS.

Antiserum: potent agglutinating or coating antibody that discriminates between the populations of RBCs within the test sample.

Dextrose: 20% wt/vol, stored below −20 C; thaw just before use.

Quality Control	Compare the results of phenotyping tests on separated and unseparated RBCs. Both "positive" and "negative" preparations should give clear-cut reactions with blood typing reagents in the separated sample, and mixed-field agglutination in the unseparated RBCs.

Procedure   Use the following steps to perform the procedure:

Step	Action
1.	Wash the RBCs three times in pH 7.3 PBS. Save an aliquot for parallel testing with the separated RBCs.
2.	Dispense 0.5 mL of RBCs into 13 × 100-mm test tubes. **Note**: Prepare a sufficient number of tubes to obtain the required quantity of each RBC population.
3.	Add an excess of antiserum (eg, 2 mL to each tube).
4.	Incubate for 15-60 minutes, with frequent gentle mixing, at the temperature appropriate for the antiserum. **Note**: Proceed immediately to Step 8 when using an agglutinating antibody.
5.	Wash the RBCs six times with large volumes of saline and completely remove the final supernate.
6.	Add 2 mL of antiglobulin serum and incubate at RT for 10 minutes with frequent gentle mixing.
7.	Wash the RBCs two times with saline using centrifugation for 30 seconds at $1000 \times g$ (or equivalent).
8.	Prepare a 20%-30% RBC suspension in saline and transfer to a Petri dish.
9.	Rock the RBCs gently for 10-15 minutes. **Note**: Initially, a large number of agglutinates will form rapidly; smaller agglutinates should begin to form after 5-10 minutes. It is important to make sure this occurs.
10.	With continuous gentle rocking of the Petri dish, carefully add 20 mL of saline to reduce the RBC concentration to 2%-3%.
11.	Gently layer this RBC suspension onto tubes containing 20% dextrose until the RBC layer is approximately 1 cm deep.

12.	Allow agglutinates to settle by gravity into the dextrose medium.
13.	Transfer the RBCs that remain in saline at the top of the dextrose column into a tube marked "negative."
14.	Transfer the RBCs in the dextrose medium into a tube marked "positive."
15.	Wash both RBC populations three times with saline.
16.	Add 1 mL AB serum to each 1 mL of "positive" RBCs.
17.	Mix and incubate at RT for 15-20 minutes (to disperse agglutination by AHG).
18.	Perform DAT with anti-IgG on both RBC populations as described in Procedure XI-A.
19.	Interpret the reactions with each cell population as follows:

If the DAT is …	Then…
negative	the cell population is suitable for phenotyping.
mixed-field	the separation is incomplete: • Repeat the procedure from Step 1.
positive	render RBCs DAT-negative using Procedure IV-D, IV-P or IV-Q before further testing.

Reference

Renton PH, Hancock JA. A method of separating agglutinated and free erythrocytes. Vox Sang 1964;9:187-90.

Effective Date

Approved by:

	Printed Name	Signature	Date
Laboratory Management			
Medical Director			
Quality Officer			

V-F. Mononuclear Cell Separation Procedure

Purpose

To provide instructions for isolating mononuclear cells from whole blood:

- For use in monocyte monolayer assays.

Background Information

Mononuclear cells (eg, monocytes and lymphocytes) can be separated from nonnucleated cells (eg, RBCs) and granulocytes in peripheral blood by centrifugation through a density gradient. Mononuclear cells, having a lower density than RBCs, are not as readily deposited as RBCs during the centrifugation process.

Limitations

Incorrect Results:

- Improper storage of reagents.

- Use of incorrect technique.

- Use of wrong reagent.

Sample Requirements

Whole blood sample, anticoagulated with heparin or EDTA; 20 mL.

Equipment/ Materials

Ficoll-Paque Plus (GE Healthcare, Piscataway, NJ).

pH 7.3 PBS.

Sterile conical centrifuge tubes: 50-mL volume.

Tissue culture medium: Roswell Park Memorial Institute 1640 medium, containing 10% (vol/vol) fetal calf serum (Sigma-Aldrich, St Louis, MO).

Quality Control

Prepare a smear of harvested WBCs and stain as described in Procedure XV-H.

Procedure   Use the following steps to perform the procedure:

Step	Action
1.	Allow reagents to warm to room temperature.
2.	Place 15 mL of whole blood into a sterile, 50-mL, conical centrifuge tube.
3.	Centrifuge at 150 $\times$ g for 10 minutes.
4.	Carefully remove the WBC/platelet-rich plasma to within 0.5 inches of the RBCs and dilute with 35 mL of pH 7.3 PBS.
5.	Using sterile technique, place 12 mL of Ficoll-Paque Plus into another sterile, 50-mL, conical centrifuge tube.
6.	Tilt the tube containing Ficoll-Paque Plus to a 30 degree angle, and slowly layer the diluted plasma onto the Ficoll-Paque Plus with a small-bore pipette, putting it as close to the meniscus as possible but without touching the Ficoll-Paque Plus.
7.	Slowly tilt the tube upright and gently transfer to a centrifuge.
8.	Centrifuge at 800 $\times$ g for 15 minutes. **Note:** Accelerate centrifuge gently to reach desired speed.
9.	Remove supernatant plasma and PBS to within 5 mL of the WBC layer.
10.	Carefully transfer WBC layer into a clean, sterile, 50-mL centrifuge tube, using a wide-bore Pasteur pipette. **Note:** WBC layer should be composed predominantly of monocytes and lymphocytes.
11.	Dilute WBCs with 40 mL of PBS. Gently mix and centrifuge at 400 $\times$ g for 10 minutes.
12.	Wash WBCs two times with PBS and centrifuge for 10 minutes each time at 400 $\times$ g. **Note:** For each wash, remove PBS to within 2.5 mL, resuspend WBCs by pipette with gentle aspiration, and dilute with 40 mL of PBS. Mix gently.
13.	Remove final wash supernate to within 0.25 mL of the WBCs. Resuspend by pipette with gentle aspiration and add tissue culture medium to the 5.0-mL mark.

14.	Determine the WBC concentration (by a hematologic method).	
15.	Proceed as follows:	
	If the WBC count is...	**Then...**
	between 3×10^6/mL and 6×10^6/mL	use immediately in MMA study as described in Section XV.
	>6×10^6/mL	dilute to between 3×10^6/mL and 6×10^6/mL with tissue culture medium before use.
	<3×10^6/mL	repeat process using blood from a different donor.

Reference

Garratty G. Predicting the clinical significance of alloantibodies and determining the in vivo survival of transfused red cells. In: Judd WJ, Barnes A, eds. Clinical and serological aspects of transfusion reactions. Arlington VA: AABB, 1982:91-119.

Effective Date

Approved by:	**Printed Name**	**Signature**	**Date**
Laboratory Management			
Medical Director			
Quality Officer			

Section VI. Alternative Serologic Methods for Antibody Detection

Because of the minute volumes of antisera required, tests in glass capillary tubes (so-called Chown capillary tubes) are well suited to the mass screening of samples against rare antisera, or to the performance of antibody detection/identification tests when sera are in short supply (eg, blood samples from neonates). The sensitivity of microplate methods permits the dilution of many rare sera beyond their sensitivity limits either in conventional test tubes or by column agglutination technology; thus, they are also useful for mass screening of samples against rare sera.

A microplate is generally considered to be either a flexible or a rigid plastic matrix of 96 short U-, V-, or flat-bottom test tubes. For most serologic testing, use of U-bottom plates permits reading of tests either by examination of RBC streaming patterns or by examination for agglutination following RBC resuspension. Some workers prefer V-bottom plates for antiglobulin testing where RBC washing is required. When compared with conventional tube procedures, microplate techniques provide 1) increased sensitivity, to the extent that some weak-D RBCs give unequivocally positive reactions in direct tests with anti-D, and 2) lower costs per test, resulting from batch testing of large numbers of samples and use of small volumes of diluted reagent antisera. The use of microplates is most commonly found in automated settings for blood grouping and antibody screening, where these plates lend themselves well to medium to high throughput.

The use of sepharose gel beads, glass beads, and other matrices in column agglutination technology has been extensively commercialized for many applications, and these kits should always be used according to the manufacturers' instructions. The advantages of column agglutination techniques are that they require smaller volumes of antisera than conventional tube tests and that the interpretation is simpler, based on the stability of the agglutination reaction, which remains fixed in the matrix. Gel-column methods have been included in this Section to provide in-house methods that, with appropriate controls, match the sensitivity of standard tube testing but require much less antisera.

Apart from the basic methods described in this section, there are innumerable modifications that experts in the field would recommend. It is at least hoped that the methods chosen for inclusion are described in sufficient detail that novices interested in applying them will find that adequate information has been provided. (See also Section II for discussion of the principles of hemagglutination and mechanisms for enhancing antigen-antibody reactions.)

The following reading list is recommended for anyone interested in applying micromethods routinely.

Suggested Reading

Chown B, Lewis M. The slanted capillary method of rhesus blood-grouping. J Clin Pathol 1951;4:464-9.

Knight RC, de Silva M. New technologies for red-cell serology. Blood Rev 1996;10:101-10.

Knight R, Poole G, eds. The use of microplates in blood group serology: A review of microplate technology in the U.K. Manchester, UK: British Society of Blood Transfusion, 1987:33-41.

Lapierre Y, Rigal D, Adam J, et al. The gel test: A new way to detect RBC antigen-antibody reactions. Transfusion 1990;30:109-13.

Scott ML. The principles and applications of solid-phase blood group serology. Transfus Med Rev 1991;5:60-72.

Sinor LT. Advances in solid-phase RBC adherence methods and transfusion serology. Transfus Med Rev 1992;6:26-31.

Weiland DL. Capillary tube techniques. In: Myers M, Reynolds A, eds. Micromethods in blood group serology. Arlington, VA: AABB, 1984:3-17.

VI-A. Capillary: Saline Agglutination Procedure

Purpose

To provide instructions for performing a capillary method for direct saline agglutination:

- RBC phenotyping.

- Antibody identification.

Background Information

The passage of RBCs through a column of serum results in multiple opportunities for antibody molecules to come into contact with their corresponding antigens. Because of this increased potential for antigen-antibody contact, capillary methods are exquisitely sensitive; IgG antibodies that cause direct agglutination in capillary techniques may react only by IAT using conventional tube methods. Capillary methods may also be used for antibody detection and identification, particularly when test sera are in short supply.

Operational Policy

Load capillary tubes individually.

Wipe tubes with tissue as each reactant is loaded, to prevent sample contamination.

Do not introduce air bubbles into the tubes because these will hinder the proper mixing of reactants.

Also see Appendix VI-1.

Limitations

Unwanted Positive Reactions:

- Serum/plasma contains a cold-reactive antibody.

- Capillary tubes are not clean.

Unwanted Negative Reactions:

- An air bubble has been introduced that prevents mixing of the reagents.

- Slant angle of the capillary tube is too steep.

- Reagents have been stored improperly.

- Reagents are contaminated.

- A test component has been omitted.

Sample Requirements

Test RBCs, washed three times and diluted to a 25%-30% suspension in PBS.

Equipment/ Materials

Capillary tubes: 0.4 mm ID × 90 mm (eg, Friedrich and Dimmock, Millville, NJ, or Thermo Fisher Scientific, Waltham, MA).

Control RBCs: positive (single-dose) and negative samples appropriate for the reagent antiserum; 25%-30% PBS suspensions. Mix immediately before use.

Magnifying glass: 7× to 10× magnification.

Reagent/test antiserum: free from particulate matter.

Sealant (eg, VWR, Batavia, IL).

Quality Control

Include antigen-positive and antigen-negative RBCs with each test.

Procedure

Use the following steps to perform the procedure:

Step	Action
1.	For each RBC sample to be tested, load a capillary tube with 2 cm of serum. Wipe off excess serum.
2.	Dip the charged end of a loaded capillary tube into a well-mixed RBC sample and allow an equal volume of RBCs to enter the tube.
3.	Invert the tube, secure the uncharged end in sealant, and place at an angle that approximates 55 degrees.
4.	Similarly, set up tests with the other RBC samples, including controls.
5.	Incubate all tubes at RT until the reaction with the positive control RBCs is complete. Use a magnifying glass to observe reactions.
6.	When the RBCs have settled to the bottom of the capillary tube, the tube may be inverted to permit additional passages of RBCs through the serum.
7.	Read and record reactions in all other tubes, using reactions in the positive and negative control tubes for comparative purposes.

8.	Interpret the reactions as follows:	
	If agglutination is...	**Then the test result is...**
	present	positive.
	absent	negative.

References   Chown B, Lewis M. Further experience with the slanted capillary method for Rh typing of red blood cells. Can Med Assoc J 1946;55:66-9.

Chown B, Lewis M. The slanted capillary method of rhesus blood-grouping. J Clin Pathol 1951;4:464-9.

**Effective
Date**

Approved by:	**Printed Name**	**Signature**	**Date**
Laboratory Management			
Medical Director			
Quality Officer			

VI-B. Capillary: Albumin One-Layer Procedure

Purpose

To provide instructions for performing a capillary method for direct albumin-enhanced agglutination—one layer technique:

- RBC phenotyping, especially Rh antigens.

Background Information

The passage of RBCs through a column of serum results in multiple opportunities for antibody molecules to come into contact with their corresponding antigens. Because of this increased potential for antigen-antibody contact, capillary methods are exquisitely sensitive and require use of only small volumes of reagent antisera. IgG antibodies that cause direct agglutination in capillary techniques may react only by IAT using conventional tube methods. The addition of BSA provides a potentiating reagent that further enhances the sensitivity of the capillary test. Thus, capillary methods are particularly suited to large-scale phenotyping of donor RBCs.

Operational Policy

Load capillary tubes individually.

Wipe tubes with tissue as each reactant is loaded, to prevent sample contamination.

Do not introduce air bubbles into the tubes because these will hinder the proper mixing of reactants.

Also see Appendix VI-1.

Limitations

Unwanted Positive Reactions:

- Serum/plasma contains a cold-reactive antibody.
- Capillary tubes are not clean.

Unwanted Negative Reactions:

- An air bubble has been introduced that prevents mixing of the reagents.
- Slant angle of the capillary tube is too steep.
- Reagents have been stored improperly.
- Reagents are contaminated.
- A test component has been omitted.

Sample Requirements

Test RBCs, washed three times and diluted to a 50% suspension in PBS.

Equipment/ Materials

30% BSA.

Capillary tubes: 0.4 mm ID × 90 mm (eg, Friedrich and Dimmock, Millville, NJ, or Thermo Fisher Scientific, Waltham, MA).

Control RBCs: positive (single-dose) and negative samples appropriate for the reagent antiserum; washed three times and diluted to a 50% suspension with PBS. Mix immediately before use.

Magnifying glass: 7× to 10× magnification.

Reagent/test antiserum: free from particulate matter.

Sealant (eg, VWR, Batavia, IL).

Quality Control

Include antigen-positive and antigen-negative RBCs with each test.

Procedure

Use the following steps to perform the procedure:

Step	Action
1.	Mix equal volumes of serum and 30% BSA in a test tube.
2.	For each RBC sample to be tested, load a capillary tube with 2 cm of serum-BSA. Wipe off excess serum.
3.	Dip the charged end (end containing serum) of a loaded capillary tube into a well-mixed RBC sample and allow an equal volume of RBCs to enter the tube.
4.	Invert the tube, secure the uncharged end in sealant, and place at an angle that approximates 55 degrees.
5.	Set up tests with the other test RBC samples and controls, following Steps 1-4.
6.	Incubate all tubes at RT until the reaction with the positive control RBCs is complete. Use a magnifying glass to observe reactions.
7.	When the RBCs have settled to the bottom of the capillary tube, the tube may be inverted to permit additional passages of RBCs through the serum.

8.	Read and record reactions in all other tubes, using reactions in the positive and negative control tubes for comparative purposes.	
	If agglutination is…	**Then the test result is…**
	present	positive.
	absent	negative.

Reference

Crawford MN, Gottman FE, Rogers LC. Capillary tube testing and enhancement with 30% albumin. Vox Sang 1976;30:144-8.

**Effective
Date**

Approved by:	**Printed Name**	**Signature**	**Date**
**Laboratory
Management**			
**Medical
Director**			
**Quality
Officer**			

VI-C. Capillary: Albumin Two-Layer Procedure

Purpose

To provide instructions for performing a capillary method for direct albumin-enhanced agglutination—two layer technique:

- RBC phenotyping, especially Rh antigens.

Background Information

The passage of RBCs through a column of serum results in multiple opportunities for antibody molecules to come into contact with their corresponding antigens. Because of this increased potential for antigen-antibody contact, capillary methods are exquisitely sensitive and require use of only small volumes of reagent antisera. IgG antibodies that cause direct agglutination in capillary techniques may react only by IAT using conventional tube methods. The addition of BSA provides a potentiating reagent that further enhances the sensitivity of the capillary test. Thus, capillary methods are particularly suited to large-scale phenotyping of donor RBCs.

Operational Policy

Load capillary tubes individually.

Wipe tubes with tissue as each reactant is loaded, to prevent sample contamination.

Do not introduce air bubbles into the tubes because these will hinder the proper mixing of reactants.

Also see Appendix VI-1.

Limitations

Unwanted Positive Reactions:

- Serum/plasma contains a cold-reactive antibody.
- Capillary tubes are not clean.

Unwanted Negative Reactions:

- An air bubble has been introduced that prevents mixing of the reagents.
- Slant angle of the capillary tube is too steep.
- Reagents have been stored improperly.
- Reagents are contaminated.
- A test component has been omitted.

Sample Requirements

Test RBCs, washed three times and diluted to a 50% suspension in PBS.

Equipment/ Materials

30% BSA.

Capillary tubes: 0.4 mm ID × 90 mm (eg, Friedrich and Dimmock, Millville, NJ, or Thermo Fisher Scientific, Waltham, MA).

Control RBCs: positive (single-dose) and negative samples appropriate for the reagent antiserum; washed three times and diluted to a 50% suspension with PBS. Mix immediately before use.

Magnifying glass: 7× to 10× magnification.

Reagent/test antiserum: free from particulate matter.

Sealant (eg, VWR, Batavia, IL).

Quality Control

Include antigen-positive and antigen-negative RBCs with each test.

Procedure

Use the following steps to perform the procedure:

Step	Action
1.	For each RBC sample to be tested, load a capillary tube with 2 cm of serum. Wipe off excess serum.
2.	Allow an equal volume of 30% BSA to enter the tube and wipe tube again.
3.	Dip the charged end (end containing serum) of a loaded capillary tube into a well-mixed RBC sample and allow an equal volume of RBCs to enter the tube.
4.	Invert the tube, secure the uncharged end in sealant, and place at an angle that approximates 55 degrees.
5.	Set up tests with the other test RBC samples and controls, following Steps 1-4.
6.	Incubate all tubes at RT until the reaction with the positive control RBCs is complete. Use a magnifying glass to observe reactions.
7.	When the RBCs have settled to the bottom of the capillary tube, the tube may be inverted to permit additional passages of RBCs through the serum.

8.	Read and record reactions in all other tubes, using reactions in the positive and negative control tubes for comparative purposes.	
	If agglutination is…	**Then the test result is…**
	present	positive.
	absent	negative.

Reference   Crawford MN, Gottman FE, Rogers LC. Capillary tube testing and enhancement with 30% albumin. Vox Sang 1976;30:144-8.

**Effective
Date**

Approved by:	Printed Name	Signature	Date
Laboratory Management			
Medical Director			
Quality Officer			

VI-D. Capillary: Papain One-Stage Procedure

Purpose

To provide instructions for performing a protease-modified capillary test with papain:

- RBC phenotyping.
- Antibody identification.

Background Information

The passage of RBCs through a column of serum results in multiple opportunities for antibody molecules to come into contact with their corresponding antigens. Because of this increased potential for antigen-antibody contact, capillary methods are exquisitely sensitive and require use of only small volumes of reagent antisera. IgG antibodies that cause direct agglutination in capillary techniques may react only by IAT using conventional tube methods, particularly when the test RBCs are pretreated with a proteolytic enzyme. Capillary methods may also be used for antibody detection and identification, particularly when test sera are in short supply.

Operational Policy

Load capillary tubes individually.

Wipe tubes with tissue as each reactant is loaded, to prevent sample contamination.

Do not introduce air bubbles into the tubes because these will hinder the proper mixing of reactants.

Also see Appendix VI-1.

Limitations

Unwanted Positive Reactions:

- Serum/plasma contains a cold-reactive antibody.
- Capillary tubes are not clean.

Unwanted Negative Reactions:

- An air bubble has been introduced that prevents mixing of the reagents.
- Slant angle of the capillary tube is too steep.
- Reagents have been stored improperly.

- Protease is inactive.

- Reagents are contaminated.

- A test component has been omitted.

Sample Requirements   Test RBCs, washed three times and diluted to a 25%-30% suspension in PBS.

Equipment/ Materials   Capillary tubes: 0.4 mm ID × 90 mm (eg, Friedrich and Dimmock, Millville, NJ, or Thermo Fisher Scientific, Waltham, MA).

Control RBCs: positive (single-dose) and negative samples appropriate for the reagent antiserum; washed three times and diluted to a 25%-30% PBS suspension with saline. Mix immediately before use.

Magnifying glass: 7× to 10× magnification.

Papain: 1% wt/vol.

Reagent/test antiserum: free from particulate matter.

Sealant (eg, VWR, Batavia, IL).

Quality Control   Include antigen-positive and antigen-negative RBCs with each test.

Procedure   Use the following steps to perform the procedure:

Step	Action
1.	For each RBC sample to be tested, load a capillary tube with 2 cm of serum. Wipe off excess serum.
2.	Allow an equal volume of 1% papain to enter the tube and wipe tube again.
3.	Dip the charged end of a loaded capillary tube into a well-mixed RBC sample and allow 2 cm of RBCs to enter the tube.
4.	Invert the tube, secure the uncharged end in sealant, and place at an angle that approximates 55 degrees.
5.	Similarly, repeat Steps 1 through 4 with the other RBC samples, including controls.

6.	Incubate all tubes at RT until the reaction with the positive control RBCs is complete. Use a magnifying glass to observe reactions.
7.	When the RBCs have settled to the bottom of the capillary tube, the tube may be inverted to permit additional passages of RBCs through the serum.
8.	Read and record reactions in all other tubes, using reactions in the positive and negative control tubes for comparative purposes.

If agglutination is…	Then the test result is…
present	positive.
absent	negative.

Reference

Lewis M, Kaita H, Chown B. Kell typing in the capillary tube. J Lab Clin Med 1958;52:163-8.

Effective Date

Approved by:	Printed Name	Signature	Date
Laboratory Management			
Medical Director			
Quality Officer			

VI-E. Capillary: Ficin One-Stage Procedure

Purpose

To provide instructions for performing a protease-modified capillary test—ficin:

- RBC phenotyping.

- Antibody identification.

Background Information

The passage of RBCs through a column of serum results in multiple opportunities for antibody molecules to come into contact with their corresponding antigens. Because of this increased potential for antigen-antibody contact, capillary methods are exquisitely sensitive and require use of only small volumes of reagent antisera. IgG antibodies that cause direct agglutination in capillary techniques may react only by IAT using conventional tube methods, particularly when the test RBCs are pretreated with a proteolytic enzyme. Capillary methods may also be used for antibody detection and identification, particularly when test sera are in short supply.

Operational Policy

Load capillary tubes individually.

Wipe tubes with tissue as each reactant is loaded, to prevent sample contamination.

Do not introduce air bubbles into the tubes because these will hinder the proper mixing of reactants.

Also see Appendix VI-1.

Limitations

Unwanted Positive Reactions:

- Serum/plasma contains a cold-reactive antibody.

- Capillary tubes are not clean.

Unwanted Negative Reactions:

- An air bubble has been introduced that prevents mixing of the reagents.

- Slant angle of the capillary tube is too steep.

- Reagents have been stored improperly.

- Protease is inactive.

- Reagents are contaminated.

- A test component has been omitted.

Sample Requirements

Test RBCs, washed three times and diluted to a 50% suspension in PBS.

Equipment/ Materials

Capillary tubes: 0.4 mm ID × 90 mm (eg, Friedrich and Dimmock, Millville, NJ, or Thermo Fisher Scientific, Waltham, MA).

Control RBCs: positive (single-dose) and negative samples appropriate for the reagent antiserum; 50% suspensions. Mix immediately before use.

Ficin: 4% (wt/vol).

Magnifying glass: 7× to 10× magnification.

pH 7.3 PBS.

Reagent/test antiserum: free from particulate matter.

Sealant (eg, VWR, Batavia, IL).

Quality Control

Include antigen-positive and antigen-negative RBCs with each test.

Procedure

Use the following steps to perform the procedure:

Step	Action
1.	For each donor sample to be tested, mix 2 large drops (approximately 100 µL) of 50% RBCs with 1 small drop (approximately 25 µL) of 4% ficin.
2.	Incubate at RT for at least 10 minutes.
3.	For each ficin-treated RBC sample thus prepared, load a capillary tube with 2 cm of serum. Wipe off excess serum.
4.	Dip the charged end of a loaded capillary tube into a well-mixed ficin-treated RBC sample and allow an equal volume of RBCs to enter the tube.
5.	Invert the tube, secure the uncharged end in sealant, and place at an angle that approximates 55 degrees.

6.	Similarly, set up tests with the other RBC samples, including controls.
7.	Incubate all tubes at RT until the reaction with the positive control RBCs is complete. Use a magnifying glass to observe reactions.
8.	When the RBCs have settled to the bottom of the capillary tube, the tube may be inverted to permit additional passages of RBCs through the serum
9.	Read and record reactions in all other tubes, using reactions in the positive and negative control tubes for comparative purposes.

If agglutination is…	Then the test result is…
present	positive.
absent	negative.

Reference   Crawford MN. Rapid testing of ficinized cells in capillary tubes (abstract). Transfusion 1978;18:598.

Effective Date

	Printed Name	Signature	Date
Approved by			
Laboratory Management			
Medical Director			
Quality Officer			

VI-F. Capillary: IAT on Precoated RBCs Procedure

Purpose   To provide instructions for performing an IAT in capillary tubes:

- RBC phenotyping.

- Antibody identification.

Background Information   The passage of RBCs through a column of serum results in multiple opportunities for antibody molecules to come into contact with their corresponding antigens. Because of this increased potential for antigen-antibody contact, capillary methods are exquisitely sensitive and require use of only small volumes of reagent antisera. This procedure is particularly suited to large-scale phenotyping of donor RBCs using antisera that react by the indirect antiglobulin technique. The procedure may also be used for antibody detection and identification, particularly when test sera are in short supply.

Operational Policy   Load capillary tubes individually.

Wipe tubes with tissue as each reactant is loaded, to prevent sample contamination.

Do not introduce air bubbles into the tubes because these will hinder the proper mixing of reactants.

Also see Appendix VI-1.

Limitations   Unwanted Positive Reactions:

- Serum/plasma contains an autoantibody.

- Capillary tubes are not clean.

- AHG reagent contains heterophile antibodies.

Unwanted Negative Reactions:

- An air bubble has been introduced that prevents mixing of the reagents.

- Slant angle of the capillary tube is too steep.

- Coated RBCs have been washed insufficiently.

- Reagents have been stored improperly.

- Reagents are contaminated.

- A test component has been omitted.

Sample Requirements

Test RBCs, washed three times and diluted to a 50% suspension in pH 7.3 PBS.

Equipment/ Materials

AHG: anti-IgG.

Capillary tubes: 0.4 mm ID × 90 mm (eg, Friedrich and Dimmock, Milville, NJ, or Thermo Fisher Scientific, Waltham, MA).

Laboratory film: Parafilm (eg, VWR, Batavia, IL).

Magnifying glass: 7× to 10× magnification.

Control RBCs: positive (single-dose) and negative samples appropriate for the reagent antiserum; washed three times with saline.

Reagent/test antiserum: free from particulate matter.

Sealant (eg, VWR, Batavia, IL).

Quality Control

Include antigen-positive and antigen-negative RBCs with each test.

Procedure

Use the following steps to perform the procedure:

Step	Action
1.	For each RBC sample, mix 10 µL of serum and 5 µL of RBCs in appropriately labeled 10 or 12 × 75-mm test tubes.
2.	Cover tubes with Parafilm to prevent evaporation and incubate tests at RT for 2 hours.
3.	Wash the RBCs four times with saline. Decant the final wash supernate to leave a 25%-30% RBC suspension.
4.	For each washed RBC sample to be tested, load a capillary tube with 2 cm of AHG. Wipe off excess AHG.
5.	Dip the charged end of a loaded capillary tube into a well-mixed RBC sample and allow an equal volume of RBCs to enter the tube.
6.	Invert the tube, secure the uncharged end in sealant, and place at an angle that approximates 45 degrees.
7.	Similarly, set up tests with the other RBC samples, including controls.
8.	Incubate all tubes at RT until the reaction with the positive control RBCs is complete. Use a magnifying glass to observe reactions.

9.	When the RBCs have settled to the bottom of the capillary tube, the tube may be inverted to permit additional passages of RBCs through the serum.	
10.	Read and record reactions in all other tubes, using reactions in the positive and negative control tubes for comparative purposes.	
	If agglutination is…	**Then the test result is…**
	present	positive.
	absent	negative.

Reference   Weiland DL. Capillary tube techniques. In: Myers M, Reynolds A, eds. Micromethods in blood group serology. Arlington, VA: AABB, 1984:3-17.

Effective Date

Approved by

	Printed Name	**Signature**	**Date**
Laboratory Management			
Medical Director			
Quality Officer			

VI-G. Capillary: Precoating for IAT Procedure

Purpose

To provide instructions for performing a capillary method for precoating RBCs for the IAT:

- RBC phenotyping.

- Antibody identification.

Background Information

The passage of RBCs through a column of serum results in multiple opportunities for antibody molecules to come into contact with their corresponding antigens. Because of this increased potential for antigen-antibody contact, capillary methods are exquisitely sensitive and require use of only small volumes of reagent antisera. This procedure is particularly suited to phenotyping RBCs using antisera that react by the indirect antiglobulin technique. The procedure may also be used for antibody detection and identification, particularly when test sera are in short supply.

Operational Policy

Load capillary tubes individually.

Wipe tubes with tissue as each reactant is loaded, to prevent sample contamination.

Do not introduce air bubbles into the tubes because these will hinder the proper mixing of reactants.

Also see Appendix VI-1.

Limitations

Unwanted Positive Reactions:

- Serum/plasma contains an autoantibody.

- Capillary tubes are not clean.

Unwanted Negative Reactions:

- An air bubble has been introduced that prevents mixing of the reagents.

- Slant angle of the capillary tube is too steep.

- Coated RBCs have been washed insufficiently.

- Reagents have been stored improperly.

- Reagents are contaminated.

- A test component has been omitted.

Sample Requirements	Test RBCs, washed three times and diluted to a 50% suspension in PBS.

Equipment/ Materials	AHG: anti-IgG.
	Capillary tubes: 0.4 mm ID × 90 mm (eg, Friedrich and Dimmock, Millville, NJ, or Thermo Fisher Scientific, Waltham, MA).
	Control RBCs: positive (single-dose) and negative samples appropriate for the reagent antiserum; washed three times and diluted to a 50% suspension with saline. Mix immediately before use.
	pH 7.3 PBS.
	Reagent/test antiserum: free from particulate matter.
	Sealant (eg, VWR, Batavia, IL).

Quality Control	Include antigen-positive and antigen-negative RBCs with each test.

Procedure   Use the following steps to perform the procedure:

Step	Action
1.	For each RBC sample to be tested, load a capillary tube with 2 cm of serum. Wipe off excess serum.
2.	Dip the charged end of a loaded capillary tube into a well-mixed RBC sample and allow an equal volume of RBCs to enter the tube.
3.	Invert the tube, secure the uncharged end in sealant, and place at an angle that approximates 60 degrees.
4.	Similarly, set up tests with the other RBC samples, including controls.
5.	Incubate all tubes at RT for 15 minutes.
6.	Invert the sealant tray and place at an angle that approximates 60 degrees for a further 15 minutes to allow the RBCs to pass through the serum a second time.
7.	Place capillary tubes (unsealed end downwards) into appropriately labeled 10 or 12 × 75-mm test tubes, each containing approximately 1 mL of PBS.
8.	Centrifuge at 1000 × g for 2 minutes (or equivalent).

9.	Remove empty capillary tubes and discard. If tubes still contain RBCs, carefully break off sealed end and recentrifuge.
10.	Wash the RBCs three to four times with PBS and completely decant the final wash supernate.
11.	To the dry RBC buttons, add AHG according to the manufacturer's directions.
12.	Centrifuge as for hemagglutination tests (see Appendix VI-2).
13.	Examine the RBCs macroscopically. Grade and record the results as follows.

If agglutination is...	Then...
present	test result is positive.
negative	proceed to Step 14.

14.	Add IgG-coated RBCs to all negative tests. Recentrifuge and examine the tests macroscopically for mixed-field agglutination.

If agglutination is...	Then the test result is...
present	negative.
absent	invalid: • Repeat the test.

Reference Graves B. Application of the antiglobulin phase to capillary tube testing (letter). Transfusion 1981;21:373.

Effective Date

Approved by:

	Printed Name	Signature	Date
Laboratory Management			
Medical Director			
Quality Officer			

VI-H. Microplate: ABO and Rh Typing Procedure

Purpose

To provide instructions for ABO and Rh typing of human blood using microplates:

- Pretransfusion testing.
- Perinatal testing.

Background Information

ABO blood types are determined by the presence or absence of A and/or B antigens on RBCs and by the presence or absence of anti-A and/or anti-B in the serum.

Rh-positive and Rh-negative phenotypes are determined by the presence or absence of D antigen on RBCs.

In adults, there is a reciprocal relationship between the A and/or B antigens on RBCs and A and/or B antibodies in the serum/plasma; eg, if A antigen is absent on the RBCs, anti-A is expected to be present in the serum/plasma.

Operational Policy

Samples from infants less than 6 months old will not regularly contain expected anti-A or anti-B; therefore, only RBC ABO typing is required.

When Rh-typing patient samples, only DATs are required.

When Rh-typing newborns of Rh-negative women (to determine maternal RhIG candidacy) or allogeneic blood donors, the method for Rh typing must be capable of detecting weak expression of D antigen. See Procedure I-D.

When agglutination occurs in routine tests, reactions equal to or greater than 2+ are expected; observation of weaker reactions necessitates further study before valid conclusions can be made. See Section XIII and Procedure I-D when weak or discrepant findings are encountered.

For electronic crossmatching, two concordant ABO types are required: one type on a current sample and one historical type, or both on a current sample. When practical, the two blood types on a current sample should be performed by different technologists using different manufacturers' reagents.

Microplates must be clean and static-free.

The microplate centrifuge must be calibrated appropriately.

Also see Appendix VI-2.

A second Rh type, incorporating an inert Rh control reagent and following reidentification of the sample, shall be performed on all patients without a historical record.

Note: Wording in reagent manufacturers' product circulars may impose further limitations on the age and type of samples used for ABO and Rh typing.

Also see Appendix VI-2.

Limitations

Unwanted Positive Reactions:

- Auto- or alloantibodies.

- Contaminated reagent or sample.

- Microplates are not clean.

Additional Reactivity:

- Anti-A$_1$ in an A$_2$ or A$_2$B individual.

- Passive antibody.

- Antibody to reagent constituent.

- Acquired-B phenomenon.

- B(A) phenomenon.

Note: T and Tn polyagglutination should not cause a typing discrepancy with currently available monoclonal typing reagents.

Unwanted Negative Reactions:

- Omission of reagent or test sample.

- Contaminated or inactive reagent.

- Contaminated sample (eg, excess soluble blood group substance from a ruptured ovarian cyst).

Missing Reactivity:

- Leukemia.

- Minor cell population (eg, transplant, genetic chimera).

- Non-ABO-type-specific plasma infusions.

- Newborn sample.

- Impaired immune response.

**Sample
Requirements**

EDTA-anticoagulated blood as a source of plasma and RBCs. Prepare RBCs as a 2%-5% suspension in saline or pH 7.3 PBS.

Note: If used for pretransfusion testing and the patient has been transfused with RBCs or has been pregnant within the preceding 3 months, or if the history is uncertain or unavailable, the sample must be obtained within 3 days of scheduled transfusion.

**Equipment/
Materials**

Anti-A and anti-B (only monoclonal products are currently available in the United States).

Anti-D: low-protein, monoclonal IgM anti-D blended with polyclonal or monoclonal IgG anti-D.

3% BSA.

Microplate equipment: flexible U-bottom microplates (eg, Spectrocell, Oreland, PA).

Sorvall T1 centrifuge with microplate rotor and carriers (eg, Thermo Fisher Scientific, Waltham, MA).

RBCs: 2%-5% suspensions of reagent group A_1 (pool of 3 donors) and B RBCs (pool of 3 donors) in EDTA saline. All donors should be Rh negative.

**Quality
Control**

Daily, for each lot of reagents in use, demonstrate that:

- Anti-A agglutinates (4+, score 12) group A_1 reagent RBCs, but not group B reagent RBCs.

- Anti-B agglutinates (4+, score 12) group B reagent RBCs but not group A_1 reagent RBCs.

- Anti-D agglutinates (3+ to 4+, score 10-12) Rh-positive RBCs (group O, R_1R_1 RBCs from Procedure I-B) but not Rh-negative RBCs (group A_1 or B reagent RBCs).

Alternatively, document daily that all samples from previously tested patients react according to the blood type of record and all discrepancies with prior results and between RBC and serum/plasma ABO types were resolved.

Note: Discrepancies between RBC and serum/plasma results must be resolved before the ABO type can be concluded. See Section XIII.

Procedure   Use the following steps to perform the procedure:

Step	Action
1.	For each sample to be tested, dispense 1 25-35 µL drop of reagent anti-A, anti-B, anti-D, and 3% BSA into microplate wells An, Bn, Cn, and Dn, respectively, where n = the sample row number for the specimen being tested.
2.	Similarly, dispense 1 drop of reagent A_1 and B RBCs into wells En and Fn.
3.	Add 1 drop of 2%-5% test RBCs to rows A-D.
4.	Add 1 drop of test serum/plasma to rows E and F.
5.	Gently tap the side of the microplate to mix sera and RBCs.
6.	Centrifuge as for microplate hemagglutination tests (see Appendix VI-2).
7.	Stand the microplates at a 45- to 50-degree angle for 3-5 minutes and observe for agglutination. Record the results.
8.	Interpret the reactions as follows:

If…	Then the test result is…
RBCs stream from the center of the well to the edge	negative.
a tight button remains in the center of the well but there is some streaming of RBCs	positive.
RBCs remain as a tight button in the center of the well	strongly positive.

9.	Interpret the blood type as follows:						
	If RBCs react...				**And serum reacts...**		**Then type is...**
	Anti-A	**Anti-B**	**Anti-D**	**BSA**	**A₁ RBCs**	**B RBCs**	
	0	0	≥2+	0	≥2+	≥2+	O Rh+
	0	0	0	0	≥2+	≥2+	O Rh–
	≥2+	0	≥2+	0	0	≥2+	A Rh+
	≥2+	0	0	0	0+	≥2+	A Rh–
	0	≥2+	≥2+	0	≥2+	0	B Rh+
	0	≥2+	0	0	≥2+	0	B Rh–
	≥2+	≥2+	≥2+	0	0	0	AB Rh+
	≥2+	≥2+	0	0	0	0	AB Rh–

If...	**Then...**
mixed-field or different reactions are observed.	see Section XIII.

Note: If discrepant reactions are observed and transfusion is necessary before resolution, only group O RBCs shall be issued. If sample is from a blood donor, discrepancies shall be resolved before release.

References

Code of federal regulations. Title 21 CFR Parts 606 and 660. Washington, DC: US Government Printing Office, 2008 (revised annually).

Price TH, ed. Standards for blood banks and transfusion services. 25th ed. Bethesda, MD: AABB, 2008 (or current edition).

Roback J, Combs MR, Grossman B, Hillyer C, eds. Technical manual. 16th ed. Bethesda, MD: AABB, 2008 (or current edition).

**Effective
Date**

Approved by:	Printed Name	Signature	Date
Laboratory Management			
Medical Director			
Quality Officer			

VI-I. Microplate: Antibody Detection Using LISS Procedure

Purpose
To provide instructions for antibody screening in a microplate using LISS:

- Antibody detection.
- Antibody identification.

Background Information
Antibodies to RBC antigens may cause direct agglutination or lysis of RBCs or may coat RBCs with globulins (eg, IgG, C3). Direct agglutination and/or lysis can be observed following centrifugation of RBC/serum mixtures. Antibody coating may be accelerated in a low-ionic environment; hence, the use of LISS. RBCs incubated with serum/plasma in the presence of LISS at 37 C are washed to remove unbound globulins and tested with AHG. Agglutination by AHG indicates that the RBCs are coated with globulins. This procedure is suitable for screening large numbers of sera for unexpected antibodies.

Operational Policy
Microplates must be clean and static-free.

The microplate centrifuge must be calibrated appropriately.

Also see Appendix VI-2.

Limitations
Unwanted Positive Reactions:

- Incorrect reagents or RBCs used.
- Microplates are not clean.

Unwanted Negative reactions:

- Incorrect reagents or RBCs used.
- Reagents are contaminated.

Sample Requirements
Clotted or EDTA-anticoagulated blood as a source of serum/plasma and RBCs.

Note: If used for pretransfusion testing and the patient has been transfused with RBCs or has been pregnant within the preceding 3 months, or if the history is uncertain or unavailable, the sample must be obtained within 3 days of scheduled transfusion.

Note: Wording in reagent manufacturers' product circulars may impose further limitations on the age and type of samples used for ABO and Rh typing.

**Equipment/
Materials**

6% BSA + Tween 20 (Sigma-Aldrich, St Louis, MO).

AHG: anti-IgG; need not be heavy-chain specific.

IgG-coated RBCs: see Section VII.

LISS solution.

Microplate equipment: U- or V-bottom microplates (eg, Spectrocell, Oreland, PA).

Sorvall T1 centrifuge with microplate rotor and carrier (eg, Thermo Fisher Scientific, Waltham, MA).

RBCs: Phenotyped group O, R_1R_1 and R_2R_2 RBCs, diluted to a 0.5% suspension with LISS; use within 6 hours of preparation.

Note: As defined in the CFR, RBCs used in pretransfusion testing to detect unexpected antibodies must carry the following antigens: D, C, c, E, e, K, k, Fy^a, Fy^b, Jk^a, Jk^b, Le^a, Le^b, M, N, S, s, and P_1.

Weakly (2+) reactive antibody (eg, dilute human IgG anti-D).

**Quality
Control**

Daily, for each lot of reagents in use, demonstrate that the weakly reactive antibody reacts appropriately with the reagent R_1R_1 and R_2R_2 RBCs.

Daily, for each lot of reagents in use, demonstrate that 6% BSA does not react with the reagent R_1R_1 and R_2R_2 RBCs.

Confirm all negative reactions with IgG-coated RBCs (see Steps 8-10 below).

Procedure

Use the following steps to perform the procedure:

Step	Action
1.	For each sample to be tested, dispense 1 drop (35 μL) of serum/plasma into 2 microplate wells.
2.	To 1 well of each serum sample, add an equal volume of 0.5% R_1R_1 RBCs in LISS. Similarly, set up tests with the R_2R_2 RBCs.
3.	Mix and incubate at 37 C for 15-20 minutes.

4.	Wash the RBCs four times with 6% BSA + Tween 20 wash solution. **Note:** Use 0.2-mL volumes for each wash. "Flick off" the supernate following each centrifugation.	
5.	Add 1 drop of AHG to each test well.	
6.	Mix and centrifuge as for microplate hemagglutination tests.	
7.	Stand the microplates at a 45- to 50-degree angle for 3-5 minutes and observe for agglutination. Record the results.	
	If...	**Then...**
	RBCs remain as a tight button in the center of the well	result is positive.
	a tight button remains in the center of the well but there is some streaming of RBCs	result is positive.
	hemolysis is present	result is positive.
	RBCs stream from the center of the well to the edge	add IgG-coated RBCs to all negative test wells: • Recentrifuge and examine the tests macroscopically for mixed-field agglutination.
8.	Add 1 drop IgG-coated RBCs to each negative test.	
9.	Mix and centrifuge as for microplate hemagglutination tests.	
10.	Interpret the reactions with the IgG-coated RBCs as follows:	
	If...	**Then the test result is...**
	a tight button remains in the center of the well but there is some streaming of RBCs	negative.
	RBCs stream from the center of the well to the edge	invalid and must be repeated.

References

Ball M. Procedures for blood grouping, antibody screening and rare phenotype screening in microplates. In: Knight R, Poole G, eds. The use of microplates in blood group serology: a review of microplate technology in the UK. Manchester, UK: British Society of Blood Transfusion, 1987:33-41.

Code of federal regulations. Title 21 CFR Parts 606 and 660. Washington, DC: US Government Printing Office, 2008 (revised annually).

Löw B, Messeter L. Antiglobulin tests in low-ionic strength salt solutions for rapid antibody screening and crossmatching. Vox Sang 1974;26:53-61.

Effective Date

Approved by:

	Printed Name	Signature	Date
Laboratory Management			
Medical Director			
Quality Officer			

VI-J. Microplate: LIP Technique Procedure

Purpose

To provide instructions for antibody screening using Polybrene (Sigma-Aldrich, St Louis, MO):

- Antibody detection.

- Antibody identification.

Background Information

Cationic polymers such as Polybrene cause aggregation of normal RBCs that can be dispersed with sodium citrate. However, sodium citrate does not disperse Polybrene-induced aggregation of antibody-coated RBCs. In the low-ionic Polybrene (LIP) procedure, RBCs are first incubated with serum under low-ionic conditions to facilitate antibody uptake. Aggregation of RBCs is induced by Polybrene, if antibody has coated the RBCs, immunoglobulin molecules form bridges between adjacent RBCs, which persist after sodium citrate is added. This procedure is suitable for large-scale phenotyping of donor blood samples.

Operational Policy

Microplates must be clean and static-free.

The microplate centrifuge must be calibrated appropriately.

Also see Appendix VI-2.

Limitations

Unwanted Positive Reactions:

- Incorrect reagents or RBCs used.

- Microplates are not clean.

- Dilution of Polybrene is incorrect.

Unwanted Negative Reactions:

- Incorrect reagents or RBCs used.

- Reagents are contaminated.

Sample Requirements

Clotted or EDTA-anticoagulated blood as a source of serum or plasma.

Note: If used for pretransfusion testing and the patient has been transfused with RBCs or has been pregnant within the preceding 3 months, or if the history is uncertain or unavailable, the sample must be obtained within 3 days of scheduled transfusion.

Equipment/ Materials

Pipettors with disposable tips to deliver 25-100 μL (eg, VWR, Batavia, IL).

AB serum lacking unexpected antibodies.

Low-ionic medium.

Microplate equipment: U- or V-bottom microplates (eg, Spectrocell, Oreland, PA).

Polybrene working solution.

Polybrene neutralizing reagent.

Sorvall T1 centrifuge with microplate rotor and carrier (eg, Thermo Fisher Scientific, Waltham, MA).

RBCs: phenotyped group O, R_1R_1 and R_2R_2 RBCs, diluted to a 0.5% suspension with LISS; use within 6 hours of preparation.

Note: As defined in the CFR, RBCs used in pretransfusion testing to detect unexpected antibodies must carry the following antigens: D, C, c, E, e, K, k, Fy^a, Fy^b, Jk^a, Jk^b, Le^a, Le^b, M, N, S, s, and P_1.

Weakly (2+) reactive antibody (eg, dilute human IgG anti-D).

Quality Control

Daily, for each lot of reagents in use, demonstrate that the weakly reactive antibody reacts appropriately with the reagent R_1R_1 and R_2R_2 RBCs.

Daily, for each lot of reagents in use, demonstrate that AB serum does not react with the reagent R_1R_1 and R_2R_2 RBCs.

Procedure

Use the following steps to perform the procedure:

Step	Action
1.	For each sample to be tested, dispense 25 μL of antiserum and 100 μL of low-ionic medium into a microplate well.
2.	Add 25 μL of 1% test RBCs and mix on a plate shaker for 15 seconds.
3.	Incubate at RT for 1 minute.
4.	Add 25 μL of Polybrene solution to each well and mix.
5.	Incubate for 15 seconds.
6.	Centrifuge at $300 \times g$ for 1 minute.
7.	Decant the supernate and add 25 μL of resuspending solution to each well.

8.	Agitate the plate by hand to resuspend the RBCs.	
9.	Examine the RBCs macroscopically for agglutination, using an illuminated background, and record the results.	

If...	Then the test result is...
RBCs are evenly suspended	negative.
RBCs remain as a tight button in the center of the well	strongly positive.
a tight button remains in the center of the well but there is some resuspension of RBCs	positive.

Reference

Malde R, Redman M. Low-ionic Polybrene technique. In: Knight RV, Poole G, eds. The use of microplates in blood group serology: A review of microplate technology in the UK. Manchester, UK: British Society of Blood Transfusion, 1987:42-43.

Effective Date

Approved by:	Printed Name	Signature	Date
Laboratory Management			
Medical Director			
Quality Officer			

VI-K. Gel: Preparing Buffered Gel Columns

Purpose

To provide instructions for preparing Sephadex gel columns for serologic testing:

- Antibody detection.
- Antibody identification.

Background Information

Sephadex gel is a porous gel composed of alkaline dextran cross-linked with epichlorohydrin and hydrated with a buffer such as PBS or LISS. The gel beads used (Sephadex G100), have a fractionation range from a molecular weight of 4000 to 150,000, which will permit the free passage of single RBCs but not the passage of RBC agglutinates. Lapierre et al described the use of Sephadex gel for conventional saline and enzyme techniques in a simple inert buffer.

Also see Appendix VI-3.

Operational Policy

The centrifuge should be calibrated appropriately to permit even packing of the gel suspension.

Limitations

Unwanted Positive Reactions:

- Gel is unevenly packed.
- Fibrin is present in the test plasma.
- Reagents are prepared incorrectly.

Unwanted Negative Reactions:

- Gel is unevenly packed.
- Supernatant buffer has not been decanted sufficiently.
- Reagent volumes are incorrect.

Sample Requirements

IgM anti-M and anti-D reagents.

Equipment/ Materials	6 × 50-mm clear polystyrene test tubes: Precipitin tubes (#5070-000, Elkay Co, Basingstoke, UK).
	10 × 5-hole precipitin test tube racks.
	Variable-volume pipettes: 5-50 μL and 200-1000 μL (VWR, Batavia, IL).
	Benchtop centrifuge with a swing-out rotor.
	Sephadex G100 superfine powder.
	0.1% BSA-LISS.
	Reagent RBCs diluted to a 1% suspension in LISS.

Quality Control	All columns must be visually inspected to ensure that the gel is packed evenly before use.

Column Preparation Procedure

Use the following steps to prepare the columns:

Step	Action
1.	Prepare the gel suspension by mixing 0.5 g of Sephadex G100 superfine powder in 10 mL of 0.1% BSA-LISS.
2.	Mix thoroughly to ensure even hydration and suspension of the beads.
3.	Pipette 350 μL of the Sephadex gel solution into 6 × 50-mm test tubes. Centrifuge at 1000 × g for 60 seconds to remove air bubbles and pack the gel.
4.	Columns may be used immediately, or store columns, covered with Parafilm, upright at 2-8 C for a maximum of 14 days.
5.	Evaluate the columns as follows:

If...	Then...
the top of the column is level	the tubes are ready to use.
the top of the column is uneven	recalibrate the centrifuge, resuspend the gel column, and recentrifuge.
the gel column "trails" down the side of the tube	ensure that a swing-out rotor is in use: • Recalibrate the centrifuge, resuspend the gel column, and recentrifuge.

**Quality
Control
Procedure**   Use the following steps to quality-control the columns:

Step	Action
1.	Take 22 gel columns from the refrigerator and allow them to warm to room temperature.
2.	Prepare a doubling dilution of anti-M and anti-D in PBS/1% BSA to a dilution of 1 in 512.
3.	Visually inspect the columns to confirm that the gel suspension is level.
4.	Decant the supernatant buffer on the columns by a rapid "flick" into a waste container.
5.	Mark two series of 10 tubes: 1, 2, 4, 8, 16, 32, 64, 128, 256, 512.
6.	Mark 2 tubes with "1" for the negative controls.
7.	Add 30 µL of M+N+ 1% RBCs to each of 10 tubes.
8.	Add 30 µL of M– RBCs to the negative control tube.
9.	Add 30 µL of each dilution to the appropriately marked tube.
10.	Repeat 7-9 with D+ and D– RBCs and the anti-D dilutions.
11.	Centrifuge at $300 \times g$ for 10 minutes.
12.	Read the tests macroscopically over a light box. Grade tests from 0 (negative) to 4+ (see Appendix VI-4 for representative agglutination patterns).
13.	Determine the required dilutions of anti-M and anti-D for positive controls as follows:

If...	Then...
there is a dilution that yields a 2+ reaction	select that dilution for a positive control.
all dilutions are strongly reactive	prepare and test higher antibody dilutions.
no dilutions are reactive	select a different example of antibody to titrate.

Reference   Lapierre Y, Rigal D, Adam J, et al. The gel test: A new way to detect RBC antigen-antibody reactions. Transfusion 1990;30:109-13.

**Effective
Date**

Approved by:	Printed Name	Signature	Date
Laboratory Management			
Medical Director			
Quality Officer			

VI-L. Gel: Preparing Anti-IgG Columns

Purpose

To provide instructions for preparing Sephadex gel columns for serologic testing:

- Antibody detection.
- Antibody identification.

Background Information

Sephadex gel is a porous gel composed of alkaline dextran cross-linked with epichlorohydrin and hydrated with a buffer such as PBS or LISS. The gel beads used (Sephadex G100), have a fractionation range from a molecular weight of 4000 to 150,000, which will permit the free passage of single RBCs but not the passage of RBC agglutinates. Lapierre et al. described the use of Sephadex gel for conventional saline and enzyme techniques in a simple inert buffer, but they also demonstrated that by incorporating anti-IgG into the gel buffer, a single-stage IAT test could be performed with no washing step. This is due to the entrapment of the unbound plasma IgG in the very top layer of gel beads.

Also see Appendix VI-3.

Operational Policy

The centrifuge should be calibrated appropriately to permit even packing of the gel suspension.

Limitations

Unwanted Positive Reactions:

- Gel is unevenly packed.
- Fibrin is present in the test plasma.
- Reagents are prepared incorrectly.

Unwanted Negative Reactions:

- Gel is unevenly packed.
- Supernatant buffer has not been decanted sufficiently.
- Reagent volumes are incorrect.

Sample Requirements

IgG anti-Jk^a and anti-D reagents.

Equipment/ Materials

6 × 50-mm clear polystyrene test tubes: Precipitin tubes (#5070-000, Elkay Co, Basingstoke, UK).

10 × 5-hole precipitin test tube racks.

Variable-volume pipettes: 5-50 μL and 200-1000 μL (VWR, Batavia, IL).

Benchtop centrifuge with a swing-out rotor.

Sephadex G100 Superfine (GE Healthcare).

EDTA-LISS.

Anti-human IgG, diluted 1:10 in 0.1% BSA-LISS.

LISS wash solution.

Antigen-positive RBCs.

Quality Control

All columns must be visually inspected to ensure that the gel is packed evenly prior to use.

Column Preparation Procedure

Use the following steps to prepare the columns:

Step	Action
1.	Prepare the gel suspension by mixing 0.5 g of Sephadex G100 superfine powder in 10 mL of EDTA-LISS/anti-IgG.
2.	Mix thoroughly to ensure even hydration and suspension of the beads.
3.	Pipette 350 μL of the Sephadex gel solution into 6 × 50-mm test tubes. Centrifuge at 1000 × g for 60 seconds to remove air bubbles and pack the gel.
4.	Store columns at 2-8 C for a maximum of 14 days.

5.	Evaluate the columns as follows:	
	If…	**Then…**
	the top of the column is level	the tubes are ready to use.
	the top of the column is uneven	recalibrate the centrifuge, resuspend the gel column, and recentrifuge.
	the gel column "trails" down the side of the tube	ensure that a swing-out rotor is in use: • Recalibrate the centrifuge, resuspend the gel column, and recentrifuge.

Quality Control Procedure

Use the following steps to quality-control the columns:

Step	Action
1.	Take 22 gel columns from the refrigerator and allow them to warm to room temperature.
2.	Prepare a doubling dilution of anti-Jk^a and anti-D in PBS/1% BSA to a dilution of 1 in 512.
3.	Visually inspect the columns to confirm that the gel suspension is level.
4.	Decant the supernatant buffer on the columns by a rapid "flick" into a waste container.
5.	Mark two series of 10 tubes: 1, 2, 4, 8, 16, 32, 64, 128, 256, 512.
6.	Mark 2 tubes with "1" for the negative controls.
7.	Add 30 μL of Jk(a+b+) 1% RBCs to each of 10 tubes.
8.	Add 30 μL of Jk(a–) RBCs to the negative control tube.
9.	Add 30 μL of each dilution to the appropriately marked tube.
10.	Repeat Steps 7-9 with D+ and D– RBCs and the anti-D dilutions.
11.	Incubate at 37 C for 15 minutes.
12.	Centrifuge at 300 × g for 10 minutes.

13.	Read the tests macroscopically over a light box. Grade tests from 0 (negative) to 4+ (see Appendix VI-4 for representative agglutination patterns).	
14.	Determine the required dilutions of anti-Jk^a and anti-D for positive controls as follows:	
	If…	**Then…**
	there is a dilution that yields a 2+ reaction	select that dilution for a positive control.
	all dilutions are strongly reactive	prepare and test higher antibody dilutions.
	no dilutions are reactive	select a different example of antibody to titrate.

Reference   Lapierre Y, Rigal D, Adam J, et al. The gel test: A new way to detect RBC antigen-antibody reactions. Transfusion 1990;30:109-13.

Effective Date

Approved by:	Printed Name	Signature	Date
Laboratory Management			
Medical Director			
Quality Officer			

VI-M. Gel: Detecting Antibodies Using Buffered Gel Columns

Purpose

To provide instructions for using Sephadex gel for serologic testing:

- Antibody detection.
- Antibody identification.

Background Information

Sephadex gel is a porous gel composed of alkaline dextran cross-linked with epichlorohydrin and hydrated with a buffer such as PBS or LISS. The gel beads used (Sephadex G100), have a fractionation range from a molecular weight of 4000 to 150,000, which will permit the free passage of single RBCs but not the passage of RBC agglutinates. Lapierre et al. described the use of Sephadex gel for conventional saline and enzyme techniques in a simple inert buffer.

Also see Appendix VI-3.

Operational Policy

The centrifuge should be calibrated appropriately to permit even packing of the gel suspension.

Limitations

Unwanted Positive Reactions:

- Gel is unevenly packed.
- Fibrin is present in the test plasma.
- Reagents are prepared incorrectly.

Unwanted Negative Reactions:

- Gel is unevenly packed.
- Supernatant buffer has not been decanted sufficiently.
- Reagent volumes are incorrect.

Sample Requirements   EDTA-anticoagulated blood as a source of plasma and RBCs.

Equipment/ Materials

Buffered gel columns.

10 × 5-hole precipitin test tube racks.

Variable-volume pipettes: 5-50 μL (VWR, Batavia, IL).

Benchtop centrifuge with a swing-out rotor.

Reagent RBCs diluted to 0.1% BSA-LISS.

Quality Control   Test diluted anti-M and diluted anti-D as described in Procedure VI-K with single-dose anti-positive RBCs on each day of use.

Procedure   Use the following steps to perform the procedure:

Step	Action
1.	Equilibrate the appropriate number of gel columns at RT before testing.
2.	Visually inspect the columns to confirm that the gel suspension is level.
3.	Decant the supernatant buffer on the columns by a rapid " flick" into a waste container.
4.	Add 30 μL of 1% reagent RBCs to labeled columns.
5.	Add 30 μL of test plasma to each column.
6.	Incubate at 37 C for 15 minutes.
7.	Centrifuge at 300 × g for 10 minutes.

8.	Read reactions macroscopically over a light box. Interpret the reactions as follows:	
	If...	**Then the test result is...**
	all RBCs have sedimented to the bottom of the tube	negative.
	there is a single band of RBCs at the top of the gel column	strongly positive.
	there are agglutinates throughout the gel	positive.
	there is a strong band at the top of the tube but also a sedimented population of RBCs	mixed-cell agglutination.
	the antigen-negative RBCs are agglutinated	invalid: • Recalibrate the centrifuge.

Reference   Lapierre Y, Rigal D, Adam J, et al. The gel test: A new way to detect RBC antigen-antibody reactions. Transfusion 1990;30:109-13.

Effective Date

Approved by:	Printed Name	Signature	Date
Laboratory Management			
Medical Director			
Quality Officer			

VI-N. Gel: Detecting Antibodies Using Anti-IgG Columns

Purpose

To provide instructions for using Sephadex gel for serologic testing:

- Antibody detection.

- Antibody identification.

Background Information

Sephadex gel is a porous gel composed of alkaline dextran cross-linked with epichlorohydrin and hydrated with a buffer such as PBS or LISS. The gel beads used (Sephadex G100), have a fractionation range from a molecular weight of 4000 to 150,000, which will permit the free passage of single RBCs but not the passage of RBC agglutinates. Lapierre et al. described the use of Sephadex gel for conventional saline and enzyme techniques in a simple inert buffer, but they also demonstrated that by incorporating anti-IgG into the gel buffer, a single-stage IAT test could be performed with no washing step. This is due to the entrapment of the unbound plasma IgG in the very top layer of gel beads.

Also see Appendix VI-3.

Operational Policy

The centrifuge should be calibrated appropriately to permit even packing of the gel suspension.

Limitations

Unwanted Positive Reactions:

- Gel is unevenly packed.

- Fibrin is present in the test plasma.

- Reagents are prepared incorrectly.

Unwanted Negative Reactions:

- Gel is unevenly packed.

- Supernatant buffer has not been decanted sufficiently.

- Reagent volumes are incorrect.

Sample Requirements

EDTA-anticoagulated blood as a source of plasma and RBCs.

Equipment/
Materials

Gel columns containing anti-IgG.

$10 \times$ 5-hole precipitin test tube racks.

Variable-volume pipettes: 5-50 µL (VWR, Batavia, IL).

Benchtop centrifuge with a swing-out rotor.

Reagent RBCs diluted to 0.1% BSA-LISS.

Quality
Control

Test diluted anti-Jk[a] and diluted anti-D as described in Procedure VI-L with single-dose anti-positive RBCs on each day of use.

Procedure

Use the following steps to perform the procedure:

Step	Action
1.	Equilibrate the appropriate number of gel columns at RT before testing.
2.	Visually inspect the columns to confirm that the gel suspension is level.
3.	Decant the supernatant buffer on the columns by a rapid "flick" into a waste container.
4.	Add 30 µL of 1% reagent RBCs to labeled columns.
5.	Add 30 µL of test plasma to each column.
6.	Incubate at 37 C for 15 minutes.
7.	Centrifuge at $300 \times g$ for 10 minutes.

8.	Read reactions macroscopically over a light box. Interpret the reactions as follows:	
	If...	**Then the test result is...**
	all RBCs have sedimented to the bottom of the tube	negative.
	there is a single band of RBCs at the top of the gel column	strongly positive.
	there are agglutinates throughout the gel	positive.
	there is a strong band at the top of the tube but also a sedimented population of RBCs	mixed-cell agglutination.
	the antigen-negative RBCs are agglutinated	invalid: • Recalibrate the centrifuge.

Reference   Lapierre Y, Rigal D, Adam J, et al. The gel test: A new way to detect RBC antigen-antibody reactions. Transfusion 1990;30:109-13.

Effective Date

Approved by:	Printed Name	Signature	Date
Laboratory Management			
Medical Director			
Quality Officer			

Appendix VI-1. Capillary Methods: General Considerations

Capillary tests are quick and simple to perform. However, the following should be undertaken to ensure optimal results:

1. Load capillaries individually. It may appear expedient to fill several tubes together; however, such an approach is not significantly quicker and uses more reagents than loading tubes individually.

2. Avoid introducing air bubbles into the tubes because these will hinder the proper mixing of reactants.

3. Wipe tubes with tissue as each reactant is loaded, to prevent sample contamination.

4. Use only reagents that are free of particulate matter. If necessary, filter through a 0.45-μ filter using microfiltration equipment: 5-mL syringe with disc filter assembly (Acrodisc, Pall Corp, East Hills, NY). Avoid using lipemic sera.

5. Dilute raw human sera with phosphate-buffered saline if necessary to avoid unwanted reactions due to cold-reactive autoagglutinins.

6. Use RBCs washed free of native plasma to prevent fibrin formation.

7. Inspect tubes carefully before use; dirty tubes may lead to spurious results.

8. The angle at which capillary tubes are slanted is important; too steep an angle in some procedures may cause RBCs to sediment too rapidly.

9. Process samples in batches of 10 during mass-screening projects.

10. Invert tubes for additional passages of RBCs through the serum to enhance reactions.

11. Observe tests frequently. Some reactions will be noticeable almost immediately, whereas other tests may manifest only subtle changes.

Appendix VI-2. Microplate Tests: General Considerations

Notes

Strict attention to the details outlined below is required to obtain reliable results when using microplates for serologic testing:

1. Normally, 25 to 35-µL volumes of reagents and RBCs are used. Cover microplates to prevent drying when processing large numbers of samples.

2. RBC suspensions should be prepared accurately. Required concentrations are between 0.2% and 1%, depending upon the procedure.

3. RBCs may be enzyme treated to enhance reactivity or permit dilution of reagent antisera. However, as with any enzyme procedure, an increase in sensitivity results in a decrease in specificity (see Section III). Thus, adequate controls are essential when enzyme-treated RBCs are used.

4. Some commercially available antisera are suitable for use in microplates, but it may be necessary to reduce the viscosity of others (eg, modified-tube anti-D) by dilution. Again, diluted reagents require use of appropriate controls.

5. Sera should be free of particulate matter. If necessary, filter through a 0.45-µ filter using microfiltration equipment: 5-mL syringe with disc filter assembly (Acrodisc, Pall Corp, East Hills, NY). Avoid using lipemic sera.

6. A standard protocol must be adopted to ensure accurate sample identification. This is facilitated by the A-H letters and 1-12 numbers etched on microplates by the manufacturer, and this system may be used as a template.

7. Microplates should be clean and free of static, which can be eliminated by one of the following:

    a. Soaking the plate in distilled or deionized water. Excess wash solution should be removed and the plates air-dried in an inverted position over paper towels before use.

    b. Rinsing with 0.1% bovine serum albumin (BSA) in saline (22% BSA, 1 mL; saline, 219 mL). Excess wash solution should be removed and the plates air-dried in an inverted position over paper towels before use.

    c. Placing the plates on damp paper towels to set up tests.

    d. Wiping the bottom of the plate with a damp cloth.

    e. Lightly flaming the bottom of the plate.

8. Although marketed as disposable, microplates may be washed and reused. Appropriate infectious disease precautions must, however, be maintained. Residual test reactants must be removed first by flicking inverted plates into a liquid waste receptacle that meets local safety requirements. The washing process is as follows:

    a. Immerse plates in 2.5% NaClO (bleach).

b. Soak in mild household detergent (eg, dilute dishwashing liquid).

c. Rinse three times with tap water.

d. Rinse three times with distilled water.

e. Invert plates over paper towels and air dry.

f. Inspect plates before use.

References

Knight R, Poole G, eds. The use of microplates in blood group serology: A review of microplate technology in the UK. Manchester, UK: British Society of Blood Transfusion, 1987:33-41.

Roback J, Combs MR, Grossman B, Hillyer C, eds. Technical manual. 16th ed. Bethesda, MD: AABB, 2008 (or current edition).

Centrifugation and Microplate Methods

The desired acceleration of gravity (g) and centrifugation time must be established for each centrifuge used for microplate testing. When g and time are correct, a distinct RBC button and clear supernate will be obtained, but the streaming of unagglutinated RBCs should not be impaired by overcentrifugation.

Flexible U-Bottom Microplates:

For hemagglutination tests: $700 \times g$ for 1-5 seconds.

For washing for IAT: $700 \times g$ for 20 seconds.

Rigid U-Bottom Microplates:

For hemagglutination tests: $700 \times g$ for 1-10 seconds, or $40 \times g$ for 45 seconds.

For washing for IAT: $700 \times g$ for 40 seconds, or $40 \times g$ for 3 minutes.

Flexible V-Bottom Microplates:

For hemagglutination tests: $700 \times g$ for 10 seconds.

For washing for IAT: $700 \times g$ for 20 seconds.

Rigid V-Bottom Microplates:

For IAT hemagglutination tests except the IAT: $900 \times g$ for 40 seconds.

For IAT hemagglutination: $900 \times g$ for 10 seconds.

For washing for IAT: $180 \times g$ for 2 minutes.

Appendix VI-3. Sephadex Gel Beads: Background Information

Sephadex (GE Healthcare Biosciences, Piscataway, NJ) gel has been used in immuno-chemistry for the fractionation of proteins for many years. It is a porous gel composed of al-kaline dextran cross-linked with epichlorohydrin and hydrated with a buffer such as PBS or LISS. Proteins are separated according to size. Large molecules above the exclusion limit cannot enter the gel pores and remain in the solute around the beads. Smaller molecules can pass into the gel freely.

Gel was first described for use in immunohematology in 1990 by Lapierre et al. The gel beads used (Sephadex G100) have a fractionation range from a molecular weight of 4000 to 150,000, which will permit the free passage of single RBCs but not the passage of RBC ag-glutinates. Lapierre et al described the use of Sephadex gel for conventional saline and en-zyme techniques in a simple inert buffer, but they also demonstrated that by incorporating anti-IgG into the gel buffer, a single-stage IAT test could be performed with no washing step. This is due to the entrapment of the unbound plasma IgG in the very top layer of gel beads. As a result of subsequent commercialization of the technology and development of plastic multicolumn cards by DiaMed AG (Cressier-sur-Morat, Switzerland), gel "column agglutina-tion" technology is used worldwide for many serologic applications.

Suggested Reading

Johnstone A, Thorpe R. Immunochemistry in practice. 2nd ed. Oxford, UK: Blackwell Scien-tific Publications, 1987.

Lapierre Y, Rigal D, Adam J, et al. The gel test: A new way to detect RBC antigen-antibody reactions. Transfusion 1990;30:109-13.

Voak D. The status of new methods for the detection of RBC agglutination. Transfusion 1999;39:1037-40.

Appendix VI-4. Agglutination Reactions in Gel Columns

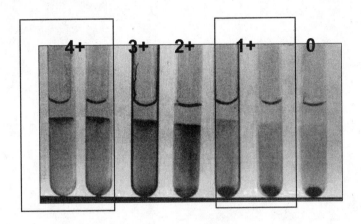

Section VII. Reagent RBCs (Non-Enzyme-Treated)

This section includes methods for the preparation of globulin-coated RBCs (immunoglobulins and complement components) for use in the quality control of antiglobulin tests, as described throughout this text. They may also be used to assess the reactivity of antihuman globulin (AHG) reagents to determine the comparative behavior of different lots of AHG reagents from various manufacturers. Such studies were popular in the late 1970s and early 1980s; however, they are rarely undertaken today, largely because less importance is given to the need for anti-C3 in AHG reagents used for pretransfusion antibody detection, and the available sources of AHG are considerably fewer than they were 20 years ago. Further applications of globulin-coated RBCs entail the use of C4-coated RBCs in the investigation of anti-Ch and -Rg (see Section IX), which are antibodies directed toward epitopes on the fourth component of human complement, C4.

Also included in this section are methods to freeze RBCs for long-term storage and subsequently thaw them for serologic testing. This enables facilities to establish an inventory of rare RBC phenotypes that can be used to resolve complex antibody problems such as those involving multiple alloantibodies and antibodies to high-prevalence antigens.

In yet other methods, RBCs are modified by chemicals that denature specific blood group antigens. Loss of reactivity with chemically modified RBCs can provide valuable clues to the antibody's specificity. See Section IX.

For further information, the interested reader is referred to the sources listed below.

Suggested Reading

Roback J, Combs MR, Grossman B, Hillyer C, eds. Technical manual. 16th ed. Bethesda, MD: AABB, 2008 (or current edition).

Issitt PD, Smith TR. Evaluation of antiglobulin reagents. In: Myhre BA, ed. A seminar on performance evaluation. Washington, DC: AABB, 1976:25-73.

VII-A. Preparing C3b/C4b-Coated RBCs

Purpose

To provide instructions for coating RBCs with C3b and C4b for use in the following:

- Quality control of negative test results with anti-C3 reagents.

Background Information

Under low-ionic conditions, C3b and C4b are bound to RBCs without prior attachment of antibody molecules (ie, via the alternative pathway).

Operational Policy

When performing comparative evaluations of different lots of AHG reagents, vary the ratio of fresh normal serum to RBCs (eg, 5:1, 4:1, 3:1, 2:1, 1:1).

Note: Some IgG may also be bound by this method.

Limitations

Unwanted Positive Reactions:

- Positive DAT on donor RBCs.

- Improper storage of reagents or coated RBCs.

- Use of incorrect technique.

- Use of wrong reagent.

Unwanted Negative Reactions:

- Improper storage of reagents or coated RBCs.

- Use of incorrect technique.

- Use of wrong reagent.

Sample Requirements

Group O whole blood collected into ACD, CPD, or CPD-A1.

Note: Before coating, RBCs should have a negative DAT using poly-specific AHG.

**Equipment/
Materials**

10% sucrose.

Anti-C3 reagent known to detect intact C3b.

Note: Some monoclonal anti-C3d will not detect intact C3b.

Anti-IgG.

Alsever's solution.

Pipettors with disposable tips to deliver 1 mL and 10 mL (eg, VWR, Batavia, IL).

**Quality
Control**

Test the coated RBCs vs anti-IgG and anti-C3.

Procedure

Use the following steps to perform the procedure:

Step	Action
1.	Mix 1 mL of whole blood with 10 mL of sucrose.
2.	Incubate at 37 C for 15 minutes.
3.	Wash the RBCs three times with saline. (The RBCs are now coated with C3b and C4b.)
4.	Resuspend the coated RBCs to a 3%-5% suspension with Alsever's solution.
5.	Test the coated RBCs with anti-IgG and anti-C3 as specified by the manufacturer.
6.	Interpret the reactions as follows:

If test results with anti-C3 are...	And/or test results with anti-IgG are...	Then...
>2+	negative	RBCs may be used: • Store refrigerated.
≤2+	positive or negative	do not use RBCs: • Repeat C3b/C4b coating procedure. • Consider inactive anti-C3 reagent.

Or, when validating negative antiglobulin test results:

If C3-coated RBCs...	Then...
give a mixed-field reaction	negative antiglobulin test result is valid.
are nonreactive	negative antiglobulin test result is invalid: • Repeat antiglobulin test. • Consider inadequate washing before addition of AHG or inactive AHG.

Reference Garratty G, Petz LD. Quality control of antiglobulin serum (letter). Transfusion 1975;15:397.

Effective Date

Approved by:	Printed Name	Signature	Date
Laboratory Management			
Medical Director			
Quality Officer			

VII-B. Preparing IgM/C3b-Coated RBCs

Purpose

To provide instructions for coating RBCs with IgM and C3b for use in the following:

- Evaluation/standardization of AHG reagents.

- Quality control of negative test results with anti-C3 reagents.

Background Information

Le (Lewis) antibodies are used to coat RBCs with C3b via the classical pathway.

Operational Policy

The proportions of RBCs and serum may need to be changed depending on the strength of the Le antibody. However, maintain the ratio of 0.25 mL of K_2EDTA to 2 mL of serum.

To assess the anti-C3 activity in AHG reagents, it will be necessary to subtract the results of tests with the IgM-coated RBCs from those obtained with the C3b-coated RBCs.

Anti-Le prepared in goats has been shown to be unsuitable for use in this procedure. Use human or rabbit anti-Le sera.

C3b-coated RBCs may be converted to C3d-coated RBCs, either by extended incubation (2 hours) in 20 volumes of freshly collected normal human serum or by treatment of the RBCs with crude trypsin, as described in Section III.

Limitations

Unwanted Positive Reactions:

- Positive DAT on donor RBCs.

- Improper storage of reagents or coated RBCs.

- Use of incorrect technique.

- Use of wrong reagent.

Unwanted Negative Reactions:

- Improper storage of reagents or coated RBCs.

- Use of incorrect technique.

- Use of wrong reagent.

**Sample
Requirements**

Anti-C3 reagent under evaluation.

**Equipment/
Materials**

Alsever's solution.

Antibody: anti-Le^a or anti-Le^{a+b}; 2 mL.

Anti-C3 reagent known to detect C3b.

Note: Some monoclonal anti-C3d will not detect intact C3b.

6% BSA.

4.45% wt/vol K$_2$EDTA.2H$_2$O.

Human complement: freshly collected, normal human serum known to lack unexpected antibodies; 16 mL.

RBCs: packed group O, Le(a+b−) RBCs, washed three times with saline; 2 mL.

Pipettors with disposable tips to deliver 200-500 µL and 2 mL (eg, VWR, Batavia, IL).

**Quality
Control**

Test with reactive anti-C3 and 6% BSA.

Procedure

Use the following steps to perform the procedure:

Step	Action
1.	Mix 250 µL of EDTA with 2 mL of antibody-containing serum. Incubate at RT for 15 minutes.
2.	Add 2 mL of saline to the serum and prepare serial twofold dilutions of the serum with saline. The dilution range should be from 1 in 2 to 1 in 256 (8 tubes), and 2-mL volumes should be prepared.
3.	Add 0.2 mL of washed Le(a+b−) RBCs to each dilution.
4.	Mix and incubate at 37 C for 60-90 minutes.
5.	Wash the RBCs four times with saline. (The RBCs are now coated with IgM.)
6.	Dilute an aliquot to a 3%-5% suspension with Alsever's solution and save for later testing.
7.	To the washed antibody-coated RBCs, add 2 mL of complement.

8.	Mix and incubate at 37 C for 15-20 minutes.
9.	Wash the RBCs four times with saline and dilute to a 3%-5% suspension with Alsever's solution. (The RBCs are now coated with C3.) Store refrigerated when not in use.
10.	Test the IgM- and C3-coated RBCs with AHG reagents, as specified by the manufacturer, and by the same technique with 6% BSA.
11.	Interpret the reactions of the C3-coated RBCs as follows:

If test results with anti-C3 are...	And/or test results with 6% BSA are...	Then...
positive	negative	highest dilution giving 1+ reaction = titer of anti-C3.
negative with RBCs coated at all dilutions	negative	do not use RBCs: • Repeat C3b coating procedure. • Consider inactive anti-C3 reagent.
positive or negative	positive	RBCs are unsuitable for use as C3-coated RBCs: • Higher serum dilution required.

Interpret the reactions of the IgM-coated RBCs as follows:

If test results with 6% BSA are...	Then...
positive	highest dilution giving 1+ reaction = titer of IgM anti-Le.

Reference Issitt PD, Smith TR. Evaluation of antiglobulin reagents. In: Myhre BA, ed. A seminar on performance evaluation. Washington, DC: AABB, 1976:25-73.

**Effective
Date**

Approved by:	Printed Name	Signature	Date
Laboratory Management			
Medical Director			
Quality Officer			

VII-C. Preparing C3b-Coated RBCs: Fruitstone Method

Purpose	To provide instructions for coating RBCs with C3b for use in the following:
	• Evaluation/standardization of AHG reagents.

Background Information	Under low-ionic conditions, the complement components C3b and C4b are bound to RBCs without prior attachment of antibody molecules (ie, via the alternative pathway). Under the strict conditions of temperature and pH specified in this procedure, only C3b is bound. The C3b-coated RBCs may be used in the evaluation of AHG reagents.

Operational Policy	Use dual electrode meters when pH-testing EDTA solutions, because single electrode meters will give erroneous pH values with EDTA solutions.

Limitations	Unwanted Positive Reactions:
	• Positive DAT on donor RBCs.
	• Improper storage of reagents or coated RBCs.
	• Use of incorrect technique.
	• Use of wrong reagent.
	Unwanted Negative Reactions:
	• Improper storage of reagents or coated RBCs.
	• Use of incorrect technique.
	• Use of wrong reagent.

Sample Requirements	Freshly collected whole blood: anticoagulated with ACD, CPD, or CPD-A1.

Equipment/ Materials	Alsever's solution, chilled to 4 C.
	Anti-C3 reagent known to detect C3b.
	Note: Some monoclonal anti-C3d will not detect intact C3b.

50-mL graduated measuring cylinder (eg, VWR, Batavia, IL).

Pipettors with disposable tips to deliver 100 μL and 1.2 mL (eg, VWR, Batavia, IL).

0.63 m $MgCl_2$.

Magnetic stirrer with stirring bar.

pH meter with dual electrode (eg, Thermo Fisher Scientific, Waltham, MA).

Sucrose sensitizing diluent.

Quality Control

Test the coated RBCs with anti-C3.

Procedure

Use the following steps to perform the procedure:

Step	Action
1.	Place 23.8 mL of sensitizing diluent in a container suitable for use with a magnetic stirrer.
2.	Place the vessel in an ice bath on a magnetic stirrer. Mix gently until the diluent temperature falls to 0-1 C.
3.	Add 1.2 mL of whole blood to the chilled diluent.
4.	Immediately add 0.1 mL of $MgCl_2$.
5.	Incubate at 0 C for 1 hour.
6.	Wash the RBCs four times with chilled Alsever's solution and store in Alsever's solution in a refrigerator.
7.	Test the C3-coated RBCs with AHG reagents, as specified by the manufacturer, and by the same technique with 6% BSA.
8.	Interpret the reactions as follows:

If test results with anti-C3 are...	And/or test results with 6% BSA are...	Then...
>2+	negative	RBCs may be used: • Store at 4 C.
≤2+	positive or negative	do not use RBCs: • Repeat C3b coating procedure. • Consider inactive anti-C3 reagent.

References   Chaplin H Jr. Characterization of red blood cells strongly coated in vitro with C3 via the alternate pathway. Transfusion 1980;20:256.

Fruitstone MJ. C3b-sensitized erythrocytes (letter). Transfusion 1978;18: 125.

**Effective
Date**

Approved by:	Printed Name	Signature	Date
Laboratory Management			
Medical Director			
Quality Officer			

VII-D. Preparing C4b-Coated RBCs

Purpose	To provide instructions for coating RBCs with C4b for use in the following: • Evaluation of polyspecific AHG reagents. • Studies with Ch/Rg antibodies.
Background Information	Under low-ionic conditions, C3b and C4b are bound to RBCs without prior attachment of antibody molecules (ie, via the alternative pathway). The addition of EDTA to the sucrose prevents the uptake of C3b, leaving RBCs coated only with C4b. Also, C4b-coated RBCs can be converted into C4d-coated RBCs and used for identifying anti-Ch/Rg (see Section IX).
Operational Policy	Use for the evaluation of polyclonal anti-C3 reagents. Monoclonal anti-C3 should not cross-react with C4.
Limitations	<u>Unwanted Positive Reactions:</u> • Positive DAT on donor RBCs. • Improper storage of reagents or coated RBCs. • Use of incorrect technique. • Use of wrong reagent. <u>Unwanted Negative Reactions:</u> • Improper storage of reagents or coated RBCs. • Use of incorrect technique. • Use of wrong reagent.
Sample Requirements	Polyspecific AHG reagents under evaluation.
Equipment/ Materials	ACD-anticoagulated whole blood, freshly collected. Sucrose K_3EDTA. 6% BSA. Pipettors with disposable tips to deliver 1 mL and 10 mL (eg, VWR, Batavia, IL).

Procedure   Use the following steps to perform the procedure:

Step	Action
1.	Mix 1 mL of ACD-anticoagulated whole blood with 10 mL of sucrose K_3EDTA.
2.	Incubate at 37 C for 15 minutes.
3.	Wash the RBCs three times with saline. (The RBCs are now coated with C4b.)
4.	Resuspend the coated RBCs to a 3%-5% suspension with Alsever's solution. Store refrigerated when not in use.
5.	Test the C4b-coated RBCs with polyspecific AHG reagents, as specified by the manufacturer, and by the same technique with 6% BSA.
6.	Interpret the reactions as follows: See table below.

If test results with AHG are…	And/or test results with 6% BSA are…	Then…
positive	negative	AHG contains anti-C4.
negative	negative	AHG lacks anti-C4.
positive or negative	positive	RBCs are unsuitable for use: • Repeat C4b coating.

Reference   Garratty G, Petz LD. Quality control of antiglobulin serum (letter). Transfusion 1975;15:397.

**Effective
Date**

Approved by:	Printed Name	Signature	Date
Laboratory Management			
Medical Director			
Quality Officer			

VII-E. Preparing Immunoglobulin-Coated RBCs

Purpose

To provide instructions for coating RBCs with immunoglobulins for use in the following:

- Evaluation of antiglobulin reagents.

- Preparation of antiglobulin-coated RBCs in solid-phase assays.

Background Information

Pure IgA and nonagglutinating IgM antibodies to RBC antigens are rare. Consequently, the use of antibodies to human RBC antigens is not a practical approach to preparing IgA/IgM-coated RBCs. Also, RBCs coated with AHG are required for solid-phase adherence assays. In this procedure, immunoglobulins are coupled to RBCs using chromic chloride.

Operational Policy

Chromium salts are generally considered highly toxic. Avoid ingestion and inhalation of dust. Wear gloves and goggles.

Note: Because this method uses a buffer, the "age" and color of the stock $CrCl_3$ solution is not important, as it is in other, less reliable methods.

The order of adding the reagents is most important. The active coupling species of the $CrCl_3$ is a complex ion that forms above pH 5.0. In the absence of protein, it precipitates and will not couple, but will directly agglutinate the RBCs. In the absence of RBCs, it will cross-link the protein.

Limitations

Unwanted Positive Reactions:

- Positive DAT on donor RBCs.

- Improper storage of reagents or coated RBCs.

- Use of incorrect technique.

- Use of wrong reagent.

Unwanted Negative Reactions:

- Improper storage of reagents or coated RBCs.

- Use of incorrect technique.

- Use of wrong reagent.

Sample Requirements

Group O packed RBCs, washed six times with saline.

Note: Use RBCs that are more than 24 hours old but less than 8 days old.

Equipment/ Materials

Antiglobulin reagents (anti-IgA, -IgG, -IgM, and -C3), as required for quality control purposes.

Chromic chloride: dilute stock 1% solution 1 in 40 with normal saline before use to yield a final $CrCl_3$ concentration of 0.25 mg/mL.

Pipettors with disposable tips to deliver 25-, 50-, and 75-μL volumes (eg, VWR, Batavia, IL).

IgA from human colostrum: lyophilized (Sigma-Aldrich, St Louis, MO). Dilute to 2 mg/mL with normal saline and dialyze overnight against normal saline. Aliquot in plastic tubes and store below −20 C.

IgM from human serum: lyophilized (Sigma-Aldrich). Dilute to 2 mg/mL with normal saline and dialyze overnight against normal saline. Aliquot in plastic tubes and store below −20 C.

IgG-coated RBCs (see Procedure V-E).

pH 7.0 PBS.

Piperazine-buffered saline.

Plastic tubes: 12 × 75 mm, with caps.

Rabbit antihuman IgG: γ-chain specific; 2 mg/mL (Sigma-Aldrich). Dialyze overnight against normal saline. Aliquot in plastic tubes and store below −20 C.

Rotating mixer.

Trypsin for $CrCl_3$ coupling.

Trypsin inhibitor: 2.5 mg/mL. Dilute 1 part with 99 parts of normal saline before use.

Vortex mixer.

Quality Control

Test the coated RBCs with antiglobulin reagents and with saline by immediate-spin technique and after 5 minutes incubation at room temperature (see Procedure XI-B).

If an antibody has been coupled to RBCs, add the coated RBCs to doubling dilutions of the antigen that the antibody recognizes. The titer will give a measure of the success of the coupling.

If an antigen has been coupled to RBCs, add the coated RBCs to doubling dilutions of the antibody that recognizes the antigen. The titer will give a measure of the success of the coupling.

Trypsin Treatment Procedure

Use the following steps to treat the RBCs with trypsin:

Step	Action
1.	Prepare a 10% suspension of RBCs in pH 7.0 PBS and warm to 37 C for 10 minutes.
2.	Add an equal volume of trypsin.
3.	Incubate at 37 C for 30 minutes, inverting periodically to mix.
4.	Wash the RBCs twice with saline.
5.	Resuspend the RBCs in trypsin inhibitor.
6.	Mix and incubate at RT for 10 minutes.
7.	Wash the RBCs three times with saline.
8.	Completely discard the final wash supernate and save the packed treated RBCs for coupling.

Coupling Procedure

Use the following steps to couple the RBCs with immunoglobulins:

Step	Action
1.	Add 75 μL piperazine-buffered saline to a 12 × 75 mm plastic tube.
2.	Add 25 μL of trypsin-treated RBCs and 25 μL of immnoglobulin to be coupled. Mix well.
3.	Add 50 μL of dilute $CrCl_3$ solution dropwise with constant vortex mixing and continue mixing for 30 seconds.
4.	Cap the tube and rotate at approximately 60 degrees horizontally for 60 minutes at RT.
5.	Wash the RBCs three times with saline.
6.	Dilute to a 3%-5% suspension with Alsever's solution and store refrigerated.

Testing Procedure

Perform tests for spontaneous agglutination as follows:

Step	Action
1.	To 1 drop of 3%-5% coated RBCs, add 2 drops of saline and mix.
2.	Centrifuge.
3.	Examine the RBCs macroscopically for agglutination; grade and record the results.
4.	Interpret the reactions as follows:

If agglutination is...	Then...
absent	• Test immunoglobulin-coated RBCs against antiglobulin reagents as described in Section XI. • Test anti-IgG-coated RBCs vs IgG-coated RBCs as described in Section VII.
present	spontaneous agglutination has occurred: • Decrease concentration of CrCl3 by 0.05 mg/mL and repeat coupling procedure. • Alternatively, immunoglobulin may contain antibody to trypsin-treated RBCs. Adsorb with trypsin-treated RBCs and repeat procedure.

Effective Date

Approved by:	Printed Name	Signature	Date
Laboratory Management			
Medical Director			
Quality Officer			

VII-F. Preparing IgG-Coated RBCs

Purpose

To provide instructions for coating RBCs with IgG for use in the following:

- Evaluating AHG reagents.

- Validating negative test results with anti-IgG.

Background Information

When incubated together, IgG antibody coats antigen-positive RBCs with IgG. The coated RBCs can be used in the evaluation of AHG reagents and in the quality control of AHG tests.

Operational Policy

When evaluating AHG reagents, vary the proportions of RBCs and serum to prepare weakly (1+), moderately (2+), or strongly (4+) reactive RBCs for evaluating AHG reagents.

For quality control of negative antiglobulin test results, the IgG-coated RBCs should, at a minimum, give a 2+ (score 8) reaction in tests with reagents containing anti-IgG.

Limitations

Unwanted Positive Reactions:

- Positive DAT on donor RBCs.

- Improper storage of reagents or coated RBCs.

- Use of incorrect technique.

- Use of wrong reagent.

Unwanted Negative Reactions:

- Improper storage of reagents or coated RBCs.

- Use of incorrect technique.

- Use of wrong reagent.

Sample Requirements

Antiglobulin reagent under evaluation or negative antiglobulin tests with anti-IgG.

Equipment/ Materials

Alsever's solution.

Antibody: weakly reactive IgG anti-D.

Note: Use a pool of 10 anti-D sera for preparing IgG-coated RBCs for use as control RBCs in AHG tests. Alternatively, modified-tube anti-D may be used; dilute 1 in 1500 or 1 in 3000 in 6% BSA before use.

Anti-IgG.

Anti-C3d.

K_2EDTA: 4.45% wt/vol.

RBCs: group O, R_1r RBCs, washed three times with saline.

Pipettors with disposable tips to deliver 200-500 μL and 2 mL (eg, VWR, Batavia, IL).

Quality Control

Test the coated RBCs vs anti-IgG and anti-C3d.

Procedure

Use the following steps to perform the procedure:

Step	Action
1.	Mix 250 μL of EDTA with 2 mL of anti-D.
2.	Incubate at RT for 15 minutes.
3.	Add 0.2 mL of RBCs.
4.	Mix and incubate at 37 C for 15-60 minutes.
5.	Wash the RBCs four times with saline and dilute to a 3%-5% suspension with Alsever's solution. Store at 4 C.
6.	Test vs AHG reagents as described by the manufacturer. Alternatively, add to negative tests with anti-IgG reagents.

7.	Interpret the reactions as follows:		
	If test results with anti-IgG are…	**And test results with anti-C3d are…**	**Then…**
	>2+	negative	RBCs may be used: • Store at 4 C.
	≤2+	positive or negative	do not use RBCs: • Repeat IgG coating procedure. • Consider inactive AHG reagents or agglutinating anti-D.

Or, when validating negative antiglobulin test results:

If IgG-coated RBCs…	**Then…**
give a mixed-field reaction	negative antiglobulin test result is valid.
are nonreactive	negative antiglobulin test result is invalid: • Repeat antiglobulin test. • Consider inadequate washing before addition of AHG or inactive AHG.

Reference   Issitt PD, Smith TR. Evaluation of antiglobulin reagents. In: Myhre BA, ed. A seminar on performance evaluation. Washington, DC: AABB, 1976:25-73.

**Effective
Date**

Approved by:	Printed Name	Signature	Date
Laboratory Management			
Medical Director			
Quality Officer			

VII-G. Treating RBCs: AET Procedure

Purpose

To provide instructions for treating RBCs with 2-aminoethylisothiouronium bromide hydrobromide (AET):

- As an aid to antibody identification.

Background Information

AET is a reducing agent that disrupts double bonds formed between cysteine residues. These bonds contribute to the secondary structure of the antigen protein. Antibodies that recognize antigens in the context of the protein conformation will not react with AET-treated RBCs. Kell antigens are very susceptible to AET treatment. Other antigens that are affected by reducing agents such as AET are the Knops, Dombrock, Lutheran, and Cartwright antigens, as well as LW[a] and JMH.

A panel of AET-treated RBCs can be used to detect other alloantibodies such as anti-Fy[a] in the presence of an antibody to a high-prevalence Kell antigen (eg, anti-k).

Operational Policy

AET treatment of RBCs produces RBCs that are similar to those seen in paroxysmal nocturnal hemoglobinuria and that readily bind complement components nonspecifically. Use anti-IgG reagents when performing antiglobulin tests with AET-treated RBCs.

Limitations

Incorrect results:

- Improper storage of reagents.

- Use of incorrect technique.

- Use of wrong reagent or omission of AET.

Sample Requirements

Test RBCs: packed RBCs to be treated, washed three times with saline; 1 mL.

Equipment/ Materials

AET: 6% wt/vol.

Note: Prepare immediately before use.

Anti-k: from commercial source or patient sample.

Note: Other Kell antibodies (eg, anti-Kp[b], anti-Js[b]) may be used in place of anti-k.

Quality Control

Test treated and untreated RBCs with anti-k (other antibodies directed to antigens inactivated by AET may be used; however, reactivity with untreated RBCs should be 2 to 4+). Treated RBCs will be nonreactive and untreated RBCs will be positive.

Procedure

Use the following steps to perform the procedure:

Step	Action
1.	Mix 1 mL of RBCs with 4 mL of AET.
2.	Incubate at 37 C for 20 minutes.
3.	Wash RBCs three times with PBS and store refrigerated in Alsever's solution for up to 1 week.

Reference

Advani H, Zamor J, Judd WJ, et al. Inactivation of Kell blood group antigens by 2-aminoethylisothiouronium bromide. Br J Haematol 1982;51:107-15.

Effective Date

Approved by:	Printed Name	Signature	Date
Laboratory Management			
Medical Director			
Quality Officer			

VII-H. Treating RBCs: DTT Procedure

Purpose
To provide instructions for preparing RBCs treated with dithiothreitol (DTT):

- For use in antibody identification.

Background Information
DTT is a reducing agent that disrupts double bonds formed between cysteine residues. These bonds contribute to the secondary structure of the antigen protein. Antibodies that recognize antigens in the context of the protein conformation will not react with DTT-treated RBCs. Kell antigens are very susceptible to DTT treatment. Other antigens that are affected by reducing agents such as DTT are the Knops, Dombrock, Lutheran, and Cartwright antigens, as well as LW^a and JMH. Cromer antigens may be weakened, and some examples of anti-Vel do not react with DTT-treated RBCs.

Operational Policy
Not applicable.

Limitations
Incorrect results:

- Improper storage of reagents.
- Use of incorrect technique.
- Inadequate treatment of RBCs with DTT.

Sample Requirements
Test RBCs: packed RBCs to be treated, washed three times with saline; 1 mL.

Equipment/ Materials
Anti-k: from commercial source or patient sample.

Note: Other Kell antibodies (eg, anti-Kp^b, anti-Js^b) may be used in place of anti-k.

DTT: 1 M.

pH 7.3 and 8.0 PBS.

Quality Control
Test treated and untreated RBCs with anti-k. (Other antibodies directed to antigens inactivated by DTT may be used; however, reactivity with untreated RBCs should be 2 to 4+.) Treated RBCs will be nonreactive and untreated RBCs will be positive.

Procedure   Use the following steps to perform the procedure:

Step	Action
1.	Dilute 1 part 1 M DTT with 4 parts pH 8.0 PBS.
2.	Mix 4 volumes of dilute DTT with 1 volume of packed RBCs.
3.	Incubate at 37 C for 30 minutes.
4.	Wash the RBCs four times with pH 7.3 PBS.
5.	Resuspend the treated RBCs to a 3%-5% suspension with PBS and use in tests with the serum/sera under investigation. **Note:** Decrease the DTT concentration if RBC lysis occurs.

References   Branch DR, Muensch HA, Sy Siok Hian S, Petz LD. Disulphide bonds are a requirement for Kell and Cartwright (Yt^a) blood group antigen integrity. Br J Haematol 1983;54:573-8.

Konigshaus GJ, Holland TI. The effect of dithiothreitol on the LW antigen. Transfusion 1984;24:536-7.

Effective Date

Approved by:	Printed Name	Signature	Date
Laboratory Management			
Medical Director			
Quality Officer			

VII-I. Inactivating S Antigen: Sodium Hypochlorite Treatment

Purpose

To provide instructions for treating RBCs with sodium hypochlorite (NaClO). This method may subsequently be used in the following:

- To confirm the presence of anti-S by showing loss of reactivity with NaClO-treated RBCs.

- To detect the presence of concomitant alloantibodies in sera containing anti-S.

- To remove anti-A and/or anti-B from anti-S before use as an anti-S typing reagent.

Background Information

S antigen is defined by the presence of a methionine residue at position 29 of glycophorin B (GPB). Oxidation of this residue by NaClO results in a loss of S antigen expression.

Operational Policy

Not applicable.

Limitations

Incorrect results:

- Improper storage of reagents.

- Use of incorrect technique.

- Use of wrong reagent.

Sample Requirements

Packed RBCs: washed three times with saline; 1 mL.

Equipment/ Materials

NaClO: 0.001%.

Untreated S+s– RBCs: washed three times with saline.

Quality Control

Treat S+s– RBCs and test with anti-S.

Procedure   Use the following steps to perform the procedure:

Step	Action
1.	Dilute 0.1 mL RBCs to a 4% suspension with 4 mL of dilute NaClO and mix gently.
2.	Centrifuge to pack the RBCs.
3.	Wash the RBCs four times with saline before use.
4.	Test treated RBCs from Step 3 with the antibody-positive sample in question and control anti-S.
5.	Interpret the reactions as follows:

If...	Then...
treated S+s– RBCs fail to react with anti-S	NaClO treatment was effective and test is valid.
treated RBCs react with anti-S	NaClO treatment was ineffective: • Prepare fresh NaClO and repeat procedure.

Reference   Rygiel SA, Issitt CH, Fruitstone MJ. Destruction of S antigen by Clorox (abstract). Transfusion 1983;23:410.

Effective Date

Approved by:	Printed Name	Signature	Date
Laboratory Management			
Medical Director			
Quality Officer			

VII-J. Freezing RBCs: Glycerol Preservation and Recovery

Purpose

To provide instructions for freezing and thawing RBCs in glycerol for use in the following:

- Long-term preservation of RBCs of rare phenotypes for use in antibody identification.

Background Information

RBCs diluted with glycerol (to prevent membrane damage by ice crystals) may be preserved frozen for many years. Hemolysis during the thawing process is minimized by washing in solutions of decreasing salt content.

Operational Policy

If possible, freeze RBCs within 1 week of collection.

Use only brief centrifugation during washing for recovery. Overcentrifugation results in aggregation of RBCs that is difficult to disperse.

RBCs frozen in this manner may acquire a positive DAT because of C3 coating; if so, perform IATs with anti-IgG.

Limitations

Incorrect Results:

- Improper storage of reagents.
- Use of incorrect technique.
- Use of wrong reagent.

Sample Requirements

RBCs collected into ACD or preserved in Alsever's solution.

Note: Freeze as soon after collection as is practicable.

Equipment/ Materials

Alsever's solution.

Glycerolyte 57 solution (Fenwal Inc, Lake Zurich, IL).

Normal saline.

Anti-IgG: obtain commercially.

Sodium chloride, 2.5% wt/vol: NaCl, 25 g; distilled water to 1 L.

Sodium chloride, 9.0% wt/vol: NaCl, 90 g; distilled water to 1 L.

Storage tubes (eg, 3.5-mL tubes, Lake Charles Manufacturing, Lake Charles, LA).

Wooden applicator sticks (eg, #128-2, Ted Pella Inc, Redding, CA).

Quality Control

Perform DAT with anti-IgG on a frozen-recovered sample if the RBCs are to be tested by an IAT.

Either confirm rare phenotype of frozen-recovered sample or test more than one example.

Freezing Procedure

Use the following steps to freeze the RBCs:

Step	Action
1.	Centrifuge whole blood samples to pack the RBCs.
2.	Remove the supernate and save for reagent use if plasma contains a valuable antibody.
3.	Wash the RBCs twice with normal saline.
4.	Dispense up to 2 mL of RBCs into appropriately labeled storage tubes.
5.	Fill the tube with saline and centrifuge to pack the RBCs. Completely remove the supernate and discard.
6.	For each volume of packed RBCs, add 2 volumes of Glycerolyte 57 solution dropwise. Gently mix the contents of the tube during this process.
7.	Mix the contents of the tube well by inversion and store at −70 C.

Recovery Procedure

Use the following steps to recover the RBCs:

Step	Action
1.	Allow RBCs to thaw at RT.
2.	Mix the tube well by inversion and transfer an aliquot (ie, 0.5-1.0 mL or an amount sufficient for the tests to be performed) into a clean, appropriately labeled 13 × 100-mm test tube.
3.	Slowly add (dropwise with continual stirring) a volume of 9.0% NaCl equal to that of the RBC/glycerol mixture.
4.	Mix gently by inversion and allow to equilibrate at RT for at least 1 minute.
5.	Fill the tube with 2.5% NaCl and mix well by inversion.
6.	Centrifuge at 1000 × g (or equivalent) for 30 seconds.

7.	Fill the tube again with 2.5% NaCl and centrifuge at $1000 \times g$ (or equivalent) for 30 seconds.
8.	Wash the RBCs twice with normal saline or until the supernate is hemoglobin-free.
9.	Perform DAT on recovered RBCs with anti-IgG.
10.	Interpret the reactions as follows:

If the DAT is…	Then…
positive	RBCs cannot be used in antiglobulin tests: • Recover a different example of the same phenotype.
negative	RBCs can be used in antiglobulin tests: • Confirm phenotype of recovered sample. • Do not use if wrong phenotype; investigate and resolve the problem.

11.	Store refrigerated in Alsever's solution.

Reference Yagnow R, Shannon S, Weiland D. Procedure for freezing and thawing of small aliquots and segments. Red Cell Free Press 1978;3:8.

Effective Date

Approved by:

	Printed Name	Signature	Date
Laboratory Management			
Medical Director			
Quality Officer			

VII-K. Freezing RBCs: Liquid Nitrogen Preservation and Recovery

Purpose

To provide instructions for freezing and thawing RBCs in liquid nitrogen for use in the following:

- Long-term preservation of RBCs of rare phenoptypes for use in antibody identification.

Background Information

RBCs in sucrose (to prevent membrane damage by ice crystals) may be preserved frozen in liquid nitrogen for many years.

Operational Policy

If possible, freeze RBCs within 1 week of collection.

Limitations

Incorrect Results:

- Improper storage of reagents.
- Use of incorrect technique.
- Use of wrong reagent.

Sample Requirements

RBCs collected into ACD or preserved in Alsever's solution.

Note: Freeze as soon after collection as is practicable.

Equipment/ Materials

Alsever's solution.

Freezing solution.

Gloves and tongs (for handling frozen samples).

Liquid N_2 (eg, from local welding company).

Magnetic stirrer: with stirring bar.

Needles: laboratory pipetting needles with 90-degree blunt tips (eg, 6-inch, 18-gauge, #Z261351, Sigma-Aldrich, St Louis, MO).

Paper cup: with several fine holes in bottom, as a liner for the stainless steel beaker.

Stainless steel beaker: approximately 250-mL capacity (eg, VWR, Batavia, IL).

Note: Insulate with polystyrene.

Storage equipment for liquid N_2: dewars, tanks, etc (eg, Praxair, Danbury, CT).

Storage vials: plastic tubes with screw caps.

Note: Drill a small hole (1/32-inch) into the cap (from the inside) to permit liquid N_2 to escape.

Styrofoam container: with lid, about 4 inches square.

Syringes: 5-20 mL.

Vortex mixer (eg, Maxi Mix, Thermo Fisher Scientific, Waltham, MA).

Quality Control

Perform DAT with anti-IgG on a frozen-recovered sample if the RBCs are to be tested by an IAT.

Either confirm rare phenotype of frozen-recovered sample or test more than one example.

Freezing Procedure

Use the following steps to freeze the RBCs:

Step	Action
1.	Centrifuge blood samples to pack the RBCs.
2.	Remove the supernatant plasma and save for reagent use if plasma contains a valuable antibody.
3.	Wash the RBCs once with normal saline.
4.	Discard supernate and add an equal volume of freezing solution. Allow to equilibrate at RT for at least 15 minutes, but no longer than 1 hour.
5.	Disassemble the syringe; return the cap to the needle hub and invert the barrel, cap-end down.
6.	Fill the barrel with washed RBCs, holding the cap firmly in place.
7.	Gently reinsert the plunger and invert, cap-end up. Remove cap, attach needle, and remove air from the syringe.
8.	Label storage vial and place in styrofoam container.
9.	Place paper cup in stainless steel beaker.
10.	Fill the beaker with liquid N_2. **Note:** Liquid N_2 will boil rapidly, while the container cools. Add more liquid N_2 to keep the internal paper cup about ¾ full.
11.	Place the magnetic stirring rod in the paper cup and turn on stirrer gradually until a vortex forms in the liquid N_2.
12.	With blood-filled syringe in hand, switch on vortex mixer and position elbow on the foam cushion.
13.	Hold syringe (needle end down) a few inches above the swirling liquid N_2. **Note:** Do not get so close that the blood in the needle freezes.

14.	Apply pressure to the plunger so that a stream of small droplets vibrates from the needle. **Note:** Needles are very fine and, if too much pressure is applied, blood may leak from the syringe hub.
15.	When all the blood has been frozen, lift the paper cup from the beaker with tongs and drain the liquid N$_2$ into the beaker. **Note:** Remove the stirring rod and clean thoroughly before reuse.
16.	Bend the paper cup to facilitate pouring. Using tongs or gloves to hold the plastic storage tubes, pour RBC beads into the vials. Screw on caps and place vials in the styrofoam container.
17.	Place vials upright into the designated compartment of the liquid N$_2$ storage tank. **Note:** The vials should be immersed in liquid N$_2$.

Recovery Procedure

Use the following steps to recover the RBCs:

Step	Action
1.	Remove vial from storage tank with tongs.
2.	Using gloves, pour off excess liquid N$_2$ through the cap.
3.	Working quickly, unscrew the vial and pour the required number (an amount sufficient for the tests to be performed) into a saline-filled, appropriately labeled 16 × 100-mm test tube.
4.	Wash the RBCs twice with normal saline or until the supernate is hemoglobin-free.
5.	Perform DAT on recovered RBCs with anti-IgG.

6.	Interpret the reactions as follows:	
	If the DAT is…	**Then…**
	positive	RBCs cannot be used in antiglobulin tests: • Recover a different example of the same phenotype.
	negative	RBCs can be used in antiglobulin tests: • Confirm phenotype of recovered sample. • Do not use if wrong phenotype; investigate and resolve the problem.
7.	Store refrigerated in Alsever's solution.	

Effective Date

Approved by:

Laboratory Management

Medical Director

Quality Officer

	Printed Name	Signature	Date

Section VIII. Antibody Identification

The processes and procedures outlined in this section present a basic approach to the identification of unexpected alloantibodies. Guidelines are included for interpreting results of antibody identification panels. Flow diagrams and process documents are presented to illustrate the various approaches to problem solving. Additional special methods for alloantibody identification are included, as well as policies for the selection of blood for transfusion to patients with unexpected alloantibodies. Section IX deals with the investigation of antibodies to antigens of high prevalence and Section XI addresses the management of samples with autoantibodies.

Selection of any given method for antibody identification should be influenced by the antibody detection procedure used; initially, it is advisable to use those techniques by which the reactive pretransfusion tests were first encountered. Furthermore, many workers advocate the routine use of an enhancement method—for example, with polyethylene glycol (Procedure II-G) or enzyme (Procedure II-C)—in antibody identification studies because PEG enhances the reactivity of almost all clinically significant antibody specificities. Comparing PEG results with results obtained using a saline antiglobulin tube test or gel test can provide clues to the type of antibody present. In addition, enzyme techniques do not detect certain antibody specificities, while they enhance the reactivity of others. Thus, results of enzyme tests can provide important information to the specificity of antibodies under investigation. It is with these points in mind that the following approaches and procedures were developed.

Suggested Reading

Roback J, Combs MR, Grossman B, Hillyer C, eds. Technical manual. 16th ed. Bethesda, MD: AABB, 2008 (or current edition).

Rudman SV, ed. Serologic problem solving: A systematic approach for improved practice. Bethesda, MD: AABB Press, 2005.

Judd's Methods in Immunohematology
Identification of Single or Multiple Antibodies
Page 1 of 8

VIII-A. Identification of Single or Multiple Antibodies

Purpose

To provide a process for evaluating patient samples when some panel cells test positive at any phase of testing.

(Although each case is unique, this is the general process to be followed.)

Background Information

Reaction patterns should be consistent with those regularly observed for the presumed antibody specificity. For example, if anti-M is the suspected specificity:

- There should be direct agglutination of M+ RBCs.

- M+ (especially M+N–) RBCs may also react by indirect antiglobulin technique.

- Ficin-treated M+ RBCs should be nonreactive.

With few exceptions (eg, Rh-positive patient with anti-D), the autologous RBCs should lack the antigen(s) to which the serum seemingly contains antibody(ies).

Interpretation of antibody identification test results requires comprehensive knowledge of the serologic vagaries of individual antibody specificities, including:

- Temperature and test phase by which each antibody is usually reactive.

- Antibody reactivity in different detection methods—ie, PEG, LISS, gel, or solid phase.

- Anticipated behavior of certain antibodies with enzyme-treated RBCs.

- Ability of a particular antibody to bind complement or cause hemolysis.

- Propensity of some antibodies to show dosage—ie, to react more strongly with RBCs from homozygotes (double dose) than with RBCs from heterozygotes (single dose).

See Figs VIII-A-1 and VIII-A-2 and Appendix VIII-1.

Operational Policy

Reported results must be consistent with those obtained in initial studies; eg, if anti-K is the only antibody deemed to be present, only the K+ reagent RBC sample used in antibody detection tests should have been reactive.

Follow institutional SOPs regarding criteria for identifying alloantibodies and for ruling out the presence of alloantibodies.

Limitations   Failure to follow these instructions may lead to failure to obtain the correct results.

Sample Requirements   Not applicable.

Equipment/ Materials   Results of antibody identification tests using untreated RBCs and any antiglobulin procedures mentioned elsewhere in Section II.

Results of antibody identification tests by Procedure II-C, if performed.

Quality Control   All negative antiglobulin tube tests should be confirmed with IgG-coated RBCs.

To obtain statistically valid antibody identification data, and to minimize the possibility that an observed pattern of reactions is the result of chance alone, sufficient antigen-positive and antigen-negative RBC samples must be tested. See Procedure VIII-D.

Process   Complete the following stages when identifying multiple antibodies in a patient sample:

Stage	Description
1.	Evaluate results of initial antibody identification or selected cell panels using the crossing-out method (Procedure VIII-C).
2.	Results of antigen typing are evaluated as follows: <table><tr><th>When antigen typing is...</th><th>Then...</th></tr><tr><td>available</td><td>eliminate from consideration antibodies to antigens present on the autologous RBCs: • Proceed to next stage.</td></tr><tr><td>not available</td><td>proceed to next stage.</td></tr></table> **Note:** If patient has been recently transfused, phenotyping (if performed) must be interpreted with caution.
3.	Examine the reaction patterns at each test phase. Evaluate possible specificities with regard to test phase and manner of reactivity (see Table VIII-A-1 for specific details).

4.	Select cells to confirm antibodies based on laboratory SOPs.	
5.	Select cells to rule out antibodies based on laboratory SOPs.	
6.	Test selected cells using the method used in initial antibody identification panels. **Note:** Method(s) with the most sensitivity may be beneficial to detect weakly reactive antibodies.	
7.	Evaluate results of selected cell panel as follows:	
	When...	**Then...**
	antibodies are confirmed and ruled out according to SOPs	process is complete.
	antibodies are not confirmed and ruled out according to SOPs	repeat Stages 4 to 7.
8.	Phenotype patient RBCs for the antigen(s) corresponding to identified antibodies:	
	When typing has...	**Then...**
	not been completed	typing is performed.
	been confirmed in Stage 2	process is complete.
	Note: If patient has been recently transfused, phenotyping (if performed) must be interpreted with caution.	

Reference Leger RM, ed. Standards for immunohematology reference laboratories. 5th ed. Bethesda, MD: AABB, 2007 (or current edition).

**Effective
Date**

Approved by:	Printed Name	Signature	Date
Laboratory Management			
Medical Director			
Quality Officer			

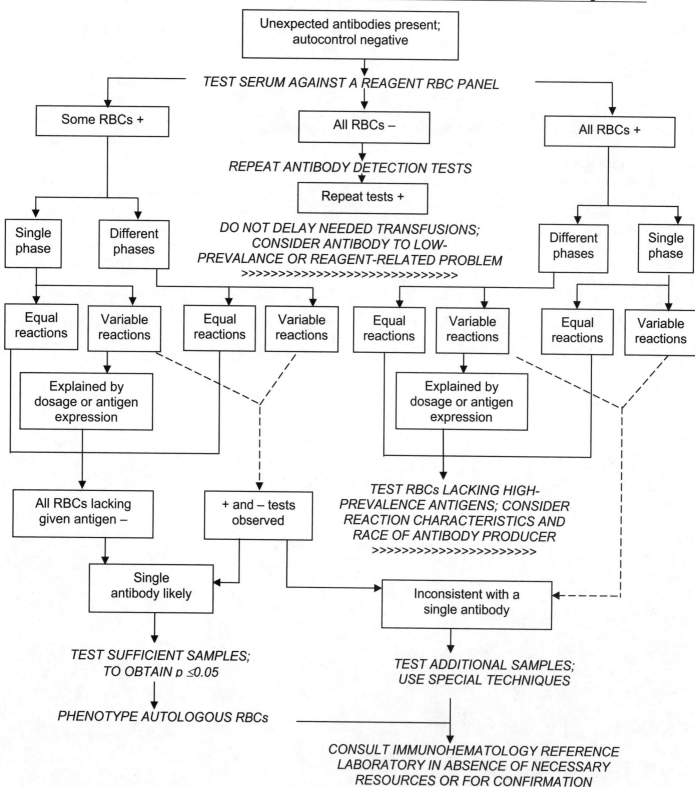

Figure VIII-A-1. Considerations in investigating unexpected antibodies.

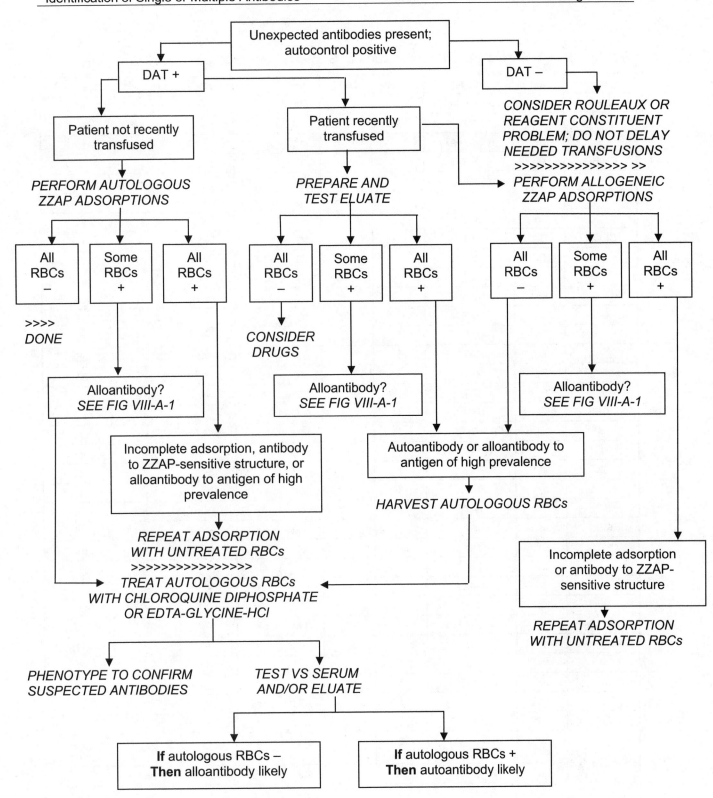

Figure VIII-A-2. Considerations in investigating blood samples with a positive autocontrol.

Table VIII-A-1. Serologic Characteristics of Some Alloantibodies to RBC Antigens

System*	Anti-	Phase†	Ficin‡	DTT§	Ig‖	C3¶	HTR#	HDFN**	% Comp††
ABO	A	RT>37-IAT	↑		M G	✓	✓	✓	56
	A₁	RT	↑		M	✓	rare	✗	64
	B	RT>37-IAT	↑		M G	✓	✓	✓	85
CH/RG	Ch	IAT	↓		G	✗	✗	✗	4
	Rg	IAT	↓		G	✗	✗	✗	2
CO	Coᵃ	IAT			G	✗	✓	✓	rare
	Coᵇ	IAT			G	rare	✓	✓	91
CROM	Crᵃ	IAT		↓	G	✗	✓	✓	rare
DI	Diᵃ	IAT			G	✗	✓	✓	>99
	Diᵇ	IAT			G	✗	✓	✗	rare
	Wrᵃ	RT-37-IAT			G M	✗	✓	✓	>99
DO	Doᵃ	IAT	↑	↓	G	✗	✓	✗	33
	Doᵇ	IAT	↑	↓	G	✗	✓	✗	13
	Hy	IAT	↑		G	✓	✓	✗	rare
FY	Fyᵃ	IAT	↓		G	rare	✓	✓	33
	Fyᵇ	IAT	↓		G	rare	✓	rare	20
GE	Ge	37<IAT	↓		G M	✓	✓	✓	rare
H	H	RT>37-IAT	↑		M G	✓	✓	✓	rare
I	I	RT>37-IAT	↑		M G	✓	✓	✗	rare
JK	Jkᵃ	IAT	↑		G M	✓	✓	✓	25
	Jkᵇ	IAT	↑		G M	✓	✓	✓	25
JMH	JMH	IAT	↓		G	✗	✗	✗	rare
KEL	Jsᵃ	IAT			G M	✗	✓	✓	>99
	Jsᵇ	IAT			G	✗	✓	✓	rare
	K	37-IAT			G M	rare	✓	✓	91
	k	37-IAT			G M	✗	✓	✓	rare
	Kpᵃ	37-IAT			G	✗	✓	✓	98
	Kpᵇ	37-IAT			G M	✗	✓	✓	rare
KNOPS	Knᵃ	IAT	↓	↓	G	✗	✗	✗	2
	McCᵃ	IAT	↓	↓	G	✗	✗	✗	2
	Slᵃ	IAT	↓	↓	G	✗	✗	✗	2
	Ykᵃ	IAT	↓	↓	G	✗	✗	✗	8
LE	Leᵃ	RT>37-IAT	↑		M G	✓	rare	✗	78
	Leᵇ	RT>37-IAT	↑		M G	✓	✗	✗	28
LU	Luᵃ	RT-37-IAT			G A	rare	✗	rare	92
	Luᵇ	RT-37-IAT		↓	G A	rare	✓	rare	rare
LW	LWᵃ	RT>37-IAT		↓	M G	✗	✓	✓	3
	LWᵇ	RT>37-IAT		↓	M G	✗	✓	✓	97

Table VIII-A-1. Serologic Characteristics of Some Alloantibodies to RBC Antigens (Continued)

System*	Anti-	Phase[†]	Ficin[‡]	DTT[§]	Ig[∥]	C3[¶]	HTR[#]	HDFN**	% Comp[††]
MNS	M	RT>37-IAT	↓		M G	✗	✗	rare	28
	N	RT>37-IAT	↓		M G	✗	rare	rare	22
	S	IAT	↓		G M	few	✓	✓	45
	s	IAT	↓		G	rare	✓	✓	11
	U	IAT			G	✗	✓	✓	rare
P	P_1	RT>37-IAT	↑		M	✓	rare	✗	22
GLOB	PP_1P^k	RT>37-IAT	↑		M G	✓	✓	✓	rare
RH	C	37<IAT	↑		G M	✗	✓	✓	30
	c	37<IAT	↑		G M	✗	✓	✓	20
	C^w	37<IAT	↑		G M	✗	✓	✓	98
	D	37<IAT	↑		G M	✗	✓	✓	85
	E	37<IAT	↑		G M	✗	✓	✓	70
	e	37<IAT	↑		G M	✗	✓	✓	2
	f(ce)	37<IAT	↑		G M	✗	✓	✓	36
SC	Sc1	IAT			G	✓	✗	✗	rare
	Sc2	IAT			G	✗	✗	✓	99
YT	Yt^a	IAT	↓	↓	G	✗	some	✗	Rare
	Yt^b	IAT	↓	↓	G	✗		✗	91

Collection*	Anti-	Phase[†]	Ficin[‡]	DTT[§]	Ig[∥]	C3[¶]	HTR[#]	HDFN**	% Comp[‡‡]
COST	Cs^a	IAT			G	✗	✗	✗	2
Series*									
901001	Vel		↑		G		✓	✗	rare
901002	Lan	IAT			G	some	✓	✓	rare
901012	Sd^a	RT			M G	✗	rare	✗	4

*ISBT notation.

[†]Optimal test phase of reactivity, where RT = room temperature, 37 = 37 C, and IAT = indirect antiglobulin test.

[‡]Effect of ficin on reactivity, where ↑ = enhancement, and ↓ = diminution.

[§]Effect of dithiothreitol (DTT) on reactivity, where ↓ = diminution.

[∥]Immunoglobulin class of antibody.

[¶]Ability of antibody to fix complement to RBCs.

[#]Antibody has caused hemolytic transfusion reactions.

**Antibody has caused hemolytic disease of the fetus and newborn.

[††]Approximate percentage of compatible donors, based mostly on antigen frequencies of European origin.

✓ = yes; ✗ = no.

VIII-B. Management of Samples and Patients with Cold Agglutinins

Purpose

To provide a process for management of samples and patients with broadly reactive cold agglutinins.

Before You Begin

Through laboratory data system, phone, or requisition, obtain patient's:

- Transfusion, transplant, and pregnancy history.
- Medical diagnoses.
- Laboratory data indicative of hemolysis.
- Drug therapy history.

Background Information

See Appendix VIII-1, Evaluation of Initial Antibody Identification Panel.

Operational Policy

Potent cold agglutinins may interfere with the results of ABO/Rh typing. Resolve as described in Process XIII-B.

Notify attending physician of significant findings.

Wash all RBCs three times in pH 7.3 PBS to minimize variation in reactivity caused by differences in pH and osmolarity among RBC diluents.

Sample Requirements

EDTA anticoagulated blood as a source of plasma and RBCs.

Note: Separate the plasma from the RBCs at 37 C.

Equipment/ Materials

Results of tests with a panel of phenotyped group O RBCs indicating the presence of a direct agglutinin reacting with all samples.

Note: The autocontrol may or may not be reactive.

Process   Complete the following stages for management of patients and samples with cold-reactive agglutinins:

Stage	Description
1.	If patient's ABO type is A_1 or A_1B, test vs A_1; A_2; O, I+; O, I– (cord); papain/ficin-treated; and autologous RBCs by Procedure II-H. Alternatively, test for specificity by Procedure XI-I. Interpret the reactions as follows:

When the antibody...	Then the specificity(ies) to consider is/are...
reacts only/preferentially with the O and A_2 RBCs	anti-HI.
reacts strongly with all samples except the O, I– RBCs	autoanti-I.
reacts with all samples except O, I– and autologous RBCs	alloanti-I.
reacts preferentially with O, I– RBCs	anti-i.
reacts with all samples except the autologous RBCs	alloantibody to high-prevalence antigen.
reacts with all samples except papain/ficin-treated RBCs	anti-Pr (or autoanti-En/ -Ge).
reacts with all samples except papain/ficin-treated RBCs and the autologous RBCs	alloanti-En and -Ge.

Stage	Description
2.	Based on specificity of the antibody, proceed as follows:

When the antibody is...	Then...
anti-HI	• Confirm A_1 status of patient RBCs. • Select A_1 RBCs for transfusion.
an autoantibody	perform autologous adsorption if saline IATs (Procedure II-I) are reactive.
alloanti-I	• Test patient RBCs for I and i antigen expression. • Rare I– blood may be indicated.
an alloantibody to a high-prevalence antigen	• Consider anti-Vel, -P, -En, -IFC, and -Ge. • Rare blood may be indicated.

3.	Use Procedure II-H to determine the need for autologous adsorption using the following criteria:	
	When tests by Procedure II-H are...	**Then...**
	strongly reactive	perform autologous adsorption (Procedure XI-J) to exclude concomitant alloantibodies.
	≤1+	no need to perform autologous adsorption; computer crossmatch may be performed.

4.	If tests by Procedure II-H so indicate, and the patient has not been recently transfused, perform Procedure XI-J. Interpret the reactions as follows:	
	When the antibody is...	**Then antibody...**
	adsorbed	is an autoantibody: • Perform crossmatch according to facility SOPs.
	not adsorbed	is an alloantibody, or the adsorption is incomplete.

5.	Evaluate clinical data relative to antibody specificity as follows:	
	When there is evidence of...	**Then consider...**
	Mycoplasma pneumoniae	autoanti-I.
	infectious mononucleosis	anti-i.
	lymphoproliferative disease	any cold autoantibody.

6.	Evaluate laboratory data as follows:	
	When there is...	**Then...**
	evidence of hemolysis	• Perform direct antiglobulin tests (Procedure XI-B). • Consider performing thermal amplitude studies (Procedure XI-G). • Notify the attending physician by telephone.
	no evidence of hemolysis	note in laboratory report.

**Effective
Date**

Approved by:	Printed Name	Signature	Date
Laboratory Management			
Medical Director			
Quality Officer			

VIII-C. Evaluation of Panel Results: Crossing Out

Purpose	To provide a process for evaluating the results of an antibody identification panel or selected cell panel to:

- Allow accurate identification of an unexpected antibody(ies).

- Determine which antibodies are ruled out.

- Determine if additional testing must be performed.

Background Information	Individuals will usually not possess the corresponding antibody in their serum if their serum did not react with antigen-positive cells.

Operational Policy	Antibodies to low-prevalence antigens such as Kp^a, Js^a, Lu^a, V, and C^w do not need to be excluded.

Process	Complete the following stages to evaluate results and cross out antigens:

Stage	Description
1.	Look at the first reagent RBC that did not react with the serum/plasma.
2.	On the top of the worksheet or on each individual panel cell, cross out the antigens present on that cell (see Fig VIII-C-1 and -2):

Use...	To cross out when the cell possesses...
two lines (**X**)	double-dose antigen (donor has a homozygous expression of the antigen).
one line (*/*)	single-dose antigen (donor has a heterozygous expression of the antigen).

Stage	Description
3.	Repeat the process for all cells in the panel that were nonreactive with the sample.

4.	Evaluate the results as follows:		
	When...	**And...**	**Then...**
	the pattern of antibody reactivity matches a pattern of antigen-positive cells not crossed off	1) all other antigens to commonly occurring antibodies have been crossed off, and 2) criteria for ruling out and identification are met as required by specific laboratory SOP	the antibody is identified and the process is complete.
	several antigens are not crossed out		proceed to Selected Cells Process (VIII-D).

Effective Date

Approved by:

Laboratory Management

Medical Director

Quality Officer

	Printed Name	Signature	Date

		Rh					MNS				Lu		P	Lewis		Kell		Duffy		Kidd		Saline		
	D	C	E	c	e	f	M	N	S	s	Lu^a	Lu^b	P₁	Le^a	Le^b	K	k	Fy^a	Fy^b	Jk^a	Jk^b	IS	37	IAT
1	+	+	0	0	+	0	+	+	+	+	0	+	0	+	0	0	+	0	+	0	+	0	0	2
2	0	0	0	+	+	+	+	0	+	0	0	+	+	0	+	+	0	+	+	+	0	0	0	0
3	0	0	+	+	0	0	0	+	0	+	0	+	+	0	+	+	+	+	0	0	+	0	0	0

Figure VIII-C-1. Antigens crossed out on the top of the antigen profile.

		Rh					MNS				Lu		P	Lewis		Kell		Duffy		Kidd		Saline		
	D	C	E	c	e	f	M	N	S	s	Lu^a	Lu^b	P₁	Le^a	Le^b	K	k	Fy^a	Fy^b	Jk^a	Jk^b	IS	37	IAT
1	+	+	0	0	+	0	+	+	+	+	0	+	0	+	0	0	+	0	+	0	+	0	0	2
2	0	0	0	+	+	+	+	0	+	0	0	+	+	0	+	+	0	+	+	+	0	0	0	0
3	0	0	+	+	0	0	0	+	0	+	0	+	+	0	+	+	+	+	0	0	+	0	0	0

Figure VIII-C-2. Antigens crossed out on each individual panel cell.

VIII-D. Selected Cells Process

Purpose

To provide a process for selecting RBCs with known phenotypes that can be used to detect, confirm, or rule out antibodies.

Background Information

It is important to keep in mind that RBCs from Black donors may not possess homozygous expressions of S, s, Fy^a, and Fy^b, even when the phenotype appears to have a double-dose antigen expression.

Operational Policy

Criteria for selecting cells:

*   In-date panels are used first.

*   If permitted by laboratory SOPs, the most recent time-expired panels are selected if no in-date panel cells fit the required antigen make-up to rule in or rule out an antibody.

*   Do not use selected cell panels older than 4 months.

*   Time-expired cells should not be the only cells used to rule out the presence of an antibody.

*   Whenever possible, when using time-expired cells to rule out, choose those that possess a homozygous expression of the antigen.

Note: Time-expired panels should be used with caution when identifying or ruling out anti-Le^a, -Le^b, or -P_1, or antibodies to Knops, Chido/Rogers, or JMH antigens because these antigens deteriorate during storage.

An alternative, preferential approach to using time-expired RBCs for the purpose of excluding alloantibodies is to issue crossmatch-compatible units known to lack the antigens corresponding to antibodies that have not been excluded. For example, if a serum contains anti-c and anti-Jk^a, but anti-K cannot be excluded, issue crossmatch-compatible units that are c–, Jk(a–), K–.

Anti-Kp^a, -Js^a, -Lu^a, -V, and -C^w are directed against low-prevalance antigens. It may not be possible to rule out these antibodies because there is a good chance there may not be an antigen-positive cell on the panel. There is no need to run additional cells positive for these antigens because the chance of a transfusion complication is minimal, and the chance of selecting a Js(a+), Lu(a+), Kp(a+), V+, or C^w+ donor unit is low.

**Equipment/
Materials**

Commercial panels (fresh are preferred, or time-expired panels).

Antibody screening cells (fresh are preferred).

Other sources when available:

- Phenotyped voluntary donors.

- Cord blood samples.

- Frozen rare cells.

- Employee voluntary donors.

**Quality
Control**

At the time of use, time-expired RBCs may be tested to demonstrate they carry adequate expression of the antigen(s) corresponding to the antibodies that need to be excluded. This can be done using anti-IgG gel columns in comparative studies between in-date and time-expired RBCs with a dilution of antibody that yields a 2+ reaction.

Process

Complete the following stages to selecting appropriate RBCs:

Stage	Description
1.	For each antibody suspected, select cells positive for the corresponding antigen and negative for the other suspected antigens, following laboratory SOPs for identification and ruling out of alloantibodies.

When...	Then select cells that are...
anti-D, -C, and -Jk^a are suspected	• **D+**C–; Jk(a–) • D–**C+**; Jk(a–) • D–C–; **Jk(a+)**

If antibodies have been previously identified, it is not necessary to select cells that are positive for those antigens.

2.	Create a worksheet using: • Commercial panel antigen profiles. • Current donor units.
3.	Test the selected cell panel.
4.	Evaluate results using a crossing out technique (see Process VIII-C).

5.	Verify criteria for identification of an antibody and ruling out of alloantibodies are met per specific laboratory SOP:	
	When criteria for ruling out and identification…	**Then…**
	are met	process is complete.
	are *not* met	repeat testing with additional selected cells until all clinically significant antibodies have been confirmed or ruled out.

Effective Date

Approved by:	**Printed Name**	**Signature**	**Date**
Laboratory Management			
Medical Director			
Quality Officer			

VIII-E. Selection of Antigen-Negative Blood for Transfusion

Purpose
To provide a process for the appropriate selection of blood for patients with alloantibodies.

Background Information
The provision of blood for patients with antibodies to blood group antigens is dependent on many factors, such as the clinical importance of the antibody, the availability of blood, and the clinical condition of the patient. In this procedure, the laboratory factors are considered.

Operational Policy
For the transfusion management of patients with unexpected alloantibodies, each antibody is placed in one of seven categories, based on reported clinical significance, frequency of the corresponding antigen, and availability of appropriate typing reagents. The categories are as follows:

- **Category I:** Potentially significant antibodies for which antigen-negative units can readily be obtained.

- **Category II:** Alloantibodies of questionable clinical significance for which crossmatch-compatible units can be obtained by screening available units.

- **Category III:** Antibodies to Knops, Ch/Rg, and JMH antigens.

- **Category IV:** Antibodies to low-prevalence antigens.

- **Category V:** Antibodies to leukocyte-related antigens.

- **Category VI:** Potentially significant alloantibodies to high-prevalence antigens.

- **Category VII:** Potentially significant antibodies for which reliable "reagent-grade" antisera are virtually nonexistent.

The category designation for specific antibodies is given in Table VIII-E-1.

When crossmatch is necessary, use the method by which antibody was best detected.

Equipment/ Materials
Valid reagent antiserum of the same specificity as the patient's alloantibody.

Donor RBCs for transfusion: 3%-5% suspensions, in saline (or as indicated in the "Instructions for Use" for the reagent antiserum).

Anti-IgG, as required in the "Instructions for Use" for the reagent antiserum.

IgG-coated RBCs as required: see Section VII, or obtain commercially.

Other reagents, as required in the "Instructions for Use" for the reagent antiserum.

Single-dose antigen-positive and antigen-negative controls (positive and negative control, respectively) for each antiserum to be tested.

Quality Control

There are no specific quality control measures applicable to this procedure. Rather, appropriate selection of blood for transfusion to the alloimmunized patient depends on accurate antibody identification, proper serologic testing of donor units (antigen typing and antiglobulin crossmatch, as appropriate), and attention to clerical details that ensure release of the correct RBC units to the right patient.

Process

To select blood for transfusion, determine the antibody category from Table VIII-E-1 and take appropriate action:

When the antibody is a...	Then...
Category I antibody	• Select antigen-negative units for transfusion regardless of current antibody strength. Units should be proven antigen-negative by testing with a valid reagent. • Perform serologic tests according to the "Instructions for Use" for the antibody in question.
Category II antibody	• Confirmation of antigen-negative status with a valid reagent is not required. If screening units by crossmatch requires too large a quantity of patient serum, reagent antisera may be used and antigen-negative units selected for compatibility testing. However, antigen-negative units (if available) should be given if a serum sample obtained within the previous 3 days reacted at IAT and subsequent massive transfusion diluted the antibody to undetectable levels. • Perform serologic tests according to the "Instructions for Use" for the antibody in question

Category III antibody	Exclude underlying clinically significant alloantibodies (See Section X).
	Issue antigobulin-crossmatch-compatible blood when possible. Issue least-reactive units if compatible blood cannot be readily found.
	Note: Anti-Ch, -Rg, and -JMH have not been reported to cause in-vivo RBC destruction. Antibodies with Knops-McCoy-related specificity and anti-Cs^a and -Yk^a may cause a slightly shortened survival of donor RBCs but have not definitively been associated with profound hemolytic transfusion reactions.
Category IV antibody	Confirm the antigen-negative status of crossmatch-compatible blood when reagent antisera are available.
	Perform serologic tests according to the "Instructions for Use" for the antibody in question.
Category V antibody	Reagent antisera are not available.
	Issue antigobulin-crossmatch-compatible units.
Category VI antibody	If antigen-negative units are available in house, confirm antigen-negative status with a commercially available reagent, where possible, or another example of the antibody. Include, at a minimum, a positive control.
	If reagent sera are not available for antigen confirmation, issue units based on crossmatch compatibility.
	If antigen-negative units are not available in house, obtain blood from other blood centers via a rare donor program (eg, American Rare Donor Program or World Health Organization).
	Confirm antigen-negative status when reagents permit, or issue units based on crossmatch compatibility.

Category VII antibody	If the patient's antibody is still demonstrable, issue units based on crossmatch compatibility.
	If the patient's antibody is not detectable, test the units with any example of the antibody available and include, at a minimum, a positive control.
	Note: If the patient has chronic transfusion needs, consider sending donor samples to a molecular testing laboratory for antigen determination.

Effective Date

Approved by:	Printed Name	Signature	Date
Laboratory Management			
Medical Director			
Quality Officer			

Table VIII-E-1. Selection of Antigen-Negative Blood for Transfusion

Anti-	Category	Anti-	Category	Anti-	Category
A_1	II	Hy	VI	M	II
Bg	V	I/i[†]	II	McC^a	III
C	I	Jk^a	I	N	II
c	I	Jk^b	I	N[‡]	VI
C^w	IV	JMH	III	P_1	II
Ch	III	Js^a	IV	P+P$_1$+P^k	VI
Cs^a	III	Js^b	VI	Rg	III
D	I	K	I	S	I
Do^a	VII	k	VI	s	I
Do^b	VII	Kn^a	III	Sd^a	III
E	I	Kp^a	IV	U	VI
e	I	Kp^b	VI	V	IV
f*	I	Lan	VI	Vel	VI
Fy^a	I	Le^a	II	Wr^a	IV
Fy^b	I	Le^b	II	Yk^a	III
Ge	VI	Lu^a	II	Yt^a	VI
H/HI/Hi[†]	II	Lu^b	VI	Xg^a	IV

*Type for c– units.

[†]Usually autoantibodies.

[‡]Antibody made by 'N'– individuals. Consider N–U– blood.

VIII-F. Determination of Probability Levels

Purpose

To provide a process to determine if antibody identification data are statistically valid. To minimize the possibility that an observed pattern of reactions is caused by chance alone, sufficient antigen-positive and antigen-negative RBC samples must be tested.

Before You Begin

Table VIII-F-1 shows the probability (p) values of various combinations of positive and negative test results. A p value of 0.05 for an anti-D (obtained by testing three Rh-positive samples and finding them to react, whereas three Rh-negative samples are nonreactive) means that an identical set of reactions caused by an antibody other than anti-D could be obtained by chance once in 20 similar studies. Thus, there is a 19:1 (95%) probability (p = 0.05) that the reactions are indeed due to anti-D.

A single reagent RBC panel may not always contain sufficient antigen-positive and antigen-negative samples to provide such a p value. For example, if the only s-negative sample on a reagent panel of 10 RBC samples is nonreactive but all other s-positive RBCs react, then there is a 10% chance (p = 0.1) that the reactions are not caused by anti-s. However, if another s-negative sample is tested and found nonreactive, then the p value improves to 0.02 (a 2% chance that an antibody other than s is involved).

The following may help in the absence of a calculator for determining factorials.

- A factorial number divided by itself = 1.

- Factorial numbers 1! and 0! can be deleted when resolving equations.

- Answers to calculations such as 4! × 6! ÷ 10! can be obtained by dividing 24 (4!) with the product of 7 × 8 × 9 × 10 (ie, those numbers up to 10 that are greater than 6).

- Factorials for 0 through 10 are as follows:

0! = 1	4! = 6 × 4 = 24	8! = 5040 × 8 = 40,320
1! = 1 × 1 = 1	5! = 24 × 5 = 120	9! = 40320 × 9 = 362,880
2! = 1 × 2 = 2	6! = 120 × 6 = 720	10! = 362880 × 10 =3,628,800
3! = 2 × 3 = 6	7! = 720 × 7 = 5040	

Operational Policy

A p level of 0.05 is the highest at which an interpretation is considered acceptable.

Because this method requires that the patient RBCs lack the antigen(s) against which the suspected antibody(ies) is/are directed, phenotype the patient RBCs with the appropriate antisera whenever practicable. Rare exceptions to this policy are cases of Rh-positive patients with a partial D antigen whose serum/plasma contains alloanti-D.

Sample Requirements

Complete results from an antibody identification panel.

Equipment/ Materials

A calculator capable of determining factorials.

Process

Complete these stages to calculate probability levels:

Stage	Description
1.	Construct a 2 × 2 table as follows:

Serum Reactions	Antigen		Total
	Present	Absent	
Positive	A	B	A+B
Negative	C	D	C+D
Total	A+C	B+D	N

where:

A = number of positive results with antigen-positive RBCs.

B = number of positive results with antigen-negative RBCs.

C = number of negative results with antigen-positive RBCs.

D = number of negative results with antigen-negative RBCs.

N = total number of RBC samples tested.

2.	Use the following equation to determine the probability level:

$$\frac{(A+B)! \times (C+D)! \times (A+C)! \times (B+D)!}{N! \times A! \times B! \times C! \times D!}$$

where ! = the symbol for factorial, the product of all whole numbers from 1 to the number involved (see Before You Begin).

Example: For a serum reacting with three S+ RBC samples but not with three S– samples, the 2 × 2 table is:

Serum Reactions	Antigen		Total
	S+	S–	
positive	3	0	3
negative	0	3	3
Total	3	3	6

The equation for p is:

$$\frac{3! \times 3! \times 3! \times 3!}{6! \times 3! \times 0! \times 3! \times 0!} = \frac{3! \times 3!}{6} = \frac{6 \times 6}{720} = 1/20 \ (0.05)$$

Note: See Table VIII-F-1 for p values for other combinations of positive and negative results.

3.	Interpret the answer as follows:

If p is...	Then the data are...
>0.05	statistically significant: • Valid conclusions can be made.
<0.05	not statistically significant: • Additional testing may be required.

References

Ellisor SS, Morel PA, eds. Statistics for blood bankers. Arlington, VA: AABB, 1983.

Moore BPL. Serological and immunological methods of the Canadian Red Cross Blood Transfusion Service. 8th ed. Toronto, ON: The Canadian Red Cross Society, 1980:200-2.

Morel PA, A handbood of biostatistical tests for immunohematologists. Alameda, CA: Associated Blood Bank Consultants, 1983.

Race RR, Sanger R. Blood groups in man. 6th ed. Oxford, UK: Balckwell Scientific Publications, 1975:480:1.

**Effective
Date**

Approved by:	Printed Name	Signature	Date
Laboratory Management			
Medical Director			
Quality Officer			

Table VIII-F-1. Probability Values

Number Tested	Number Positive	Number Negative	p
6	4	2	.067
6	3	3	.050
7	5	2	.048
7	4	3	.029
8	7	1	.125
8	6	2	.036
8	5	3	.018
8	4	4	.014
9	8	1	.111
9	7	2	.028
9	6	3	.012
10	9	1	.100
10	8	2	.022
10	7	3	.008
10	6	4	.005
10	5	5	.004

VIII-G. Acidifying Sera

Purpose

To provide instructions for identifying weak examples of anti-M and anti-Pr by acidifying serum.

Background Information

Except for anti-M and anti-Pr, the reactivity of most blood group antibodies does not vary significantly between pH 5.5 and 8.5. Some anti-M and anti-Pr react either solely or preferentially in direct agglutination tests at an acidic pH of around 6.2. This may be related to the charged carboxyl groups present on the sialoglycoproteins carrying these antigens.

Operational Policy

RBCs used in tests with acidified serum should be washed free of preservative before testing; some RBC diluents are buffered to pH 7.5.

Limitations

Failure to obtain the correct results may be caused by:

- Improper storage of reagents.
- Use of incorrect technique.
- Addition of wrong reagent.
- Omission of patient's serum or HCl.

Sample Requirements

Test serum: suspected to contain anti-M or anti-Pr; 1-2 mL.

Equipment/ Materials

0.2 N hydrochloric acid (HCl).

Litmus paper: for pH range 5.5-8.0 (eg, VWR, Batavia, IL).

Quality Control

Check pH of acidified serum with litmus paper; pH should be 6.2 or below.

Procedure   Use the following steps to perform the procedure:

Step	Action
1.	Mix 1 volume of 0.2 N HCl with 9 volumes of serum.
2.	Test the acidified serum in parallel with untreated serum by saline agglutination tests as described in Section II or by the cold antibody titration (specificity) procedure (II-H).

Reference   Beattie KM, Zuelzer WW. The frequency and properties of pH-dependent anti-M. Transfusion 1965;5:322-6.

Effective Date

	Printed Name	Signature	Date
Approved by:			
Laboratory Management			
Medical Director			
Quality Officer			

VIII-H. Using a Combined Adsorption/Elution Procedure

Purpose

To provide instructions for identifying antibodies present in multispecific sera. Combined adsorption/elution can also be used to:

- Demonstrate weakly expressed antigens on RBCs or weakly reactive antibodies present in serum/plasma.

- Aid in identification of antibody specificity, particularly when multiple antibodies are present in a given sample.

- Concentrate and purify antibodies by adsorption/elution—eg, adsorption of antibody in group O serum to high-prevalence antigen on group O RBCs, with subsequent preparation of an eluate that can be used to type RBCs of all ABO types.

Background Information

Adsorption/elution studies are usually undertaken when all other tests have failed to reveal the specificities of the antibodies present. Adsorption of antibody is best accomplished using a low serum-to-RBC ratio (eg 2:1 or less), whereas eluates are likely to yield more antibody when a high serum-to-RBC ratio is used (eg, 5:1 or more).

For antibody identification purposes, a large volume of serum is used to coat a smaller volume of RBCs—ideally a 5:1 ratio of serum and weakly reactive RBCs are used (a lower ratio, at a minimum of 2:1, may be used if the sample is limited). Bound antibody is eluted and the eluate is tested for antibody reactivity. See Section IV for principles of elution techniques. In some instances, the serum is further adsorbed, using a low serum-to-RBC ratio (eg, 2:1), and tested in parallel with the eluate and unadsorbed serum for antibody reactivity.

Pretreatment of the RBCs with proteolytic enzymes may enhance the adsorption process (see Section III and procedures for autologous adsorption in Section XI).

Operational Policy

As a general rule, a weakly reactive sample should be selected because it can be assumed this will carry only one of the blood group determinants to which the serum contains antibody. The selection of the adsorbing RBCs is of paramount importance to the success of these studies. However, this may have to be an inspired guess, based on the phenotype of the patient (if known).

To avoid dilution of the serum during the adsorption process, which may lead to loss of weak alloantibody activity, it is important to remove as much of the residual saline as possible in Step 4. This may be facilitated by placing a narrow strip of filter paper (eg, Whatman #1, Kent, UK) into the packed RBCs and allowing residual saline to soak into the paper by capillary action.

RBCs may be treated with ZZAP instead of papain or ficin (see Section III).

Limitations

Failure to obtain the correct results may be caused by:

- Improper storage of reagents.
- Use of incorrect technique.
- Use of wrong reagents.

Sample Requirements

Serum or plasma for adsorption: 4-10 mL.

RBCs for adsorption: 4-10 mL.

Note: Reserve an aliquot of unadsorbed serum for testing in parallel with the adsorbed serum.

Equipment/ Materials

Ficin or papain: 1% wt/vol.

Glycine max (syn. *soja*) lectin (eg, Immucor, Norcross, GA, or see Section XIV).

Elution reagents: acid elution or organic solvent procedures are recommended (see Section IV).

Protein refractometer (eg, QA Supplies, Norfolk, VA).

Quality Control

Confirm that the RBCs for adsorption have been treated with proteolytic enzyme (if used). Untreated RBCs should be nonreactive with *G. max*, whereas complete agglutination should be observed with protease-treated RBCs.

Using a refractometer, measure the protein content of the adsorbed and unadsorbed serum. The adsorption process should not have lowered the protein content by more than 20% of the total protein in the unadsorbed sample.

To establish that antibody detected in elution is RBC-membrane derived and does not represent unbound "free" antibody, test the final wash supernate in parallel with the eluate.

To demonstrate that the antibody was subject to adsorption/elution, test the eluate against a reserved aliquot of the adsorbing RBC sample.

Procedure   Use the following steps to perform the procedure:

Step	Action
1.	In 13 or 16 × 100-mm test tubes, wash the RBCs to be used for adsorption three times with saline. Use vacuum aspiration equipment (if available) or Pasteur pipettes to remove supernate between each wash.
2.	For enzyme treatment of RBCs, if desired for adsorption, mix 2 volumes of RBCs with 1 volume of 1% papain or 1% ficin in a 16 × 100-mm test tube. Incubate at 37 C for 30 minutes and wash three times with saline.
3.	Dispense 2-mL aliquots of RBCs (untreated or enzyme-treated) into each of 3 appropriately labeled 10 × 75-mm test tubes.
4.	Fill the tubes with saline and centrifuge to pack the RBCs (≥1000 × g for at least 5 minutes). Remove as much of the supernate as possible.
5.	To coat RBCs for subsequent eluate preparation, mix 1 volume of RBCs with 2-5 volumes of serum in a 13 × 100-mm test tube.
6.	Incubate at the appropriate temperature (eg, 4 C for agglutinating antibodies or 37 C for antiglobulin-reactive antibodies) for 30 minutes to 2 hours.
7.	Centrifuge to pack the RBCs and harvest the serum. Wash the RBCs as described in Procedure IV-A and proceed with eluate preparation (see Section IV for appropriate eluate procedure).
8.	Test the adsorbed serum with antibody screening cells by the appropriate technique (eg, RT for agglutinating antibodies or 37 C for antiglobulin-reactive antibodies).

9.	**If further adsorptions are…**	**Then…**
	required to remove antibody	mix 2-4 volumes of serum from Step 7 (or start with unadsorbed serum) with another volume of packed RBCs (untreated or protease-treated, as desired) in a 13 × 100-mm test tube: • Incubate as in Step 6. • Proceed to Step 10.
	not required	proceed to Step 12.
	Note: It is appropriate to reduce the volume of serum at this stage so that the ratio of serum to RBCs is 2:1 or less.	
10.	Centrifuge to pack the RBCs and repeat Step 9.	
11.	Centrifuge to pack the RBCs. Harvest the serum and save for testing for antibody reactivity.	
12.	Test the adsorbed serum for antibody specificity in parallel with the eluate and unadsorbed serum. Include the adsorbing RBC sample in these studies, using the method by which the antibodies were detected.	

Reference   Judd WJ. Elution of antibody from RBCs. In: Bell CA, ed. Seminar on antigen-antibody reactions revisited. Arlington, VA: AABB, 1982:175-221.

Effective Date

Approved by:

	Printed Name	Signature	Date
Laboratory Management			
Medical Director			
Quality Officer			

VIII-I. Detecting Trypsin-Resistant N_{VG} Receptors

Purpose

To provide instructions for detecting trypsin-resistant N_{VG} receptors on glycophorin B (GPB) and hybrid glycophrins.

Background Information

Normal human RBCs have an N-like determinant on the trypsin-resistant sialoglycoprotein that carries S, s, and U antigens (GPB). This determinant is referred to as 'N' (N-quotes). When untreated M+N– RBCs with a normal GPB are tested with *Vicia graminea* (anti-N_{VG}) lectin they type as N–. However, strong reactions with anti-N_{VG} will be seen after the same RBCs have been treated with trypsin. It is generally assumed that the presence of trypsin-sensitive MN-active sialoglycoprotein (GPA) sterically hinders reactivity between anti-N_{VG} and trypsin-resistant GPB; cleavage of GPA by trypsin allows for increased binding between anti-N_{VG} and 'N'.

Reactions obtained with trypsin-treated RBCs and anti-N_{VG} can be used to evaluate the presence or absence of normal glycosylation at the *N*-terminal region of GPB. Negative results may be caused by incomplete glycosylation or absence of GPB (as with S–s–U– RBCs). In the case of RBCs from individuals heterozygous for S^u and a gene complex that produces Henshaw, the amino acid at the *N*-terminal region of He-active GPB is such that attached alkali-labile tetrasaccharides are oriented in a manner that does not permit binding with anti-N_{VG}.

Operational Policy

Purified trypsin should be used for RBC treatment: crude extracts of trypsin, used to convert C3b/C4b to C3d/C4d on RBCs for tests on antiglobulin reagents or the recognition of anti-Ch or -Rg, are unsuitable for the purpose described above (see Section III).

Limitations

Failure to obtain the correct results may be caused by:

- Improper storage of reagents.
- Use of incorrect technique.
- Inadequate treatment of RBCs with trypsin.
- Use of anti-N_{VG} contaminated with bacteria, foreign matter, the contents of other reagent vials, or human serum.
- Incorrect centrifugation of tests.

Sample Requirements

Trypsin-treated RBCs: diluted to a 3%-5% suspension with saline (see Procedure III-J).

Untreated RBCs: washed three times and diluted to a 3%-5% suspension with saline.

Equipment/ Materials

Trypsin-treated M–N+S–s–U– and M+N–S+s+ RBCs: diluted to a 3%-5% suspension with saline.

Untreated M–N+S–s–U– and M+N–S+s+ RBCs: washed three times and diluted to a 3%-5% suspension with saline.

Vicia graminea (anti-N$_{VG}$) lectin: available commercially (eg, Immucor, Norcross, GA), or see Section XIV.

Quality Control

Test untreated and trypsin-treated M+N–S+s+U+ and M–N+S–s–U– RBCs with *V. graminea*.

Trypsin-treated M+N–S+s+U+ RBCs should react (>2+) with *V. graminea*; the untreated RBCs should be nonreactive.

Trypsin-treated M–N+S–s–U– RBCs should be nonreactive with *V. graminea*; the untreated RBCs should be strongly (3+ to 4+) reactive.

Procedure

Use the following steps to perform the procedure:

Step	Action
1.	Mix 1 drop of trypsin-treated RBCs and 2 drops of anti-N$_{VG}$ lectin in an appropriately labeled 10 or 12 × 75-mm test tube.
2.	Similarly, set up tests with the untreated RBCs.
3.	Incubate at 37 C for 15 minutes.
4.	Centrifuge as for hemagglutination tests.
5.	Examine the RBCs macroscopically; grade and record the results.
6.	Interpret the reactions as follows: <table><tr><td>**If anti-N$_{VG}$ and trypsin-treated RBCs are…**</td><td>**Then…**</td></tr><tr><td>negative</td><td>RBCs lack normal GPB.</td></tr><tr><td>positive</td><td>RBCs possess normal GPB.</td></tr></table>

Reference

Pavone BG, Billman R, Bryant J, et al. An auto-anti-En[a], inhibitable by MN sialoglycoprotein. Transfusion 1981;21:25-31.

Effective Date

Approved by:

	Printed Name	Signature	Date
Laboratory Management			
Medical Director			
Quality Officer			

VIII-J. Using Soluble Blood Group Substances in an Inhibition Procedure

Purpose

To provide instructions for confirming antibody specificity, recognizing additional (concomitant) antibody reactivity, or determining ABH secretor status.

Background Information

ABH, Lewis, I, P_1, and Sd^a antigens are present in a soluble form in certain body fluids or tissue extracts. Such soluble antigens can be used to inhibit antigen-antibody interactions. Table VIII-J-1 summarizes the source and specificity of some soluble blood group substances.

Human milk and urine will also contain ABH and Lewis activity according to the ABO, Lewis, and secretor status of the donor.

Operational Policy

H/Le^a/Le^b substance and avian P_1 substance are available commercially; they should be used according to the manufacturer's directions.

Limitations

Failure to obtain the correct results may be caused by:

- Improper storage of reagents.
- Use of incorrect technique.
- Use of wrong reagent.
- Omission of inhibitor.

Sample Requirements

Test serum containing antibody for inhibition: 0.5-1.0 mL.

Equipment/ Materials

Dialysis tubing: 10-mm-ID cellulose-membrane tubing with MW cutoff ≈12,400 (eg, Sigma-Aldrich, St Louis, MO).

Micro-filtration apparatus: 5-mL syringe with disc-filter assembly (eg, Acrodisc) and 0.45-μ filter pads (Pall Corp, East Hills, NY).

pH 7.3 PBS.

RBCs: washed three times and diluted to a 3%-5% suspension with saline; test a minimum of one antigen-negative and two antigen-positive samples.

Judd's Methods in Immunohematology
Using Soluble Blood Group Substances in an Inhibition Procedure
Page 2 of 4

Blood group substances (BGS):

- Human milk.
- Human saliva.
- Hydatid cyst fluid (HCF).
- Pigeon egg white (available commercially; eg, Immucor, Norcross, GA).
- Urine.

Quality Control

For each suspected antibody under investigation, test a known example of the same specificity for inhibition, if available.

The method includes a control for dilution of antibody by the addition of soluble BGS.

Procedure

Use the following steps to perform the procedure:

Step	Action
1.	Mix equal volumes of test serum and soluble BGS. Minimally, 0.2-mL volumes should be used for testing against three reagent RBC samples.
2.	Prepare a control tube containing equal volumes of serum and pH 7.3 PBS.
3.	Incubate at RT for 30 minutes.
4.	For each RBC sample to be tested, mix 1 drop of RBCs with 2-3 drops of serum + BGS in 10 or 12 × 75-mm test tubes.
5.	Set up similar tests with the control serum + PBS mixture.
6.	Test using the procedure by which the antibody preferentially reacts (eg, saline agglutination tests at RT). For anti-Sd^a, incubate at RT and wash for antiglobulin testing with polyspecific AHG.

7.	Interpret results as follows:		
	If…	**And…**	**Then there is…**
	agglutination is present	control serum + PBS mixture is reactive	no inhibition or partial inhibition.
	no agglutination is present	control serum + PBS mixture is reactive	inhibition.
	Note: See Table VIII-J-1 for specific inhibition by soluble BGS.		

Effective Date

Approved by:

	Printed Name	Signature	Date
Laboratory Management			
Medical Director			
Quality Officer			

Table VIII-J-1. Antibody Inhibition by Blood Group Substances

Anti-	Inhibited By
H	Saliva containing H substance—ie, Se, Le(a–b–), or Le(a–b+) donors
I	Human milk (inhibits natural anti-I^D more readily than pathological anti-I^F; inhibition may not be complete)
Le^a	Saliva containing Le^a substance—ie, from Le(a+b–) and Le(a–b+) donors
Le^{bH}	Saliva containing H substance—ie, Se, Le(a–b–) or Le(a–b+) donors (H substance, as well as Le^b substance, is inhibitory)
Le^{bL}	Saliva containing Le^b substance
P_1	Hydatid cyst fluid or pigeon egg white
Sd^a	Human or guinea-pig urine

VIII-K. Inhibiting Rouleaux with DIDS

Purpose

To provide instructions for inhibiting rouleaux using 4,4′-diisothiocy-anatostilbene-2,2′-disulfonic acid (DIDS):

- Management of samples with a reverse albumin-to-globulin ratio.

Background Information

Rouleaux is a phenomenon that may mimic agglutination. It is seen with sera that have an abnormal protein content, especially those with a reversed albumin-to-globulin ratio. RBCs manifesting rouleaux appear microscopically like aggregates of stacked coins. When rouleaux is marked, these aggregates can be difficult to distinguish from antibody-mediated agglutination.

DIDS inhibits rouleaux by binding irreversibly to sites on band 3 of the RBC membrane. DIDS blocks the binding of macromolecules present in rouleaux-forming serum/plasma to the same sites on band 3.

Expression of the following blood group antigens is not adversely affected by treatment of RBCs with DIDS: A, B, c, Ch, D, E, Fy^a, Fy^b, Jk^a, JMH, K, k, Le^a, Lu^b, LW^a, M, S, Wr^b, and Yt^a.

Rouleaux should not be observed at the antiglobulin phase of testing.

Operational Policy

DIDS is moist and light-sensitive. Store dessicated, in the dark at 4 C.

Limitations

Failure to obtain the correct results may be caused by:

- Improper storage of reagents.
- Use of incorrect technique.
- Use of wrong reagent.

Sample Requirements

Serum or plasma: 1 mL.

**Equipment/
Materials**

Pipettors with disposable tips to deliver 150 μL (eg, VWR, Batavia, IL).

4% dextran in normal serum: serum with negative test results for unexpected antibodies.

DIDS: $C_{16}H_8N_2O_6S_4Na_2$.

Reagent RBCs: 3%-5% suspensions of reagent RBCs (eg, RBCs for screening sera for unexpected antibodies).

**Quality
Control**

On day of use, demonstrate inhibition of rouleaux-forming properties of 4% dextran in normal serum.

Procedure

Use the following steps to perform the procedure:

Step	Action
1.	Place 1 drop of each reagent RBC suspension into three appropriately labeled 10 or 12 × 75-mm test tubes, one for DIDS-treated RBCs, one for a saline control, and one for 4% dextran.
2.	Add 150 μL DIDS (approximately 5-6 drops) to DIDS-treated RBCs tube.
3.	Add a similar volume of saline to the second tube.
4.	Add a similar volume of 4% dextran to the third tube.
5.	Mix and incubate at 37 C for 10 minutes.
6.	Wash the RBCs once with saline and decant the supernate.
7.	Test 1 drop of DIDS-treated RBCs against the serum/plasma under investigation at RT by Procedure II-H or a direct agglutination method selected from Section II.
8.	In parallel, test the untreated and dextran-treated RBCs against the test serum.
9.	Read for the presence or absence of rouleaux microscopically.

10.	Interpret the reactions as follows:			
	If RBCs + DIDS + test serum react…	**And RBCs + saline + test serum react…**	**And RBCs + DIDS + 4% dextran react…**	**Then interpret as…**
	0	+	0	rouleaux.
	+/0	+/0	+	invalid.
	+	+	0	not rouleaux.

Reference Norris S, Neff T, Wilkinson S. Serologic evaluation of a rouleaux-inhibiting chemical (abstract). Transfusion 1993;33(Suppl):65S.

Effective Date

Approved by:	Printed Name	Signature	Date
Laboratory Management			
Medical Director			
Quality Officer			

VIII-L. Identifying Anti-N$_{form}$

Purpose

To provide instructions for differentiating anti-N$_{form}$ from cold-reactive "auto" anti-N and anti-N made by MS^u/MS^u individuals and other M+N– persons whose RBCs lack 'N'.

Background Information

Patients undergoing renal dialysis on instruments cleansed with formaldehyde may develop anti-N ("dialysis" anti-N or anti-N$_{form}$). Such antibodies may be differentiated from other forms of anti-N in tests with formalin-treated RBCs.

Formalin treatment enhances serologic reactivity of anti-N$_{form}$ but does not potentiate the reactions of cold-reactive "auto" anti-N made by normal M+N– individuals, nor does it potentiate the reactions of the clinically significant anti-N seen in MS^u/MS^u individuals and other M+N– persons whose RBCs lack 'N'.

Formaldehyde is not currently used to cleanse dialysis instruments. This type of anti-N is rare.

Operational Policy

Not applicable.

Limitations

Failure to obtain the correct results may be caused by:

- Improper storage of reagents.
- Use of incorrect technique.
- Use of wrong reagent.

Sample Requirements

Test serum containing anti-N: 2 mL.

Equipment/ Materials

Known example of anti-N$_{form}$, if available.

Neutral-buffered formalin (NBF): 1%.

RBCs: M+N–, M+N+, and M–N+ phenotypes; washed three times with saline.

Note: An aliquot of these same RBCs not subjected to formalin treatment should be saved for the purpose of control tests.

Quality Control

Test a known example of anti-N$_{form}$ against treated and untreated RBCs when available.

Test untreated control RBCs in parallel with the treated RBCs.

Procedure

Use the following steps to perform the procedure:

Step	Action
1.	Mix 0.2 mL of NBF with 0.1 mL of each RBC sample.
2.	Incubate at 37 C for 15 minutes.
3.	Wash the RBCs three times with saline.
4.	Resuspend the formalin-treated RBCs to a 3%-5% suspension with saline and store at 4 C.
5.	Prepare serial twofold dilutions of the test serum in saline. The dilution range should be from 1:2 to 1:4096 (12 tubes), and the volumes prepared should be not less than 1 mL.
6.	Prepare serial twofold dilutions of a known example of anti-N$_{form}$ as in Step 5.
7.	Place 3 drops of each dilution into each of 6 labeled 10 or 12 × 75-mm test tubes.
8.	Add 1 drop of formalin-treated M+N– RBCs to 1 tube of each serum dilution. Similarly, test each dilution against the other 2 formalin-treated RBC samples and the untreated samples.
9.	Gently agitate the contents of each tube and incubate at RT for 1 hour.
10.	Centrifuge as for hemagglutination tests.
11.	Examine the RBCs macroscopically; grade and record the results.
12.	Interpret the reactions as follows: <table><tr><th>If...</th><th>Then...</th></tr><tr><td>there is a 4-tube higher titration endpoint with formalin-treated RBCs as compared to the titer with untreated RBCs</td><td>results are suggestive of anti-N$_{form}$.</td></tr><tr><td>there is not an increase in reactivity</td><td>the anti-N is unlikely to be anti-N$_{form}$.</td></tr></table>

References   Baker FJ, Silverton RE, Luckcock ED. Introduction to medical technology. 4th ed. London: Butterworths, 1966.

Judd WJ. On the recognition of N-deficient red blood cells and the selection of blood for transfusion to patients with anti-N. Immunohematology 1986;2:49-53.

Effective Date

Approved by:	Printed Name	Signature	Date
Laboratory Management			
Medical Director			
Quality Officer			

VIII-M. Detecting Complement-Fixing Antibodies by a Two-Stage EDTA-IAT

Purpose

To provide instructions for performing a two-stage EDTA-IAT:

- Detection of anti-Jk^a and -Jk^b in stored sera (that might be undetectable).
- Enhancement of the reactivity of other weakly reactive IgG antibodies that can bind C3.

Background Information

Some complement-binding anti-Jk (and presumably complement-binding antibodies of other specificities such as Le) may become undetectable if sera are stored. This loss of reactivity is caused by the formation of anti-complement activity resulting from denaturation of complement components (ie, conversion of C3b to C3c and C3d) upon storage.

To restore antibody reactivity to stored serum, an equal volume of fresh serum may be added. Alternatively, the following procedure (which uses EDTA to destroy the anticomplement properties of stored sera) can be useful in restoring antibody reactivity.

Operational Policy

Not applicable.

Limitations

Unwanted Negative Reactions:

- Failure to add serum and/or enzyme-treated RBCs.
- Use of anti-IgG contaminated with bacteria, foreign matter, the contents of other reagent vials, or human serum.
- Incorrect centrifugation of tests.
- Failure to wash RBCs free of unbound globulins.
- Failure to add active AHG.

Sample Requirements

Test serum: 2 mL.

Judd's Methods in Immunohematology
Detecting Complement-Fixing Antibodies by a Two-Stage EDTA-IAT
Page 2 of 3

Equipment/ Materials

Pipettors with disposable tips to deliver 250 µL (eg, VWR, Batavia, IL).

AHG: polyspecific.

K_2EDTA: 4.45% wt/vol.

Human complement: freshly collected, normal human serum known to lack unexpected antibodies; 2 mL.

RBCs: 2% suspensions of phenotyped allogeneic group O RBC samples, plus the autologous RBCs (to serve as an autocontrol).

Sheep RBCs: available in most clinical immunology laboratories, or obtain commercially (eg, Pel-Freez Biologicals, Rogers, AR).

Quality Control

Confirm all negative reactions with IgG-coated RBCs (see Step 9 below).

Demonstrate that EDTA solution inhibits lysis between human complement and sheep RBCs.

Procedure

Use the following steps to perform the procedure:

Step	Action
1.	Mix 250 µL of EDTA with 2 mL of the serum under investigation. Incubate at RT for 15 minutes.
2.	For each RBC sample to be tested, mix 3 drops of test serum and 1 drop of RBCs in appropriately labeled 10 or 12 × 75-mm test tubes.
3.	Incubate at 37 C for 30-60 minutes.
4.	Wash the RBCs four times with saline and completely decant the final wash supernate.
5.	To the dry RBC buttons thus obtained, add 3 drops of human complement.
6.	Incubate at 37 C for 15-20 minutes.
7.	Wash the RBCs four times with saline and completely decant the final wash supernate.
8.	To the dry RBC buttons thus obtained, add AHG according to the manufacturer's directions: • Mix and centrifuge as for hemagglutination tests. • Examine the RBCs macroscopically for agglutination and hemolysis. • Grade and record the results.

9.	Add 1 drop of IgG-coated RBCs to all tubes with negative antiglobulin results: • Mix and centrifuge. • Dislodge the cell buttons gently. • Examine macroscopically for agglutination. • Grade and record the results.	
10.	Interpret the reactions of the IgG-coated RBCs as follows:	
	If agglutination is...	**Then...**
	present	test is complete.
	absent	test is invalid: • Repeat Steps 1-9. • Consider cell washer problem or inactive AHG.

References

Issitt PD. Applied blood group serology. 3rd ed. Miami, FL: Montgomery Scientific Publications, 1985.

Issitt PD, Smith TR. Evaluation of antiglobulin reagents. In: Myhre BA, ed. A seminar on performance evaluation. Washington, DC: AABB, 1976:25-73.

Polley MJ, Mollison PL. The role of complement in the detection of blood group antibodies with special reference to the antiglobulin test. Transfusion 1961;1:9-22.

Effective Date

Approved by:

	Printed Name	Signature	Date
Laboratory Management			
Medical Director			
Quality Officer			

Appendix VIII-1. Evaluation of Initial Antibody Identification Panel

When...	And autocontrol is...	Then antibody(ies) most likely present is/are...
some panel cells are positive at any phase of testing	negative	single or multiple antibodies.
all panel cells are equally positive (2 to 4+) in the IAT	negative	an antibody to a high-prevalence antigen.
all panel cells are weakly positive (2+) in the IAT with variable reactivity	negative	Knops antibody, anti-Yt^a, anti-JMH, or anti-Ch/Rg.
all panel cells are positive	strongly positive (3 to 4+)	warm autoantibody.
all panel cells are positive, or some positive, some negative	weakly positive (2+)	multiple antibodies, in a patient experiencing a delayed transfusion reaction.
all panel cells are negative	negative	an antibody directed against a low-prevalence antigen.
all panel cells are equally positive (1 to 4+) at IS and negative or weaker at 37 C and IAT	negative or positive	cold-reactive autoantibody (anti-I, -IH).

Appendix VIII-2. Approaches to Identify/Confirm Antibody Specificity

Anti-	Approach	Procedure
Ch/Rg	• Destroy with proteases • Enhance with C4d-coated RBCs • Adsorb with C4-coated RBCs	• II-C • IX-C • IX-E
Do	Enhance with proteases or PEG	III-D, III-G, II-G
Fy	Destroy with proteases	II-C
H	Inhibit with H secretor saliva	VIII-J
HLA	Test with chloroquine-treated RBCs	IX-D
Jk	• Enhance with proteases, LISS-Ficin, or PEG, or • Enhance by two-stage EDTA-antiglobulin test	• II-C, II-F, II-G • VIII-M
JMH	Destroy with proteases and AET	II-C, VII-G
KEL	Destroy with AET/DTT	VII-G, VII-H
Kn	Destroy with AET/DTT	VII-G, VII-H
Le	Inhibit with saliva containing Le^a and/or Le^b	VIII-J
Lu	Destroy with trypsin/chymotrypsin and AET	VII-G, III-G, III-J, III-B
M	• Enhance by acidification • Destroy with proteases	• VIII-G • II-C
McC	Destroy with AET/DTT	VII-G, VII-H
N	• Destroy with proteases • Enhance Nform if patient on renal dialysis • Test for 'N' if patient is Black	• II-C • VIII-L • VIII-I
P_1	Inhibit with soluble P1 substance	VIII-J
Rg	• Destroy with proteases • Enhance with C4d-coated RBCs • Adsorb with C4-coated RBCs	• II-C • IX-C • IX-E
S	• Destroy with proteases • Destroy with NaClO	• III-D, III-G • VII-I
Sd^a	Inhibit with Sd(a+) urine	VIII-J
Yk^a	Destroy with AET/DTT	VII-G, VII-H
Yt^a	• Destroy with proteases • Destroy with AET	• II-C • VII-G

Section IX. Investigating Antibodies to High-Prevalence Antigens

The procedures used in this section are designed to aid in characterizing antibodies to high-prevalence antigens (see Tables IX-1 and IX-2 and Fig IX-1) and, in some instances, will serve to assist in the recognition of concomitant antibodies. These procedures are to be considered adjuncts to the antibody identification procedures described in Sections II and VIII. Tables IX-1 and IX-2 summarize the expected serologic reactions of many antibodies to high-prevalence antigens. The sources in Suggested Reading list provide additional information.

General Comments

It is difficult to recommend a single pathway for the identification of antibodies to high-prevalence antigens. Identification often requires access to rare reagent RBC samples and known examples of the corresponding antibodies. These resources are generally available in an immunohematology reference laboratory; however, use of a logical and considered approach in a routine blood bank laboratory with more limited resources can often provide clinically useful information. Obviously, before any testing is undertaken, it is important to demonstrate that the autologous control is nonreactive—or mixed-field, should the patient have been recently transfused (see Fig VIII-A-1 and VIII-A-2). When the autocontrol is nonreactive, a "shotgun" approach is often used, entailing testing the antibody against a battery of rare phenotypes while simultaneously testing the patient's RBCs with antisera to high-prevalence antigens. However, such an approach is time consuming and sometimes unfruitful. Before any investigation is undertaken, it is advisable to consider the following points, which can be helpful in guiding the investigation:

1) Consider the ABO phenotype of the antibody producer:

    a) Anti-H and -HI are seen in A_1 and A_1B individuals; are less common among A_2, B, and A_2B individuals; and are uncommon in O and A_2 individuals. They may initially present as antibodies to high-prevalence antigens because, unless otherwise indicated, all group O reagent RBCs will have strong expression of H and I antigens; ABO-identical RBCs usually will be compatible at 37 C and by the indirect antiglobulin technique.

    b) The rare O_h (Bombay) phenotype may present as an apparent group O with a direct agglutinin in the serum that is not an autoantibody.

2) Phenotype the autologous RBCs for Rh (C, c, D, E, and e); M, N, S, and s; K; Fy^a and Fy^b; and Jk^a and Jk^b. When an agglutinating antibody is present, phenotyping for Le^a and Le^b, and P_1 can also be helpful. Not only does this identify which antibodies to common antigens the patient can produce but also Rh phenotyping serves to recognize uncommon (eg, R_2R_2 and rare Rh-deletion) phenotypes. With these points in mind:

    a) Consider anti-e, -Hr$_o$, -Rh17, -Rh29, etc.

    b) Test for Ss and Fy antigens to recognize people of African ethnicity who may make anti-U or other antibodies to high-prevalence antigens that may be absent on RBCs from individuals of this ethnic group (eg, anti-Js^b, -Hy, -At^a, or -Cr^a).

c) Test for k if RBCs are K+.

d) When Le^a and Le^b are absent from the RBCs, consider anti-Le^a/Le^{bH}/H/HI.

e) Consider the rare p phenotype if the RBCs are nonreactive with anti-P$_1$, and a direct agglutinin that is not an autoantibody is present.

3) Check the race of the antibody producer; if of African ethnicity, proceed as in 2b, above.

4) Test serum with enzyme-treated and chemically modified RBCs as described in Section III. Use "phenotypically matched" RBCs, as determined in 2 above, for these studies.

5) Perform extended phenotyping with rare antisera before thawing rare RBCs for serum testing.

6) To conserve time and resources, consider using a panel of "null" RBCs as an initial screen for specificity; include phenotypes such as Rh$_{null}$, K$_o$, Lu(a–b–); p; and O$_h$.

The Use of Proteases and Reducing Agents in Antibody Identification

The biochemical nature of the glycolipids and glycoproteins that carry blood group antigens is well understood. This knowledge can be incorporated into any approach to resolving investigations of antibodies to high-prevalence antigens. Testing a patient's plasma with aliquots of test RBCs treated either with a commonly used protease such as ficin (or papain) or with 200 mM dithiothreitol (DTT) can give a pattern of reactivity that is highly predictive of the blood group specificity (see Table IX-1). In yet other studies, purified enzymes can be used to selectively cleave blood group antigens. Loss of reactivity with RBCs treated with some enzymes but not others again provides clues to the antibody's specificity. See Section III and Table IX-2. Although the cost, preparation, and quality control of these reagents may appear burdensome at first glance, the time saved by the rapid resolution of investigations of antibodies to high-prevalence antigens ("nuisance" antibodies in particular) as well as the savings in rare reagent RBCs and antisera—not to mention staff frustration—make them worthwhile.

Serologically Difficult Antibodies with Limited Clinical Relevance

Some of the antibodies that are the most serologically difficult to identify are those with the least clinical significance. These include antibodies to Knops antigens and anti-Cs^a, -Ch, -Rg, -Yt^a, and anti-JMH. Characteristically, these antibodies react at high serum dilutions, but the observed reactions are usually ≤2+ with undiluted serum. (In contrast, other undiluted alloantibodies reacting 2+ in antiglobulin tests (eg, anti-D, -K, -Fy^a) usually have titers less than 8.) The antibodies may also demonstrate variable reactivity with the antibody identification panel RBCs and are often poorly reactive with cord RBCs. These antibodies are considered "nuisance" antibodies because they often take considerable time to identify but, with the exception of some anti-Yt^a, rarely, if ever, cause significant RBC destruction.

The Knops antigens are determinants on complement receptor 1 (CR1, C3b/C4b receptor), a glycoprotein that is involved in the clearance of immune complexes. The expression of Knops antigens varies from one person to another. Furthermore, patients whose blood is hemolyzing, or who are complement deficient for some other reason, may type as antigen negative. The Cs^a antigen, although not part of the Knops system, shows a phenotypic association with these antigens.

The Ch and Rg antigens are defined by polymorphisms on C4, the fourth component of human complement, which is deposited on the RBCs under normal physiological conditions. Thus, anti-Ch and anti-Rg react with the small amount of C4 present on normal RBCs. Moreover, this involvement with C4 facilitates recognition of anti-Ch and -Rg through the use of RBCs coated with excess C4 under low-ionic conditions in vitro or by inhibition with plasma or serum containing C4 from normal Ch+, Rg+ individuals.

Titration tests are widely used to differentiate these nuisance antibodies from alloantibodies with a greater potential to cause immune hemolysis. However, it should be noted that not all antibodies with the above specificities are necessarily of high titer, and other, potentially more clinically significant antibodies (eg, anti-Hy) may sometimes manifest similar characteristics.

Suggested Reading

Daniels G. Effect of enzymes on and chemical modifications of high-frequency red cell antigens. Immunohematology 1992;8:53-7.

Garratty G. Evaluating the clinical significance of blood group alloantibodies that are causing problems in pretransfusion testing. Vox Sang 1998;74(Suppl 2):285-90.

Giles C. Serologically difficult red cell antibodies with special reference to Chido and Rodgers blood groups. In: Mohn JK, ed; International Convocation on Immunology (5th:1976:Buffalo); State University of New York at Buffalo; Center for Immunology. Human blood groups. Basel; New York: Karger, 1977.

Reid ME, Lomas-Francis C. Blood group antigen factsbook. 2nd ed. San Diego, CA: Academic Press, 2004.

Rolih SD, ed. High-titer, low avidity antibodies: Recognition and resolution. Washington, DC: AABB, 1979.

Storry JR. A review: Modification of the red blood cell membrane and its application in blood group serology. Immunohematology 2000;16:101-4.

Table IX-1. Effect of Papain and Thiol Reagents on Reactions of Antibodies to High-Prevalence RBC Antigens

Papain	200 mM DTT/AET	Possible Specificity
0	+	MNS, Ge, Fy, Xg^a, Ch/Rg
0	0	In, JMH
+	+/w	Cromer, Knops, Lu, Do, AnWj, Raph
+/0	0	Yt
+	0	Kell, LW, Sc
+	+	ABO, P$_1$, Rh, Le, Jk, Fy3, Di, Co, Ge3, Ok^a, Ii, P, At^a, Cs^a, Emm, Er^a, Jr^a, Lan, Sd^a, PEL, MAM, ABTI
+	+/0	Vel
+	++	Kx

DTT = dithiothreitol; AET = 2-aminoethylisothiouronium bromide hydrobromide; 0 = antibody nonreactive; + = antibody reactive; +/w = some examples reactive, others show weakened reactions (weak antibodies may be nonreactive); +/0 = some examples reactive, others nonreactive; ++ = enhanced reactivity.

Table IX-2. Effects of Enzymes and Chemicals on Reactions of Antibodies to High-Prevalence RBC Antigens

Anti-	Enzyme/Chemical						Anti-	Enzyme/Chemical					
	TRY	CHY	PAP	PRO	NEU	DTT		TRY	CHY	PAP	PRO	NEU	DTT
ABTI	+	+	+	+	+	+	Kn[a]	0	0	+	+	+	0
AnWj	+	+	+	+	+	+	Kp[b]	+	+/w	+	+	+	0
At[a]	+	+	+	+	+	+	KTIM	+	+/w	+	+	+	0
Ch	0	0	0	0	+	+	Ku	+	w	+	+	+	0
Co3	+	+	+	+	+	+	Kx	+	+	+	+	+	+
Co[a]	+	+	+	+	+	+	Lan	+	+	+	+	+	+
Cr[a]	+	0	+	+	+	w	Lu3	0	0	+	0	+	0
CRAM	+	0	+	+	+	w	Lu4	0	0	+	0	+	0
CROV	+	0	+	+	+	w	Lu5	0	0	+	0	+	0
Cs[a]	+	+	+	+	+	+	Lu6	0	0	+	0	+	0
Di[b]	+	+	+	+	+	+	Lu8	0	0	0	0	+	0
Dr[a]	+	0	+	+	+	w	Lu12	0	0	+	0	+	0
Emm	+	+	+	+	+	+	Lu13	0	0	+	0	+	0
En[a]FR	+	+	+	+	+	+	Lu14	0	0	+	0	+	0
En[a]FS	+	+	0	0	+	+	Lu17	0	0	+	0	+	0
En[a]TS	0	+	0	0	+/0	+	Lu20	0	0	+	0	+	0
Er[a]	+	+	+	+	+	+	Lu21	0	0	+	0	+	0
Es[a]	+	0	+	+	+	w	Lu[b]	0	0	+	0	+	0
Fy3	+	+	+	+	+	+	Luke	+	+	+	+	+	+
Fy6	+	0	0	0	+	+	LW[a]	+	w	+	0	+	0
Ge2	0	w	0	0	+/0	+	LW[ab]	+	w	+	0	+	0
Ge3	0	+	+	0	+	+	MAM	+	+	+	+	+	+
Ge4	0	+	0	0	+	+	McC[a]	0	0	+/0	w	+	0
GIL	+	+	+	+	+	+	MER2	0	0	+	0	+	w
GUTI	+	0	+	+	+	w	Ok[a]	+	+	+	+	+	+
Gy[a]	w	+	+	w	+	w	RAZ	+	+/w	+	+	+	0
H	+	+	+	+	+	+	P	+	+	+	+	+	+
Hy	+	+	+	+	+	w	PEL	+	+	+	+	+	+
I	+	+	+	+	+	+	Rg	0	0	0	0	+	+
i	+	+	+	+	+	+	Rh17	+	+	+	+	+	+
IFC	+	0	+	+	+	w	Rh29	+	+	+	+	+	+
In[b]	0	0	0	0	+	0	Sc1	+	+	+	0	+	+
INFI	0	0	0	0	+	0	Sc3	+	+	+	0	+	+
INJA	0	0	0	0	+	0	SCER	+	+	+	0	+	+
JK3	+	+	+	+	+	+	SCAN	+	+	+	0	+	+
JMH	0	0	0	+/0	+	0	SERF	+	0	+	+	+	w
Jo[a]	0	w	+	w	+	+/0	STAR	+	+	+	0	+	+
Jr[a]	+	+	+	+	+	+	Tc[a]	+	0	+	+	+	w
Js[b]	+	*+/w	+	+	+	0	TOU	+	+/0	+	+	+	0
k	+	+/w	+	+	+	0	U	+	+	+	+	+	+
K11	+	+/w	+	+	+	0	UMC	+	0	+	+	+	w
K12	+	+/w	+	+	+	0	Vel	+	+	+	+	+	+
K13	+	+/w	+	+	+	0	Wes[b]	+	0	+	0	+	w
K14	+	+/w	+	+	+	0	Wr[b]	+	+	+	+	+	+
K18	+	+/w	+	+	+	0	Xg[a]	0	0	0	0	+	+
K19	+	+/w	+	+	+	0	Yk[a]	0	0	+	+	0	0
K22	+	+/w	+	+	+	0	Yt[a]	+	0	0	0	+	0
KALT	+	+/w	+	+	+	0	ZENA	+	0	+	+	+	w

TRY = trypsin-treated RBCs; CHY = chymotrypsin-treated RBCs; PAP = papain- or ficin-treated RBCs; PRO = pronase-treated RBCs; NEU = neuraminidase-treated RBCs; DTT = RBCs treated with dithiothreitol or 2-aminoethylisothiouronium bromide hydrobromide (AET); + = antibody reactive; 0 = antibody nonreactive; w = reactions weakened (weak antibodies may be nonreactive); +/0 = some examples reactive, others nonreactive; +/w = some examples reactive, others show weakened reactions.

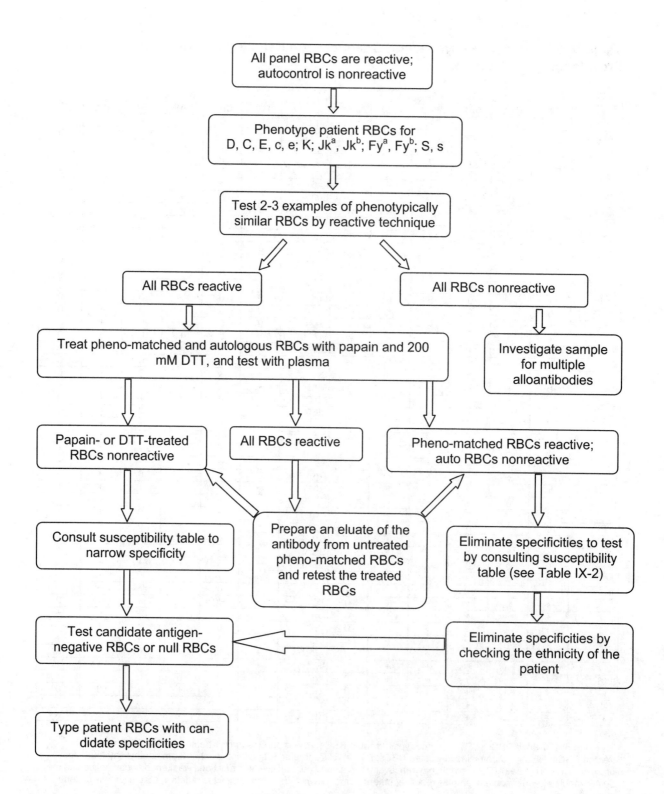

Figure IX-1. Investigation of antibodies to high-prevalence antigens.

IX-A. Inhibiting Antibodies with Pooled Plasma or Serum

Purpose

To provide instructions for the inhibition of blood group antibodies by soluble plasma antigens:

- Inhibition of antibodies to high-prevalence antigens in the Cromer blood group system.

Background Information

Anti-Ch and anti-Rg, which are directed against polymorphisms on the C4 component of human complement, are inhibited by plasma or serum containing C4 from Ch+, Rg+ individuals. This procedure may be used for the identification of anti-Ch and anti-Rg and may permit recognition of other, concomitant antibodies in sera containing anti-Ch or anti-Rg.

Antigens of the Cromer blood group system are carried on decay accelerating factor (DAF, or CD55), which is present in plasma/serum. This procedure can also be used in the identification and investigation of antibodies to Cromer antigens.

Operational Policy

A pool of at least 6 donor plasma samples should be used to ensure that Ch and Rg antigens are well represented.

Use 6% BSA as a dilution control.

Limitations

Unwanted Positive Reactions:

- Antibodies to leukocyte antigens (eg, anti-Bg^a) may also be partially inhibited by plasma.

Unwanted Negative Reactions:

- A test component has been omitted.
- The plasma pool is Ch/Rg negative.

Sample Requirements

Plasma: 1 mL.

Equipment/ Materials

AHG: polyspecific or anti-IgG.

6% BSA.

pH 7.3 PBS.

Normal plasma: pooled from 6 or more samples known to lack unexpected antibodies.

Group O reagent RBCs: 3%-5% suspensions from previously tested samples. Select three samples based on the strength of observed reactions (eg, 2+, 1+, and ±).

Pipettors with disposable tips to deliver 0.3 mL to 1 mL (eg, VWR, Batavia, IL).

Quality Control

Perform parallel titrations of patient's plasma/serum with 6% BSA as a negative (dilution) control.

Confirm all negative reactions with IgG-coated RBCs.

Procedure

Use the following steps to perform the procedure:

Step	Action
1.	Prepare serial twofold dilutions of test plasma in pH 7.3 PBS. The dilution range should be from 1 in 2 to 1 in 4096 (12 tubes), and the volumes prepared should not be less than 0.3 mL for each RBC sample to be tested.
2.	For each RBC sample to be tested, place 2 or 3 drops of each dilution into 2 appropriately labeled 10 or 12 × 75-mm test tubes.
3.	To 1 tube, add 2 or 3 drops of pooled plasma.
4.	To the other tube, add 2 or 3 drops of 6% BSA.
5.	Gently agitate the contents of each tube and incubate at RT for at least 30 minutes.
6.	Add 1 drop of 3% RBCs to each tube.
7.	Gently agitate the contents of each tube and incubate at 37 C for 1 hour.
8.	Wash the RBCs three to four times with saline and completely decant the final wash supernate.
9.	To the dry RBC buttons, add AHG and centrifuge according to the manufacturer's directions.
10.	Examine the RBCs for agglutination; grade and record the results.

11.	Interpret the reactions as follows:	
	If…	**Then…**
	the titration endpoint for both plasma and 6% BSA series is the same (±1 tube)	no inhibition has occurred.
	the titration endpoint for the plasma series is >2 tubes shorter than the 6% BSA series	specific inhibition of the patient's antibody has occurred.
	the titration endpoint for the 6% BSA series is >2 tubes shorter than the plasma series	no blood-group-specific inhibition has occurred. The patient's plasma may contain additional antibodies to caprylate.
12.	Add IgG-coated RBCs to all negative tests. Centrifuge and examine the tests macroscopically for mixed-field agglutination. Repeat tests when tests with IgG-coated RBCs are nonreactive.	

Reference Reid ME, Lomas-Francis C. Blood group antigen factsbook. 2nd ed. San Diego, CA: Academic Press, 2004.

Effective Date

Approved by:

	Printed Name	Signature	Date
Laboratory Management			
Medical Director			
Quality Officer			

IX-B. Identifying Anti-Ch/Rg: Rapid Procedure

Purpose

To provide instructions for coating RBCs in vitro with C4d for the rapid detection of Ch/Rg antibodies.

Background Information

Anti-Ch and anti-Rg are directed against polymorphisms on the C4d fragment of human complement. These antibodies usually react only weakly in antiglobulin tests with the trace amount of C4d present on normal RBCs. However, they cause direct agglutination of RBCs coated in vitro with excess C4d. Such RBCs are prepared by incubation of Ch+, Rg+ plasma in a low-ionic medium containing EDTA. Under these conditions, C4b is bound nonimmunologically to RBCs. The bound C4b is converted to C4d by trypsin treatment of the coated RBCs.

Operational Policy

Do not refreeze enzyme solutions.

Limitations

Unwanted Positive Reactions:

- AHG contains anti-C3d.

- Washing of antiglobulin tests was insufficient.

Unwanted Negative Reactions:

- RBCs were insufficiently coated with C4.

- Enzyme treatment was ineffective.

Sample Requirements

Serum/plasma suspected to contain anti-Ch/Rg: 0.3 mL.

Equipment/ Materials

Anti-Ch or -Rg, as a control reagent.

AHG: anti-IgG; need not be heavy-chain specific.

RBCs: coated with C4b by incubation of whole blood with sucrose/EDTA (see Section VII) and subsequent treatment with trypsin to convert to C4d-coated RBCs (see Section III); store in Alsever's solution at 4 C. Coated RBCs may also be frozen (see Section VII).

Note: Prepare trypsin-treated RBCs from the same donor used for C4 coating, but do not subject these RBCs to prior treatment with sucrose/EDTA.

Quality Control

Test known anti-Ch or anti-Rg in parallel with the test sample. Expected reactions with C4d-coated RBCs are ≥2+ by direct agglutination and 3+ to 4+ with anti-IgG, with negative or weak (1+) reactions with trypsin-treated control RBCs.

Confirm all negative reactions with IgG-coated RBCs.

Procedure

Use the following steps to perform the procedure:

Step	Action
1.	Mix 2 drops of test serum with 1 drop of C4d-coated RBCs.
2.	Similarly test the non-C4-coated, trypsin-treated (control) RBCs.
3.	Incubate at RT for 5 minutes.
4.	Centrifuge as for hemagglutination tests.
5.	Examine the RBCs macroscopically; grade and record the results.
6.	Interpret the reactions as follows:

If agglutination is…	Then…
present with C4d-coated RBCs but absent with trypsin-treated control RBCs	result is positive.
absent with both C4d-coated and control RBCs	result is negative.
present with both C4d-coated and trypsin-treated RBCs	result is caused by anti-trypsin or other alloantibodies.

Step	Action
7.	Wash the RBCs three to four times with saline and completely decant the final wash supernate.
8.	To the dry RBC buttons, add anti-IgG and centrifuge according to the manufacturer's directions.
9.	Examine the RBCs macroscopically; grade and record the results.

10.	Interpret the reactions as follows:	
	If agglutination is...	**Then...**
	present with C4d-coated RBCs but absent with trypsin-treated control RBCs	result is positive.
	absent with both C4d-coated and control RBCs	result is negative.
	present with both C4d-coated and trypsin-treated RBCs	result is caused by anti-trypsin or other alloantibodies.
11.	Add IgG-coated RBCs to all negative tests. Centrifuge and examine the tests macroscopically for mixed-field agglutination. Repeat when tests with IgG-coated RBCs are nonreactive.	

Reference

Judd WJ, Kraemer K, Moulds JJ. The rapid identification of Chido and Rodgers antibodies using C4d-coated red blood cells. Transfusion 1981;21:189-92.

Effective Date

Approved by:	Printed Name	Signature	Date
Laboratory Management			
Medical Director			
Quality Officer			

IX-C. Recognizing Antibodies To HLA Determinants

Purpose

To provide a method for stripping residual HLA antigens from RBCs using chloroquine diphosphate.

Background Information

Chloroquine diphosphate can be used to strip HLA antigens from platelets and neutrophils without removing neutrophil- and platelet-specific antigens. The same applies to RBCs; antibodies to HLA A2, A28, B7, B15, B17, and others may react with RBCs that express the corresponding HLA antigen. The same RBCs are nonreactive following exposure to chloroquine diphosphate, whereas erythrocyte blood group antigens are unaffected. Although the mechanism by which chloroquine diphosphate removes HLA determinants from cells is not known, this procedure can be used to verify that RBC incompatibility is caused by HLA antibodies and may help in antibody identification tests with sera containing multispecific antibodies.

Operational Policy

Not applicable.

Limitations

Unwanted Positive Reactions:

• The treatment was not performed correctly.

Unwanted Negative Reactions:

• Antigen-negative RBCs were selected for treatment.

• Tests were not washed sufficiently.

• Serum/plasma was omitted inadvertently.

Sample Requirements

Plasma/serum suspected to contain antibodies to HLA antigens: 2 mL.

Equipment/ Materials

AHG: polyspecific or anti-IgG.

22% or 30% BSA.

Chloroquine diphosphate: 20% wt/vol.

IgG-coated RBCs: see Section VII, or obtain commercially.

Antigen-positive RBCs for chloroquine treatment: 0.1 mL packed, pheno-typed, homologous group O RBC samples (ie, those used for antibody detection/identification; washed three times before use.

Untreated control RBCs: 3%-5% suspensions in saline or commercially prepared diluent.

Quality Control

Test a known example of HLA antibody (eg, anti-Bg), if available, in parallel with the serum under investigation.

Confirm all negative reactions with IgG-coated RBCs.

Procedure

Use the following steps to perform the procedure:

Step	Action
1.	In appropriately labeled 10 or 12 × 75-mm test tubes, mix 0.1 mL of each RBC sample to be treated with 0.4 mL of chloroquine diphosphate.
2.	Incubate at RT for 90 minutes.
3.	Wash the RBCs three times and dilute to a 3%-5% suspension with saline. Label to indicate treatment with chloroquine diphosphate.
4.	For each RBC sample to be tested (treated and untreated), mix 3 drops of test serum, 2 drops of BSA, and 1 drop of RBCs in appropriately labeled 10 or 12 × 75-mm test tubes.
5.	Incubate at 37 C for 30 minutes.
6.	Wash the RBCs three to four times with saline and completely decant the final wash supernate.
7.	To the dry RBC buttons, add AHG and centrifuge according to the manufacturer's directions.
8.	Examine the RBCs macroscopically; grade and record the results.

9.	Interpret the reactions as follows:	
	If agglutination is...	**Then...**
	present with both treated and untreated RBCs	the antibody is not directed at an HLA antigen.
	absent with treated RBCs but positive with the untreated control RBCs	an HLA antibody is present.
10.	Add IgG-coated RBCs to all negative tests. Centrifuge and examine the tests macroscopically for mixed-field agglutination. Repeat when tests with IgG-coated RBCs are nonreactive.	

Reference Swanson J, Sastamoinen R. Chloroquine stripping of HLA A,B antigens from red cells (letter). Transfusion 1985;25:439-40.

Effective Date

Approved by:	Printed Name	Signature	Date
Laboratory Management			
Medical Director			
Quality Officer			

Judd's Methods in Immunohematology
Using Allogeneic C4 for Adsorption of Anti-Ch/Rg
Page 1 of 3

IX-D. Using Allogeneic C4 for Adsorption of Anti-Ch/Rg

Purpose

To provide instructions for the adsorption of anti-Ch/Rg from patient plasma using autologous RBCs coated with C4 from inert allogeneic plasma.

Background Information

Anti-Ch and anti-Rg are directed against C4, the fourth component of human complement. Large amounts of C4 can be bound to RBCs by incubation of RBCs with normal plasma under low-ionic conditions. In this procedure, allogeneic C4 is used to coat autologous RBCs from patients with anti-Ch and -Rg. These RBCs are used to adsorb the anti-Ch/Rg and permit recognition of other, concomitant alloantibodies.

Operational Policy

Adsorption studies should be performed after the plasma antibody has been identified to be either anti-Ch or anti-Rg.

Limitations

Unwanted Positive Reactions:

- Antibody specificity is not directed against Ch/Rg antigens.

- Coating plasma is Ch/Rg negative.

- Plasma specificity is directed against a Ch/Rg antigen variant lacking in the coating plasma.

- Autologous RBCs are coated incompletely with C4.

Unwanted Negative Reactions:

- The patient's plasma has been diluted during the adsorption procedure.

Sample Requirements

Test serum containing anti-Ch/Rg: 2 mL.

**Equipment/
Materials**

Autologous RBCs: washed three times with saline; 2 mL.

Ch+, Rg+ plasma: from anticoagulated (ACD, CPD, or CPD-A1) whole blood known to lack unexpected antibodies.

Known anti-Ch or anti-Rg, if available.

Protein refractometer (eg, #47752-872, VWR, Batavia, IL).

Sucrose/EDTA.

**Quality
Control**

Test known anti-Ch or anti-Rg, against the C4-coated RBCs to demonstrate coating with C4. See Procedure IX-B for details.

Using a refractometer, measure the protein content of the adsorbed and unadsorbed serum. The adsorption process should not have lowered the protein content by more than 20% of the total protein in the unadsorbed sample.

Procedure

Use the following steps to perform the procedure:

Step	Action
1.	Divide the RBCs into 1-mL aliquots and dispense into 16 × 100-mm test tubes.
2.	Add 1 mL of plasma and 10 mL of sucrose/EDTA to each tube.
3.	Mix well and incubate at 37 C for 15 minutes.
4.	Wash the RBCs four times with saline.
5.	Transfer the RBCs into a 13 × 100-mm test tube and centrifuge to pack the RBCs ($\geq$1000 × g for at least 5 minutes); discard the supernate. The RBCs are now coated with C4.
6.	To 1 tube of C4-coated RBCs, add 2 mL of serum to be adsorbed.
7.	Incubate at 37 C for 1 hour.
8.	Centrifuge to pack the RBCs ($\geq$1000 × g for at least 5 minutes) and transfer the supernate to the second tube of C4-coated RBCs.
9.	Incubate at 37 C for 1 hour.
10.	Centrifuge to pack the RBCs and transfer the adsorbed serum into a clean test tube.
11.	Test by the saline-antiglobulin technique described in Section II.

12.	Examine the RBCs macroscopically; grade and record the results.	
13.	Interpret the reactions as follows:	
	If agglutination is…	**Then…**
	present	the plasma most likely contains an additional alloantibody: • Proceed with routine antibody identification (Section VIII) using the adsorbed plasma.
	absent	proceed to Step 14.
14.	Add IgG-coated RBCs to all negative tests. Centrifuge and examine the tests macroscopically for mixed-field agglutination.	
15.	Interpret the reactions as follows:	
	If agglutination is…	**Then…**
	present	the plasma does not contain additional alloantibodies.
	absent	the result is invalid: • Repeat the IAT.

Reference   Ellisor SS, Shoemaker MM, Reid ME. Absorption of anti-Chido from serum using autologous red blood cells coated with homologous C4. Transfusion 1982;22:243-5.

Effective Date

Approved by:	Printed Name	Signature	Date
Laboratory Management			
Medical Director			
Quality Officer			

IX-E. Using 2 M Urea for the Screening/Confirmation of Jk(a–b–) RBCs

Purpose

To provide instructions for using 2 M urea to screen for and identify Jk(a–b–) phenotype RBCs.

Background Information

The Jk antigens are carried on the RBC urea transporter. RBCs that lack the urea transporter have the Jk(a–b–) phenotype and are resistant to lysis by 2 M urea. This phenotype is found in all populations but is more commonly found in individuals of Polynesian descent and of Finnish descent. Therefore screening donor RBCs with a rapid 2 M urea lysis test in areas where the phenotype is likely is a quick and inexpensive method for identifying these rare donors. The 2 M urea lysis test can also be used to confirm the Jk(a–b–) phenotype.

Operational Policy

Not applicable.

Limitations

Unwanted Positive Reactions:

- The urea concentration is incorrect.
- Water was used instead of urea.

Unwanted Negative Reactions:

- PBS was used instead of 2 M urea.

Sample Requirements

Washed RBCs from anticoagulated blood samples, resuspended to 2% in PBS.

Equipment/ Materials

Control Jk(a–b–) and Jk(a+b+) RBCs, suspended to 2% in PBS.

2 M urea aqueous solution.

Distilled or deionized water.

Spectrophotometer set at 540 nm (optional).

Pipettors with disposable tips to deliver 250 µL and 1 mL volumes (eg, VWR, Batavia, IL).

Quality Control

The procedure includes tests with Jk(a–b–) RBCs.

Confirmation Procedure

Use the following steps to confirm the Jk(a–b–) phenogype:

Step	Action
1.	Dispense 250 µL of control and test RBCs into each of 2 appropriately labeled 12 × 75-mm glass test tubes.
2.	Centrifuge to pack the RBCs, and decant the supernate.
3.	To one tube, add 1 mL of water; to the other tube, add 1 mL 2 M urea.
4.	Mix the contents in each tube and incubate at RT for 2 minutes.
5.	At 2 minutes, centrifuge the tubes to pack any remaining cells.
6.	Transfer an aliquot of each supernate to clean, labeled tubes for visual analysis.
7.	Resuspend the RBCs and allow to stand at RT for 15 minutes.
8.	Centrifuge and transfer the supernates to clean, labeled test tubes for visual analysis.
9.	Evaluate the results as follows:<table><tr><td>**If hemolysis is...**</td><td>**Then...**</td></tr><tr><td>present in the water control but absent with the 2 M urea</td><td>the RBCs lack the urea transporter.</td></tr><tr><td>present in the water control and with 2 M urea</td><td>the RBCs have a functional urea transporter; the Jk(a–b–) phenotype maybe transient.</td></tr></table>
10.	If recording the degree of hemolysis is required, measure the amount of hemolysis in each tube using a spectrophotometer set at 540 nm.
11.	Calculate the percentage of hemolysis, setting the water control as 100%.

Screening Procedure

Use the following steps to screen for the Jk(a–b–) phenotype:

Step	Action
1.	Dispense 250 µL of control and test RBCs into an appropriately labeled 12 × 75-mm glass test tube.
2.	Centrifuge to pack the RBCs, and decant the supernate.
3.	Add 1 mL of 2 M urea to each tube. Mix well and allow to stand at RT for 15 minutes.
4.	Centrifuge to pack the RBCs, and inspect the tubes visually.
5.	Interpret the reactions as follows:

If hemolysis is...	Then...
present	RBCs have a functional urea transporter.
absent	RBCs might lack the urea transporter: • Test RBCs with anti-Jk^a and anti-Jk^b according to local procedure.

References

Edwards-Moulds J, Kasschau MR. The effect of 2 molar urea on Jk(a-b-) red cells. Vox Sanguinis 1988;55:181-5

Edwards-Moulds J, Kasschau MR. Methods for the detection of Jk heterozygotes: Interpretations and applications. Transfusion 1988;28:545-8.

Effective Date

	Printed Name	Signature	Date
Approved by:			
Laboratory Management			
Medical Director			
Quality Officer			

Section X. Prenatal and Perinatal Testing

The procedures described in this section are essential to the appropriate management of hemolytic disease of the fetus and newborn (HDFN) and prevention of RhD alloimmunization during pregnancy. Included are titration tests to determine the titer of potentially harmful alloantibodies, methods to screen for and quantify fetal RBCs in the maternal circulation [as a means of determining the required dose of Rh Immune Globulin (RhIG) to administer to Rh-negative women who deliver Rh-positive infants], and a procedure for measuring bilirubin in amniotic fluid (as a means of predicting the severity of HDFN). Guidelines are given for the extent of required testing during the various stages of pregnancy.

See Suggested Reading at the end of this introduction for a detailed discussion of serologic findings in HDFN.

The following recommendations for prenatal and perinatal testing have been compiled from a publication of the AABB Scientific Section Coordinating Committee.

ABO and Rh Typing

Initial Visit

All women, regardless of the results of tests performed elsewhere, should have blood drawn for serologic testing as early as possible during each pregnancy. This testing should include ABO and RhD typing and tests for unexpected serum antibodies. However, ABO and Rh typing need not be repeated at the initial visit for subsequent pregnancies, provided that the testing facility has records of concordant results on two or more samples obtained on different occasions, and the patient's Rh status is noted on the clinical records for each admission.

Initial Rh testing need not include a test for weak D when direct agglutination tests with anti-D are nonreactive. Patients whose RBCs do not react in direct tests with anti-D can be regarded as Rh-negative and treated as such.

During Pregnancy

Repeat tests for ABO and Rh are recommended for all women during their first pregnancy, ideally at 26 to 28 weeks' gestation, including those that initially type as Rh positive. Otherwise, it is not necessary to repeat ABO or Rh typing during pregnancy, except when pretransfusion tests are requested. Provided that the testing facility has concordant results on two or more samples obtained on different occasions, and the patient's Rh status is noted on the current clinical record, repeat-testing for Rh upon admission for amniocentesis, antepartum RhIG therapy, or abortion is unnecessary.

At Delivery

It is necessary to retest for ABO and Rh at delivery when pretransfusion tests are requested. The Rh type should be determined on all women admitted for delivery. However, unless there is a request for transfusion, Rh testing is not necessary when the testing facility has concordant results on two or more samples obtained on different occasions, and the patient's Rh status is noted on the current clinical record.

Tests for Unexpected Antibodies

Initial Visit

At their first visits to the obstetrician, all pregnant women, regardless of Rh type, should be tested during each pregnancy for unexpected serum antibodies. Antiglobulin testing should be performed with anti-IgG to detect, preferentially, those antibodies with the potential to cause HDFN. The use of enzyme-treated RBCs and/or polyspecific antihuman globulin (AHG) is not advocated.

During Pregnancy: Rh-Negative Patients

At 26 to 28 weeks' gestation, before RhIG is given, samples should be obtained from all Rh-negative women for testing for unexpected antibodies. RhIG need not be withheld pending the results of antibody detection tests.

During Pregnancy: Rh-Positive Patients

Unless pretransfusion tests have been requested or there is a history of significant antibodies, previous blood transfusions, or traumatic deliveries, Rh-positive patients should be screened for antibodies once during pregnancy, at the initial visit.

At Delivery

Antibody detection tests are necessary when pretransfusion tests are requested and when a maternal sample is needed for neonatal pretransfusion testing or investigation for HDFN.

Antibody Identification

All Visits

If test results for unexpected antibodies are positive at any time during pregnancy, the antibody should be identified.

Following RhIG Therapy

It should not be assumed that an antibody present in an Rh-negative woman is anti-D, even following RhIG therapy. In such instances, tests with a limited reagent RBC panel should be performed to exclude the presence of other antibodies.

At Delivery

Antibodies detected at delivery should be identified. If a woman has received RhIG during pregnancy, antibody identification tests may be performed with a limited panel of Rh-negative RBCs to exclude clinically significant antibodies other than D.

Antibody Titration

Initial Visit

Titration of Rh antibodies early in pregnancy is appropriate to ascertain the presence of significant antibody levels that may lead to HDFN and, for low-titer antibodies, to establish a baseline for comparison to titers found later in pregnancy. Titration of non-Rh antibodies should be undertaken only after discussion with the obstetrician regarding the significance of the results. The purpose of titration is not to diagnose HDFN; instead, it is to regulate the use of more definitive studies such as amniotic fluid analysis or measurement of middle cerebral arterial flow by Doppler (MCAD).

During Pregnancy

Repeat-titration of Rh antibodies, at 2 to 4 week intervals after 18 weeks' gestation, is appropriate, provided that the data are used to indicate the need for fetal monitoring by other means (eg, measurement of MCAD or cordocentesis). Once such other means have been applied, no further titrations are warranted. Titration of non-Rh antibodies should be undertaken only after discussion with the obstetrician about how the data will be used in the clinical management of the pregnancy.

At Delivery

Antibodies detected at delivery should not be titrated. In particular, the practice of titrating passive anti-D following antenatal or postpartum RhIG therapy should be discontinued. Rather, anti-D not detected earlier in pregnancy should be assumed to be caused by RhIG therapy until proven otherwise. Evidence for active immunity to D can best be obtained by performing antibody detection tests 6 months after delivery or at the initial visit for the next pregnancy.

RhIG Therapy

First Trimester

Rh-negative women who abort during the first trimester may be treated with a 50-μg dose of RhIG. This is the only situation for which a 50-μg dose is appropriate. Rh-negative women who undergo an invasive procedure during the first trimester, such as chorionic villus sampling (CVS), or who approach miscarriage but the pregnancy continues, should receive a 300-μg dose of RhIG.

Antepartum ≥13 Weeks' Gestation

All Rh-negative women showing no evidence of active immunization to the D antigen should receive a 300-μg dose of RhIG at 26 to 28 weeks' gestation. A 300-μg dose of RhIG should also be administered following trauma, amniocentesis, or any other procedure that could cause fetomaternal hemorrhage (FMH), such as CVS or cordocentesis, unless it can be shown that the fetus is Rh negative.

Note: During the third trimester, there is the potential for excessive FMH (ie, fetal bleeding >15 mL RBCs, requiring treatment with more than a single 300-μg dose of RhIG). Accordingly, the need to quantitate the extent of the FMH, particularly in cases of trauma, should be considered. Also, any woman receiving antepartum RhIG therapy should receive additional 300-μg doses every 12 weeks until delivery; this particularly applies to women who receive RhIG during the first trimester and to women who receive RhIG at 26-28 weeks' gestation but whose pregnancy extends beyond 12 weeks thereafter.

Postpartum ≥13 Weeks' Gestation

Rh-negative women should receive the standard 300-μg dose of RhIG, preferably within 72 hours after delivery or abortion, unless it can be shown that the fetus is Rh negative or the patient has anti-D not related to antenatal RhIG administration. This recommendation applies to all abortions, whether spontaneous or induced.

FMH Testing

When an Rh-positive infant or fetus is delivered beyond 20 weeks' gestation, or if the Rh status of the infant/fetus is not known, the mother, if Rh negative, should be tested for excessive FMH. The test for FMH should not be performed selectively. Ideally, a maternal blood sample should be obtained approximately 1 hour after delivery of an Rh-positive baby to perform a screening test for excessive FMH. Recommended screening tests include the rosette test and the enzyme-linked antiglobulin test (ELAT); microscopic examination of weak D tests is not an acceptable method for the purpose of detecting excessive FMH. If the test result for FMH is positive, the extent of the bleeding should be determined; an ELAT, a Kleihauer-Betke test, or a flow-cytometric procedure is an acceptable quantitative method. After quantifying the hemorrhage, any appropriate additional doses of RhIG should be administered as soon as possible, preferably within 72 hours of delivery.

Cord Blood Testing

All Deliveries

In the absence of clinically significant unexpected antibodies in the maternal serum, no testing of cord blood samples is required except to aid in diagnosis, assist in neonatal care, or determine RhIG candidacy of Rh-negative mothers.

Infants of Rh-Negative Mothers

Blood from infants born to Rh-negative mothers should be tested for RhD. Rh-negative mothers of infants found to be Rh-positive, either by direct or indirect testing (for weak D), are candidates for RhIG therapy, as are women whose infants' Rh status is unknown.

Infants of Mothers with Significant Unexpected Antibodies

ABO and Rh typing and a direct antiglobulin test (DAT) should be performed on cord blood samples from infants of women with clinically significant unexpected antibodies. Routine eluate preparation and testing is not encouraged, provided that confirmatory antibody identification tests were performed on the maternal serum within 72 hours of delivery. When maternal blood is not available, the infant's blood should be used for compatibility testing.

Infants Who Become Jaundiced

In the absence of detectable maternal alloantibodies, serologic studies should focus on establishing an immune basis for jaundice. The differential diagnoses include fetomaternal ABO incompatibility (ABO HDFN) and HDFN caused by antibody to a low-prevalence (paternal) antigen. Other considerations include prematurity, infection, and rare hematologic abnormalities such as hereditary spherocytosis. Serologic investigation can be limited to a DAT and an RBC ABO type on a cord blood sample; a test for unexpected antibodies should be performed if the mother was not tested during pregnancy. The potential for ABO HDFN exists when the infant's ABO type is incompatible with that of the mother, regardless of the DAT result. If no ABO incompatibility exists and the DAT is positive because of IgG coating, testing the maternal serum/plasma, or an eluate from the cord blood sample, against paternal RBCs may be informative.

Reference

Judd WJ, for the 2003-2004 Scientific Section Coordinating Committee. Guidelines for prenatal and perinatal immunohematology. Bethesda, MD: AABB, 2005.

Suggested Reading

Garratty G, ed. Hemolytic disease of the newborn. Arlington, VA: AABB, 1984.

Klein HG, Anstee DJ, eds. Mollison's blood transfusion in clinical medicine. 11th ed. Oxford, UK: Blackwell Publishing, 2005.

Roback J, Combs MR, Grossman B, Hillyer C. Technical manual. 16th ed. Bethesda, MD: AABB, 2008 (or current edition).

X-A. Tests During Pregnancy

Purpose	To provide a process for testing during pregnancy.

Before You Begin

Through laboratory data system, phone, or requisition, obtain:

- Patient's transfusion and pregnancy history.
- Gestational age of current pregnancy.
- Past prenatal/pretransfusion test results.

Sample Requirements

EDTA-anticoagulated or clotted whole blood.

Operational Policy

Use R_2R_2 RBCs when titrating anti-D, -c, and -E; use double-dose RBCs if readily available when titrating other alloantibodies (not for anti-C or anti-K).

Do not titrate anti-D if passive from RhIG therapy.

Do not titrate if critical titer has been reached and HDFN is being monitored by nonserologic means.

If anti-C and anti-D are present, and anti-C titer vs r'r RBCs is greater than or equal to the anti-D titer vs R_2R_2, consider anti-G. For conclusive evidence of anti-G and absence of anti-D, testing vs rare DIIIb RBCs may be required. In the absence of such RBCs, consider RhIG therapy.

Process

Review the stages below to determine the appropriate timing for testing required during pregnancy:

Stage	Description	
1.	Perform ABO and Rh typing according to the following criterion:	
	When...	**Then...**
	ABO and Rh typing is performed at initial visit, ideally during the first trimester	repeat typing: • At 26-28 weeks' gestation. • When pretransfusion tests are requested.

2.	Perform tests for unexpected antibodies according to the following criterion:	
	When...	**Then...**
	tests for unexpected antibodies are performed at initial visit, ideally during the first trimester	repeat tests: • At 26-28 weeks' gestation on Rh– women (optional). • When pretransfusion tests are requested.
3.	Perform antibody identification according to the following criterion:	
	When...	**Then...**
	tests for unexpected antibodies are positive	perform antibody identification: • Upon receipt of samples for titration studies. • When pretransfusion tests are requested.
4.	Perform antibody titration according to the following criterion:	
	When...	**Then...**
	antibodies capable of causing HDFN are identified	perform antibody titration: • At regular intervals after 18 weeks' gestation. • Until critical titer (eg, 8) is reached.

Reference   Judd WJ, for the 2003-2004 Scientific Section Coordinating Committee. Guidelines for prenatal and perinatal immunohematology. Bethesda, MD: AABB, 2005.

**Effective
Date**

Approved by:	Printed Name	Signature	Date
Laboratory Management			
Medical Director			
Quality Officer			

X-B. Rh Immune Globulin Administration

Purpose

To provide a process for administering RhIG during pregnancy and at delivery:

- All pregnant women.

(Also see Fig X-B-1).

Before You Begin

Through requisition or phone, and from records of prenatal tests, obtain:

- Results of direct tests with anti-D.
- Gestational age of current pregnancy.

Sample Requirements

EDTA-anticoagulated or clotted whole blood from mother, preferably collected 1 hour after delivery.

Cord blood sample.

Operational Policy

Both 50-μg and 300-μg doses of RhIG are available. Do not administer the 50-μg dose unless the pregnancy terminates during the first trimester. In all other situations, 300-μg doses are indicated.

Weak expression of D may be indicative of a partial D phenotype. Do not perform a test for weak D unless otherwise stipulated (see Stage 2 below).

Indications for RhIG therapy during pregnancy, or for termination after the first trimester, include amniocentesis, CVS, antepartum hemorrhage, cordocentesis, blunt abdominal trauma, ectopic pregnancy, fetal death, and spontaneous or therapeutic abortion.

Process

Review the stages below to complete the process for determining RhIG candidacy during pregnancy and at delivery:

Stage	Description	
1.	Evaluate the results of prenatal Rh typing according to the following criterion:	
	When...	**Then...**
	reactions with anti-D are ≤1+ by tube or ≤2+ by gel	administer a 300-μg dose of RhIG at 26-28 weeks' gestation.

2.	At delivery, determine RhIG candidacy according to the following criterion:	
	When...	**Then...**
	mother is Rh– by the criterion in Stage 1 and cord blood types as Rh+ **Note:** Test cord blood RBCs for weak expression of D if nonreactive in direct tests with anti-D (see below).	administer a 300-μg dose of RhIG within 72 hours of delivery. perform a rosette test on maternal blood for evidence of FMH in excess of 15 mL of fetal RBCs.
3.	At delivery, quantify FMH according to the following criterion:	
	When...	**Then...**
	cord blood types as Rh+ only in the test for weak D or rosette test is positive	quantify FMH by the Kleihauer-Betke test (see Procedure X-G).
4.	Within 72 hours of delivery, determine RhIG candidacy according to the following criterion:	
	When...	**Then...**
	percentage of fetal RBCs is >0.2%	calculate the number of required doses of RhIG using the following equation: $[(24 \times \% \text{ fetal RBCs}) \div 15] + 1$

Reference

Judd WJ, for the 2003-2004 Scientific Section Coordinating Committee. Guidelines for prenatal and perinatal immunohematology. Bethesda, MD: AABB, 2005.

**Effective
Date**

Approved by:	Printed Name	Signature	Date
Laboratory Management			
Medical Director			
Quality Officer			

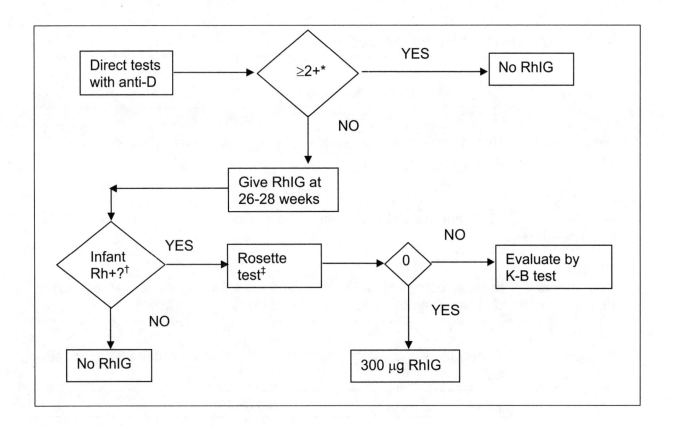

Figure X-B-1. Flow diagram for Rh Immune Globulin administration.

*By tube technique.
†Include test for weak D.
‡Proceed to K-B test when infant has weak expression of RhD.
K-B test = Kleihauer-Betke test.

X-C. Evaluation of HDFN at Delivery

Purpose   To provide a process for testing at delivery.

Before You Begin   Through laboratory data system, phone, or requisition, obtain:
- Prenatal test results.

Sample Requirements   EDTA-anticoagulated or clotted whole blood.

Operational Policy   Routine testing (ABO/Rh, DAT, and tests for unexpected antibodies) of cord blood samples should not be performed.

Process   Review the stages below to determine the recommended testing at delivery:

Stage	Description
1.	Test cord blood sample according to the following criterion:

When...	Then perform...
mother has antibodies capable of causing HDFN or there are no records of tests on maternal blood during pregnancy	• ABO and Rh type. • DAT. • Tests for unexpected antibodies.

Stage	Description
2.	Test cord blood sample according to the following criterion:

When...	Then perform...
mother types as Rh– in tests with anti-D and is not actively immunized to RhD	• ABO and Rh test for weak D when indicated. • DAT.

3.	Test cord blood sample according to the following criterion:	
	When...	**Then perform...**
	there is clinical evidence of neonatal jaundice and maternal antibody screen is negative	• ABO and Rh type. • DAT. • Tests for unexpected antibodies.

4.	According to test results in Stage 3, take the following action:	
	When...	**Then report...**
	fetomaternal ABO incompatibility exists	• DAT result. • Potential for ABO HDFN exists.

5.	Test paternal sample according to test results in Stage 3:	
	When...	**Then perform...**
	there is clinical evidence of neonatal jaundice, maternal antibody screen is negative, and there is no evidence of fetomaternal ABO incompatibility	• ABO and Rh type. • Crossmatch with maternal serum/plasma if ABO compatible. • Crossmatch with eluate from cord blood RBCs if ABO incompatible.

6.	Test maternal sample according to test results in Stage 5:	
	When...	**Then...**
	crossmatches against paternal RBCs performed in Stage 5 are positive	• Consider identifying antibody. • Report infant at risk of HDFN due to antibody to low-prevalence antigen.

Reference   Judd WJ, for the 2003-2004 Scientific Section Coordinating Committee. Guidelines for prenatal and perinatal immunohematology. Bethesda, MD: AABB, 2005.

**Effective
Date**

Approved by:	Printed Name	Signature	Date
Laboratory Management			
Medical Director			
Quality Officer			

X-D. Prenatal Antibody Titration Procedure

Purpose

To provide instructions for titrating potentially significant antibodies encountered in pregnancy:

- Prenatal management of HDFN.

Background Information

Antibody titration is a semiquantitative method of determining antibody concentration. Serial, twofold doubling dilutions of serum are prepared and tested for antibody activity. The reciprocal of the highest dilution of plasma or serum that gives a 1+ reaction is referred to as the titer (eg, for a 1 in 128 dilution, titer = 128).

In pregnancy, antibody titration is performed to ascertain whether women have significant levels of antibodies that may lead to HDFN. For anti-D, a critical titer (8-32, depending on the institution) is used to regulate the use of more definitive studies such as amniotic fluid analysis or measurement of MCAD.

Operational Policy

Because the critical titer has been established for cases of RhD HDFN, titration of non-Rh antibodies should be undertaken only after discussion with the obstetrician about how the data will be used in the clinical management of the pregnancy.

Antibodies detected at delivery should not be titrated. In particular, the practice of titrating passive anti-D following antenatal or postpartum RhIG therapy should be discontinued. Instead, anti-D not detected earlier in pregnancy should be assumed to be the result of RhIG therapy until proven otherwise. Evidence for active immunity to D can best be obtained by performing antibody detection tests 6 months after delivery or at the initial visit for the next pregnancy.

Reserve the current sample (freeze below –30 F) for comparative testing with any subsequent sample from the patient.

Use double-dose RBCs as indicator cells when practicable.

Except for patients with apparent anti-C+D, do not titrate Rh antibodies separately; eg, if anti-c and anti-E are present, test vs R_2R_2 (DcE/DcE) RBCs because the antibody may have an anti-cE (Rh27) component.

When anti-C+D are titrated vs r'r and R_2R_2 RBCs, and the titer vs r'r RBCs is greater than that with the R_2R_2 RBCs, anti-G (not anti-C+D) may be present. Consider the patient a candidate for RhIG prophylaxis unless anti-D can be shown to be present (eg, with DIIIb RBCs).

Limitations

Falsely High Titer:

- Microscopic examination of tests.

- Overcentrifugation of tests.

- Carryover from failure to use clean pipette tip for each dilution.

- Use of wrong reagent or sample, including use of enhancement media or protease-treated RBCs.

- Use of RBCs carrying strong expression of Bg antigens (HLA antigens) when titrating serum/plasma from multiparous women containing anti-Bg.

Falsely Low Titer:

- Omission of serum/plasma.

- Too heavy or too light a cell suspension.

- Use of wrong reagent or sample.

Sample Requirements

Serum or plasma, including frozen sample from previous titration study, if available.

Equipment/ Materials

13 × 75 mm test tubes

AHG: anti-IgG; need not be heavy-chain specific.

Pipettes with disposable tips to deliver 100- and 500-μL volumes (eg, VWR, Batavia, IL).

IgG-coated RBCs.

Indicator RBCs: 2% concentration in pH 7.3 PBS:

- R_2R_2 RBCs for anti-D, anti-c, anti-E, and anti-cE.

- r′r RBCs for apparent anti-C in the presence of apparent anti-D.

- R_1R_1 RBCs for anti-C, anti-e, and anti-Ce.

- Double-dose RBCs, if available, for all other antibodies.

- Consider paternal RBCs for antibodies to low-prevalence antigens.

- pH 7.3 PBS.

Quality Control

When titrating an antibody for the first time, the titration may be performed by two technologists using different indicator RBCs. Results must agree, or repeat until concordance is reached.

Test the current sample in parallel with the most recent previous sample from the patient, if available.

Confirm all negative reactions with IgG-coated RBCs.

Procedure

Use the following steps to perform the procedure:

Step	Action
1.	Using 0.5-mL volumes, prepare serial twofold dilutions of serum in pH 7.3 PBS. The initial tube should contain undiluted serum and the doubling dilution range should be from 1 in 2 to 1 in 2048 (total of 12 tubes).
2.	Place 0.1 mL of each dilution into appropriately labeled 10 or 12 × 75-mm test tubes.
3.	Add 0.1 mL of RBCs to each dilution.
4.	Gently agitate the contents of each tube. Incubate at 37 C for 1 hour.
5.	Wash the RBCs four times with saline and completely decant the final wash supernate.
6.	To the dry RBC buttons thus obtained, add anti-IgG according to the manufacturer's directions.
7.	Centrifuge as for hemagglutination tests.

8.	Examine the RBCs macroscopically; grade and record the reactions.
9.	Mix and centrifuge: • Dislodge the cell buttons gently. • Examine macroscopically for agglutination. • Grade and record the results.
10.	Add 1 drop of IgG-coated RBCs to all tubes with negative antiglobulin results: • Mix gently. • Centrifuge. • Examine macroscopically for agglutination. • Grade and record the results.
11.	Interpret the reactions as follows:

If antibody dilutions…	And negative reactions are…	Then antibody titer is…
react	confirmed	the reciprocal of the highest dilution that yields a 1+ reaction.
are nonreactive	confirmed	0.
are reactive or nonreactive	not confirmed	unknown; test is invalid: • Repeat Steps 1-10. • Consider cell washer problem or inactive AHG.

Reference   Judd WJ, for the 2003-2004 Scientific Section Coordinating Committee. Guidelines for prenatal and perinatal immunohematology. Bethesda, MD: AABB, 2005.

**Effective
Date**

Approved by:	Printed Name	Signature	Date
Laboratory Management			
Medical Director			
Quality Officer			

X-E. Screening for Fetal Rh-Positive RBCs in Maternal Rh-Negative Samples

Purpose

To provide instructions for performing a rosette test to screen for fetal Rh-positive RBCs in maternal Rh-negative blood:

- To determine if more than a single 300-μg dose of RhIG should be administered to an Rh-negative woman who has delivered an Rh-positive infant.

Background Information

When anti-D is mixed with RBCs from an Rh-negative mother of a recently delivered Rh-positive infant, the antibody binds to fetal RBCs present in the maternal sample. After removal of unbound antibody by washing, subsequently added Rh-positive enzyme-treated indicator RBCs bind to the anti-D coating the fetal RBCs to form rosettes that can be detected microscopically. This procedure is recommended for screening Rh-negative mothers of Rh-positive infants for an FMH in excess of 15 mL of RBCs (the amount above which more than a single 300-μg dose of RhIG is indicated). It can also be used to detect an FMH greater than 15 mL of RBCs following trauma during pregnancy.

Operational Policy

This is a screening method for an FMH in excess of 15 mL of fetal RBCs. Do not use this method for quantifying the FMH.

Maternal RBCs that carry weak expression of D will exhibit grossly positive results when tested by this rosette technique; however, weak D women are considered Rh-negative and are candidates for RhIG therapy. Therefore, weak D women who deliver an Rh-positive infant should be evaluated for an FMH greater than 15 mL RBCs using a non-anti-D-based method such as Procedure X-H.

When the infant's RBCs carry weak expression of D, negative results may be obtained. In such instances, evidence for an FMH greater than 15 mL should be obtained by nonserologic means such as Procedure X-H.

Limitations

Unwanted Positive Reactions:

- Inadequate washing of RBCs before adding enzyme-treated indicator RBCs.

- Maternal RBCs carry weak expression of D.

- Infant's RBCs carry weak expression of D.

Unwanted Negative Reactions:

- Inactive reagents.

- Use of wrong reagent or sample.

- Inadequate enzyme treatment of indicator RBCs.

Sample Requirements

Maternal blood sample, preferably collected 1 hour after delivery. Wash RBCs three times and dilute to a 3% suspension with saline.

Equipment/ Materials

Anti-D: Prepare chemically modified anti-D using a pool of six anti-D samples (minimum titer = 512) according to Procedure XV-C.

Indicator RBCs: 0.1 mL R_2R_2 RBCs treated with papain or ficin (two-stage method) as described in Section III; dilute to a 0.2% suspension (1 drop 4%-5% RBCs, 20-25 drops saline) just before use.

Microscope slides and coverslips (eg, VWR, Batavia, IL).

Rh– RBCs: 0.1 mL 50% O, rr RBCs, washed three times and diluted to a 3% suspension (3 mL) with saline.

Rh+ RBCs: 0.1 mL 50% O, D+ RBCs, washed three times and diluted to a 3% suspension (3 mL) with saline.

Positive control RBCs: 0.6% Rh+ RBCs in Rh– RBCs, prepared by mixing 1 drop 3% Rh+ RBCs with 16 drops 3% Rh– RBCs and diluting 1 drop of this mixture with a further 9 drops 3% Rh– RBCs.

Quality Control

The procedure includes tests with negative and positive control samples.

Procedure   Use the following steps to perform the procedure:

Step	Action
1.	Dispense 3 drops of anti-D into each of 3 appropriately labeled 12 × 75-mm test tubes.
2.	To 1 tube, add 2 drops of test RBCs; similarly, set up tests with positive and negative control RBC samples (use Rh– RBCs as negative control).
3.	Gently agitate the contents in each tube and incubate at 37 C for 30 minutes.
4.	Wash the RBCs five times with saline.
5.	Add 3 drops of 0.2% indicator R_2R_2 RBCs to each tube and mix gently but thoroughly.
6.	Incubate at 37 C for 30 minutes.
7.	Centrifuge as for hemagglutination tests.
8.	Gently resuspend the RBCs and pour a drop onto a microscope slide. Carefully place a coverslip over the drop of RBCs.
9.	Allow the RBCs to settle for 15 seconds and examine at least 10 fields microscopically at 100× magnification.
10.	Interpret the reactions as follows: <table><tr><th>If rosettes are…</th><th>Then…</th></tr><tr><td>visible (even one)</td><td>test is positive: • Quantify FMH to determine required dose of RhIG.</td></tr><tr><td>not visible</td><td>test is negative: • Administer a single 300-µg dose of RhIG.</td></tr></table>

Reference   Sebring ES, Polesky HF. Detection of fetal-maternal hemorrhage in Rh immune globulin candidates: A rosetting technique using enzyme treated Rh_2Rh_2 indicator erythrocytes. Transfusion 1982;22:468-71.

**Effective
Date**

Approved by:	Printed Name	Signature	Date
Laboratory Management			
Medical Director			
Quality Officer			

Judd's Methods in Immunohematology
Quantifying Anti-D with the Enzyme-Linked Antiglobulin Test
Page 1 of 5

X-F. Quantifying Anti-D with the Enzyme-Linked Antiglobulin Test

Purpose

To provide instructions for quantifying anti-D using an ELAT:

- Monitoring alloimmunized pregnancies for HDFN.

- Assay of RhIG preparations.

Background Information

In the ELAT, RBCs are first coated with antibody and washed as for the IAT. The coated RBCs are then incubated with an anti-IgG plus alkaline phosphatase conjugate (IgG-AP). Unbound anti-IgG-AP is removed by washing, and a substrate is added that interacts with AP to produce a yellow color, the intensity of which is measured at 405 nm. Using a constant RBC concentration, the amount of color produced can be related to antibody concentration. This procedure has been developed for determining anti-D levels in IU/mL.

Operational Policy

This procedure is contraindicated on samples collected after RhIG administration or delivery, or when HDFN is being monitored by other means such as amniocentesis or Doppler studies.

Limitations

Incorrect Results:

- Improper storage of reagents.

- Use of incorrect technique, including failure to wash RBCs free of unbound globulins and improper transfer of supernates.

- Use of wrong reagent.

- Omission of a test component.

- Use of inactive or contaminated reagents.

Sample Requirements

Anti-D: diluted in BSA-PBS; prepare duplicate sets of three different dilutions for each sample, with 1-mL minimum of each dilution.

Note: Appropriate dilution range must be determined empirically.

**Equipment/
Materials**

BSA-LISS.

BSA-PBS.

BSA-NS.

Anti-IgG conjugate: ovine (sheep) antihuman IgG conjugated with AP (eg, MP Biomedicals, Irvine, CA). Determine the appropriate dilution for the anti-IgG-AP from titration studies (using serial twofold dilutions in BSA-PBS) with Rh+ RBCs precoated with a 1000× dilution of commercially prepared modified-tube (high-protein) anti-D. Plot the optical density (OD) values against anti-IgG-AP dilution on linear graph paper. Choose a dilution of anti-IgG-AP that gives an OD value with Rh+ RBCs on the straight part of the curve, yet gives a low OD with Rh– RBCs.

Carbonate buffer: 0.05 M, pH 9.8.

Laboratory film (eg, Parafilm, VWR, Batavia, IL).

Pipettes with disposable tips to deliver 0.2-mL and 0.5-mL volumes (eg, VWR, Batavia, IL).

p-nitrophenol phosphate (PNP) substrate: PNP (eg, Sigma-Aldrich, St Louis, MO), diluted to 2 mg/mL with 0.05 M carbonate buffer just before use.

RBCs: antigen positive; pooled from four samples; group, O R_1R_1 RBCs. Use within 24 hours of collection. Wash three times with saline; then wash once and dilute to a 2% suspension with LISS-PBS.

Note: Centrifuge the last saline wash to pack the RBCs, and remove the buffy coat by vacuum aspiration before proceeding with the BSA-PBS wash.

RBCs: antigen negative; pooled from four samples; group O, rr RBCs. Prepare as described above.

NaOH: 1 N.

Spectrophotometer (eg, Spectronic 200, VWR, Batavia, IL or equivalent): at wavelength of 405 nm.

Standard anti-D dilutions: The Second International Standard for Anti-D Immunoglobulin 01/572, containing 285 IU/mL (National Institute for Biological Standards and Control, Potters Bar, Hertfordshire, UK). Dilute in BSA-PBS and prepare duplicate sets of six dilutions (eg, from 1 in 200 to 1 in 6400).

Note: Appropriate dilution range must be determined empirically.

Test tubes: glass, 12 × 75-mm. Prepare for ELAT by filling with BSA-PBS, discarding BSA-PBS after a few minutes, and inverting to drain.

Quality Control
Prepare an "in-house" standard anti-D for inclusion in each test run. Result should be within ±10% of assigned value.

Procedure
Use the following steps to perform the procedure:

Step	Action
1.	Dispense 0.5 mL of each antibody dilution to be tested into 2 appropriately labeled, precoated 12 × 75-mm glass test tubes.
2.	Add 0.5 mL of 2% group O, R_1R_1 RBCs in BSA-LISS to each tube and mix well.
3.	Similarly, set up single tests with O, rr RBCs.
4.	Prepare a "hemolysis control" tube for both R_1R_1 and rr samples by incubating 0.5 mL of RBCs with 0.5 mL of BSA-PBS.
5.	Incubate at 37 C for 15 minutes.
6.	Wash the RBCs six times with BSA-PBS and aspirate the supernates.
7.	Add 0.2 mL of anti-IgG-AP (at working concentration) to each tube.
8.	Cover the tubes with Parafilm and incubate at 37 C for 1 hour; mix periodically by gentle agitation during this time.
9.	Wash the RBCs three times with BSA-PBS and aspirate the supernates.
10.	Resuspend the RBCs in BSA-NS and transfer to clean, appropriately labeled 12 × 75-mm test tubes. (See notes in Equipment/Materials).
11.	Centrifuge to pack the RBCs, and aspirate the supernate.
12.	Add 0.2 mL BSA-NS and 0.2 mL PNP to the RBC buttons.
13.	Mix well, cover the tubes with Parafilm, and incubate at 37 C for 60 minutes.
14.	Remove Parafilm and centrifuge to pack the RBCs. (See notes in Equipment/Materials.)
15.	Transfer the supernates into clean test tubes and add 0.5 mL of 1 N NaOH (to stop the enzyme reaction).
16.	Using 1-cm cuvettes, read the OD of each supernate at 405 nm. **Note:** Read against a reagent blank consisting of PNP, 0.2 mL; BSA-NS, 0.2 mL; and 1 N NaOH, 0.5 mL.

17.	For dilutions of the International Standard anti-D, determine the corrected OD as follows: [(OD TAg+) – (OD CAg+)] – [(OD TAg–) – (OD CAg–)] where OD = optical density; T = test; Ag+ = antigen-positive RBCs; C = hemolysis control; Ag– = antigen-negative RBCs.
18.	Plot the corrected OD against the reciprocal of each dilution on linear graph paper.
19.	Determine the corrected OD for each of the three sample dilutions. If not within the range of the standard curve, test dilutions at a lower or higher serum concentration as needed.
20.	Compare the corrected OD for each dilution against the standard curve and calculate the anti-D concentration as follows: Concentration of unknown = (A × C) ÷ B where A = reciprocal of the dilution of the test sample; B = reciprocal of the International Standard dilution that gives the same corrected OD as the test sample dilution; C = concentration of the working standard.
21.	Use the average concentrations obtained with each dilution as the final anti-D concentration.
22.	Interpret the results as follows:

If antibody content is...	Then...
≥0.7 IU/mL	monitor for HDFN by a nonserologic method.
≤0.7 IU/mL	continue to measure anti-D content as requested by the obstetrician.

References

Leikola J, Perkins HA. Enzyme-linked antiglobulin test: An accurate and simple method to quantitate red cell antibodies. Transfusion 1980;20:138-44.

Postoway N, Nance SJ, Garratty G. Variables affecting the enzyme-linked antiglobulin test when detecting and quantitating IgG red cell antibodies. Med Lab Sci 1985;42:11-19.

**Effective
Date**

Approved by:	Printed Name	Signature	Date
Laboratory Management			
Medical Director			
Quality Officer			

X-G. Screening for Large Fetomaternal Hemorrhage (Modified Kleihauer-Betke Acid-Elution Test)

Purpose

To provide instructions for quantifying the extent of FMH:

- To determine the number of 300-μg doses of RhIG that should be administered to an Rh-negative woman who has delivered an Rh-positive infant.

Background Information

Fetal hemoglobin (HbF) is resistant to denaturation by both acidic and alkaline solutions, in contrast to adult hemoglobin (HbA). In this procedure, HbA is eluted from a blood smear from a postdelivery maternal blood sample. The smear is then counterstained with erythrosin to reveal fetal RBCs in a background of unstained maternal RBCs. The percentage of fetal RBCs present is determined and used to calculate the amount of RhIG to administer.

Operational Policy

This quantitative test should not be used for screening purposes; it is subject to yielding unwanted positive tests as a result of maternal synthesis of HbF during pregnancy.

To avoid RBC distortion, do not use saline to prepare 20% cell suspensions.

Prepare working buffer solution immediately before use.

Limitations

Incorrect Results:

- Maternal synthesis of HbF during pregnancy.
- Citric acid buffer at wrong pH.
- Use of wrong reagent or improper technique.
- Failure to prepare buffer immediately before use.

Sample Requirements

Maternal RBCs: 20% suspension in native serum or plasma.

Equipment/ Materials

0.1 M citric acid.

0.5 % erythrosin B.

80% ethanol.

Microscope slides (eg, VWR, Batavia, IL).

pH meter: with KCl electrode (eg, VWR, Batavia, IL).

RBCs: 20% suspensions in native plasma:

- Group O cord blood.

- Normal adult group O, preferably from a male donor.

Note: This also serves as a negative control.

- Positive control RBCs: 1% cord RBCs in adult RBCs at a concentration of 20% in ABO-compatible serum or plasma.

Working buffer at pH 3.3: 0.1 M citric acid, 147 mL; 0.2 M disodium hydrogen phosphate, 53 mL. Prepare immediately before use. Check pH and adjust, if necessary, by adding the appropriate reagent.

Note: The correct incubation time in the working buffer must be determined empirically for each batch of stock buffer solutions. Fetal RBCs in the control smear should be dark red and refractile, with clearly outlined, smooth edges; adult RBCs should appear as colorless "ghost" cells. If differentiation between fetal and adult RBCs is not clear, adjust incubation time accordingly (shorten time to increase staining intensity of fetal RBCs, or lengthen time to decrease coloration of adult RBCs).

Coplin jar (eg, VWR, Batavia, IL).

Graduated measuring cylinder: 100 mL and 250 mL (eg, VWR, Batavia, IL).

Quality Control

The procedure includes positive and negative controls.

Procedure   Use the following steps to perform the procedure:

Step	Action
1.	Place freshly prepared working buffer in a Coplin jar, first at 56 C (until the temperature reaches 35-36 C) and subsequently at 37 C.
2.	Make thin blood smears of test and control samples. Air dry and label appropriately; then place in a slide carrier.
3.	Immerse the slides in a dish of 80% ethanol and fix for 5 minutes.
4.	Transfer the slides to a dish containing cold tap water and rinse under cold running tap water.
5.	Transfer the slides into the dish of working buffer at 37 C for 5 minutes. (See note in Equipment/Materials.)
6.	Transfer the slides to a dish containing cold tap water and rinse under cold running tap water.
7.	Immerse the slides in a dish of erythrosin B for 5 minutes.
8.	Transfer the slides to a dish containing cold tap water and rinse under cold running tap water.
9.	Allow smears to dry, and examine them using a 40× microscope objective.
10.	Record the number of fetal RBCs observed during a count of 2000 adult RBC ghosts.
11.	Calculate the required dose of RhIG as follows:

If the percentage of fetal RBCs is…	Then the required number of 300-µg vials of RhIG to administer is…
≥0.3%	[(24 × % fetal RBCs) ÷ 15] + 1.
<0.3%	1.

References   Lee CL. Estimation of fetal RBCs in mother (letter). N Engl J Med 1976;
295:1080.

Mollison PL. Quantitation of transplacental hemorrhage. Br J Haematol
1972;3:31-4.

Sebring ES. Fetomaternal hemorrhage, incidence, and methods of detection and quantitation. In: Garratty G, ed. Hemolytic disease of the newborn. Arlington, VA: AABB, 1984:87-117.

Shephard MK, Weatherall DJ, Swift HH. Semi-quantitative estimation of the distribution of fetal hemoglobin in red cell populations. Bull Johns Hopkins Hosp 1977;1:313-31.

Effective Date

Approved by:	Printed Name	Signature	Date
Laboratory Management			
Medical Director			
Quality Officer			

X-H. Quantifying Fetomaternal Hemorrhage with the Enzyme-Linked Antiglobulin Test

Purpose   To provide instructions for quantifying the extent of FMH:

- To determine the number of 300-μg doses of RhIG that should be administered to an Rh-negative woman who has delivered an Rh-positive fetus.

Background Information   In the ELAT, RBCs are first coated with antibody and washed as for the IAT. The coated RBCs are then incubated with an anti-IgG plus alkaline phosphatase conjugate (IgG-AP). Unbound anti-IgG-AP is removed by washing, and a substrate is added that interacts with AP to produce a yellow color, the intensity of which is measured at 405 nm. Within certain limits, the amount of color produced is directly proportional to the antigen/antibody concentration present during the initial coating phase. This technique can be used for quantifying RBC antigens and antibodies (see procedures discussed in Section XV) and may also be applied to the estimation of minor RBC populations. This procedure is applicable to the detection of Rh-positive fetal RBCs in Rh-negative maternal blood, as a quantitative test for the recognition of FMH requiring treatment with more than a single dose of RhIG.

Operational Policy   Some women synthesize fetal hemoglobin in pregnancy. This anti-D-based procedure may be used when abnormally high fetal RBC counts are observed by the Kleihauer-Betke test (Procedure X-G).

Limitations   Incorrect Results:

- Improper storage of reagents.
- Use of incorrect technique, including failure to wash RBCs free of unbound globulins, and improper transfer of supernates.
- Use of wrong reagent.
- Omission of a test component.
- Use of inactive or contaminated reagents.

Sample Requirements

RBCs: from EDTA-, ACD-, CPD-, or A1-anticoagulated maternal blood sample, washed three times in saline and diluted to a 5% suspension with BSA-NS (see below); a minimum of 0.4 mL is required.

Note: Ideally, obtain samples 1 hour after delivery; test and administer required dose of RhIG within 72 hours after delivery.

Equipment/ Materials

BSA-LISS.

BSA-PBS.

BSA-NS.

Anti-D: commercially prepared modified-tube anti-D (human) serum, 0.1 mL; 2% BSA-PBS (see below), 2.4 mL. Prepare on day of use.

Anti-IgG conjugate: ovine (sheep) antihuman IgG conjugated with AP (eg, MP Biomedicals, Irvine, CA). Determine the appropriate dilution for the anti-IgG-AP from titration studies (using serial twofold dilutions in BSA-PBS) with Rh+ RBCs precoated with a 1000× dilution of commercially prepared modified-tube (high-protein) anti-D. Plot the OD values against anti-IgG-AP dilution on linear graph paper. Choose a dilution of anti-IgG-AP that gives an OD value with Rh+ RBCs on the straight part of the curve, yet gives a low OD with Rh– RBCs.

Carbonate buffer: 0.05 M, pH 9.8.

Graduated 5-mL pipettes (eg, VWR, Batavia, IL).

Graph paper (linear).

Laboratory film (eg, Parafilm, VWR, Batavia, IL).

Pipettes with disposable tips to deliver 0.2-mL and 0.5-mL volumes (eg, VWR, Batavia, IL).

ρ-nitrophenol phosphate (PNP) substrate: PNP (eg, Sigma-Aldrich, St Louis, MO), diluted to 2 mg/mL with 0.05 M carbonate buffer just before use.

Rh– RBCs: three examples of adult group O, rr RBCs from EDTA-, ACD-, CPD-, CPD-, or A1-anticoagulated samples. Use within 1 week of collection. Wash three times and dilute to a 5% suspension in BSA-NS.

Note: 10 mL of 5% Rh– RBCs are required for preparation of standard curve.

Rh+ cord blood RBCs: group O, R_1r or R_2r RBCs from EDTA-, ACD-, CPD-, or A1-anticoagulated cord blood samples. Use within 1 week of collection. Wash three times and dilute to a 5% suspension in BSA-NS.

1 N NaOH.

Spectrophotometer (eg, Spectronic 200, VWR, Batavia, IL or equivalent): at wavelength of 405 nm.

Test tubes: glass, 12 × 75-mm. Prepare for ELAT by filling with BSA-PBS, discarding BSA-PBS after a few minutes, and inverting to drain.

Quality Control

The procedure includes tests with negative and positive control samples.

Procedure

Use the following steps to perform the procedure:

Step	Action
1.	Prepare standard-curve Rh+ cord RBCs in 5% Rh– RBC samples as follows: <ul><li>Dilute 0.1 mL of 5% cord Rh+ RBCs with 4.9 mL 5% adult Rh– RBCs to yield a 2% concentration of cord Rh+ RBCs in adult Rh– RBCs.</li><li>Make serial twofold dilutions of the above admixture (using 0.5-mL volumes) in a 5% suspension of Rh– RBCs (yield = 1.0%, 0.5%, 0.25%, 0.125%, 0.0625%, 0.03125% and 0.0156% concentrations of cord Rh+ RBCs in Rh– RBCs).</li><li>Prepare a 1.5% concentration of cord Rh+ RBCs in Rh– RBCs by diluting 1 mL 2% Rh+ cord RBCs in Rh– RBCs with 0.5 mL of 5% Rh– RBCs.</li><li>Retain sufficient 2% Rh+ cord RBCs in Rh– RBCs and 5% Rh– RBCs for control purposes.</li></ul>
2.	For each cord RBC suspension to be tested, dispense 0.2 mL dilute anti-D into 2 appropriately labeled, prewetted test tubes.
3.	Add 0.1 mL of the 2% suspension of cord Rh+ RBCs in Rh– RBCs into the first set of 2 tubes and mix well; similarly (in duplicate), add 0.1 mL of the remaining cord RBC dilutions to the appropriate tubes.
4.	In duplicate, set up tests with 0.1 mL each of the 5% Rh– control RBC samples and dilute anti-D.
5.	Similarly, set up duplicate tests with 0.1 mL of the test RBCs and dilute anti-D.
6.	Incubate all tubes at 37 C for 30 minutes; mix periodically by gentle agitation during this time.
7.	Wash the RBCs four times with BSA-PBS and aspirate the final supernate.

8.	Add 0.2 mL of anti-IgG-AP (at working concentration) to each tube.
9.	Cover the tubes with Parafilm and incubate at 37 C for 1 hour; mix periodically by gentle agitation during this time.
10.	Wash the RBCs three times with BSA-PBS and aspirate the final supernate.
11.	Dilute the RBCs in BSA-NS and transfer to clean, appropriately labeled 12 × 75-mm test tubes.
12.	Centrifuge to pack the RBCs and aspirate the supernate.
13.	Add 0.2 mL BSA-NS and 0.2 mL PNP to the RBC buttons.
14.	Mix well and incubate at 37 C for 60 minutes.
15.	Centrifuge to pack the RBCs.
16.	Transfer the supernates into clean test tubes and add 0.5 mL 1 N NaOH (to stop the enzyme reaction).
17.	Using 1-cm cuvettes, read the OD of each supernate at 405 nm. **Note:** Read against a reagent blank consisting of PNP, 0.2 mL; BSA-NS, 0.2 mL; and 1 N NaOH, 0.5 mL.
18.	Take the mean of the two OD values of each fetal RBC dilution and prepare a standard curve on linear graph paper.
19.	Take the mean of the two OD values of the test sample(s) and determine the percentage of fetal RBCs in the test sample from the standard curve.
20.	Calculate the required dose of RhIG as follows:

If the percentage of fetal RBCs is…	Then the required number of 300-µg vials of RhIG to administer is…
≥0.3%	[(24 × % fetal RBCs) ÷ 15] + 1.
<0.3%	1.

References   Leikola J, Perkins HA. Enzyme-linked antiglobulin test: An accurate and simple method to quantitate red cell antibodies. Transfusion 1980;20:138-44.

Leikola J, Perkins HA. Red cell antibodies and low ionic strength: A study with enzyme-linked antiglobulin test. Transfusion 1980;20:224-8.

Postoway N, Nance SJ, Garratty G. Variables affecting the enzyme-linked antiglobulin test when detecting and quantitating IgG red cell antibodies. Med Lab Sci 1985;42:11-19.

Riley JZ, Ness PM, Taddie SJ, et al. Detection and quantitation of fetal maternal hemorrhage utilizing an enzyme-linked antiglobulin test. Transfusion 1982;22:472-4.

Wilson L, Wren MR, Issitt PD. Enzyme linked antiglobulin test: Variables affecting the test when measuring levels of red cell antigens. Med Lab Sci 1985;42:20-25.

**Effective
Date**

Approved by:	Printed Name	Signature	Date
Laboratory Management			
Medical Director			
Quality Officer			

X-I. Analyzing Amniotic Fluid by Spectrophotometry

Purpose
To provide instructions for determining the change in optical density at 450 nm (ΔOD_{450}) of amniotic fluid:

- Monitoring a fetus for HDFN in an alloimmunized pregnancy.

Background Information
Spectrophotometric analysis of amniotic fluid at 450 nm will reveal the presence of bilirubin. The height of the bilirubin peak above a baseline of absorbance drawn from 350 to 700 nm (ΔOD_{450}) reflects the bilirubin concentration, which when plotted against gestational age is used to predict the severity of and manage HDFN caused by maternal alloimmunization.

Note: This assay has been replaced by noninvasive Doppler studies that measure the flow rate of blood through the midcerebral artery.

Operational Policy
Collection of amniotic fluid is an invasive procedure that traditionally has been regulated by the results of titration studies. It used to be indicated when the titer of anti-D was 16 or greater, or when the titer increased at least twofold during pregnancy.

Limitations
Unwanted Positive Reactions:

- Amniotic fluid contaminated with hemoglobin or particulate matter.

Unwanted Negative Reactions:

- Improper storage of amniotic fluid.

Sample Requirements
Amniotic fluid: preferably not contaminated with blood; 3-5 mL. Store in dark (exposure to light results in loss of bilirubin pigment).

**Equipment/
Materials**

Bilirubin standard: 5 mg/dL (eg, Sigma-Aldrich, St Louis, MO).

Graph paper: semi-log scale.

Micro filtration apparatus: 5-mL syringe with disc-filter assembly (Acrodisc, Pall Corporation, East Hills, NY) and 0.45-μ filter pads.

Normal amniotic fluid: 20-30 mL pooled amniotic fluid from nonalloimmunized women (supernates from amniotic fluid obtained for genetic analysis). Centrifuge to remove particulate matter, clarify by filtration, and dispense into 2.5-3.0 mL aliquots. Store frozen at –70 C.

Spectrophotometer with optically matched 1-cm square quartz cuvettes (eg, VWR, Batavia, IL).

5-mL graduated pipettes (eg, VWR, Batavia, IL).

**Quality
Control**

Spike aliquot of normal amniotic fluid with 50 μL bilirubin. On spectrophotometric analysis, the bilirubin should demonstrate a peak at 450 nm that should not be present in normal amniotic fluid without bilirubin.

Procedure

Use the following steps to perform the procedure:

Step	Action
1.	Centrifuge the amniotic fluid to remove particulate matter.
2.	Clarify the supernate by filtration.
3.	Fill 1 cuvette with 2.5 mL of distilled water (blank).
4.	Fill a second cuvette with 2.5 mL of amniotic fluid (test).
5.	Measure OD values of the amniotic fluid at wavelengths of 350, 360, 365, 370, 380, 390, 400, 405, 410, 415, 420, 430, 440, 450, 460, 470, 480, 490, 500, 550, 600, 650, and 700 nm. **Note:** At each change of wavelength, set the blank and absorbance scale to zero.
6.	Plot OD readings (log scale) against wavelength in nm (linear scale).
7.	Draw a straight line from the 365-nm point to the 550-nm point.
8.	Determine the absorbance value at which this straight line intersects a vertical line drawn from the 450-nm point.
9.	Subtract this value from the actual OD reading obtained with the amniotic fluid at 450 nm; this figure is the ΔOD_{450}.

10.	Interpret the results as follows:	
	If ΔOD_{450} is...	**Then...**
	<0.2	• Fetus is likely Rh–. • If fetus is Rh+, in-utero death is unlikely within 2 weeks.
	0.2 to 0.34	fetus is Rh+ and probably affected with HDFN: • Because ΔOD_{450} may drop below 0.2, repeat procedure in 1 week. • A rapidly rising ΔOD_{450} and a history of a stillbirth is an indication for fetal transfusion if <30 weeks' gestation. Delivery immediately if >30 weeks' gestation.
	0.35 to 0.7	fetus is Rh+ and severely affected; may already be in congestive heart failure: • Treat by fetal transfusion if <30 weeks' gestation, or immediate delivery if >30 weeks' gestation.
	>0.7	fetus is hydropic and moribund: • Fetal death is imminent. • Immediate delivery is warranted; the prognosis is poor.
11.	Alternatively, use the Liley procedure (see Liley in reference list) to determine the significance of ΔOD_{450} and gestational age.	

References

Gambino SR, Freda VJ. The measurement of amniotic fluid bilirubin by the method of Jendrassik and Grof. Am J Clin Path 1966;46:198-203.

Liley AW. Liquor amnii analysis in the management of pregnancy complicated by rhesus sensitization. Am J Obstet 1961;82:1359-70.

Nelson GH, Talledo AE. Amniotic fluid spectral analysis in the management of patients with rhesus sensitization. Am J Clin Pathol 1961;52:363-9.

Effective Date

Approved by:	Printed Name	Signature	Date
Laboratory Management			
Medical Director			
Quality Officer			

X-J. Treating Cord Blood Contaminated with Wharton's Jelly

Purpose	To provide instructions for testing cord blood samples contaminated with Wharton's jelly:

- Receiving spontaneous aggregation of cord blood sample.

Background Information	Occasionally, cord blood samples may be contaminated with an excessive amount of Wharton's jelly that cannot be removed by routine washing of RBCs. This may result in spontaneous agglutination of the test cells, making the performance of routine serologic tests difficult or impossible. The addition of hyaluronidase to packed cord RBCs denatures Wharton's jelly and permits routine testing of cord blood samples.

Operational Policy	Not applicable.

Limitations	Incorrect Results:

- Improper storage of reagents.
- Use of incorrect technique.
- Use of wrong reagent.

Sample Requirements	Cord blood RBCs: wash four times and pack.

Equipment/ Materials	6% BSA. A_2 and B control RBCs: from clotted or anticoagulated blood, washed four times and packed. Hyaluronidase, working solution: 1 mg/mL.

Quality Control	The procedure includes tests with A_1 and B control RBCs.

Procedure   Use the following steps to perform the procedure:

Step	Action
1.	To 2-3 drops of washed packed RBCs, add 1 drop of 1 mg/mL hyaluronidase.
2.	Mix and dilute as desired for serologic testing.
3.	Test with anti-A, -B, and -D and 6% BSA as described in Section I.
4.	Interpret the reactions as follows:

If the treated RBCs…	Then…
aggregate in the presence of 6% BSA	ABO/Rh type is invalid.
do not aggregate in the presence of 6% BSA	interpret the reactions with anti-A, -B, and -D.

Reference   Killpack S. Umbilical cord blood. Lancet 1950;ii:827.

Effective Date

Approved by:

	Printed Name	Signature	Date
Laboratory Management			
Medical Director			
Quality Officer			

Section XI. Investigating Samples Containing Autoantibodies

The procedures outlined in this section are those used in the confirmation of suspected autoimmune disease states that may or may not be associated with immune hemolysis. They also are applied to the differentiation of auto- from alloantibody activity. Such studies are essential for the proper selection of blood for transfusion to patients with autoantibodies, because autoantibody may mask concomitant alloantibody activity.

A direct antiglobulin test (DAT) is a reagent test for immune hemolysis. A positive DAT on RBCs from a neonate is suggestive of hemolytic disease of the fetus and newborn (HDFN). A positive DAT on RBCs from adults is suggestive of autoimmune hemolytic anemia; however, the DAT may be positive in apparently healthy people and can be a benign finding in hospital patients. Drugs, the passive acquisition of antibodies, and alloimmune reactions to recent transfusions also can account for a positive DAT.

Classification

Autoantibodies can be classified on the basis of immunoglobulin class, optimal thermal reactivity, and blood group specificity, as discussed below.

Warm-Reactive Autoantibodies

The vast majority of warm-reactive autoantibodies are IgG proteins. They may bind C3 to RBCs both in vivo and in vitro. The following have been described as warm-reactive autoantibodies, as single antibodies and as mixtures:

1. Simple Rh antibodies with apparent anti-D, -C, -c, -E, or -e specificity.

2. Antibodies to common RhD and RhCE determinants that fail to react with Rh-deletion phenotypes.

3. Antibodies to non-Rh high-prevalence antigens in many blood group systems. Examples include anti-En^a, -U, -Wr^b, -Ge, -I^T, -Kp^b, -K13, and -LW.

4. Antibodies to non-Rh polymorphic gene products such as A, N, K, and Jk^a.

Cold-Reactive Autoantibodies

The majority of cold-reactive autoantibodies are C3-binding IgM proteins and are directed towards Ii-system antigens. Many are clinically benign; indeed, most adult human sera contain anti-I reacting only at or below 4 C and nonpathologic titers may be as high as 64 in tests incubated at RT. However, potent anti-I may cause severe RBC destruction and is seen in patients with *Mycoplasma pneumonia* infection. Anti-i is seen in infectious mononucleosis. Rare biphasic hemolysins, usually IgG autoantibodies with anti-P specificity (Donath-Landsteiner antibody), cause dramatic RBC destruction; they are associated with paroxysmal cold hemoglobinuria, a condition that was more commonly found as a complication of tertiary syphilis but now is seen rarely in young children following viral illness. Other cold-reactive autoantibody specificities have been observed, with or without associated immune-mediated hemolysis, including the following:

1. I/i-related antibodies that react preferentially with RBCs carrying a normal H antigen content (eg, anti-IH) or P_1 antigen expression (anti-IP$_1$).

2. Antibodies to the Pr series of antibodies that are sensitive to the action of proteolytic enzymes.

3. Anti-Rx (previously called anti-Sd^x).

4. Anti-Gd.

The serologic characteristics of some of these antibodies are summarized in Table XI-1.

Clinically benign cold-reactive autoantibodies are sometimes considered the "bane" of the clinical serologist, for they create a variety of problems in routine pretransfusion testing. Notably, they cause RBC agglutination and bind C3 at temperatures up to 37 C. The C3-binding is detected in antiglobulin tests using polyspecific (anti-IgG + anti-C3) antihuman globulin. This reactivity is potentiated in tests using bovine albumin or low-ionic-strength saline; both media are widely used for the detection of unexpected antibodies and crossmatching. However, test protocols have been modified to avoid their detection in most instances. Nonetheless, occasional examples continue to cause positive test results for unexpected antibodies, positive crossmatches, or discrepant ABO typing results.

It is important that the procedures employed for evaluating blood samples from patients with suspected immune hemolysis are capable of differentiating between the causes of a positive DAT mentioned earlier. For this reason, a detailed summary of the patient's diagnosis, drug therapy, and prior transfusions is invaluable. Furthermore, it is important to remember that the results of serologic tests are not diagnostic and do not prove that a patient has immune-mediated hemolysis. Rather, the significance of the data obtained must be evaluated in light of the patient's clinical condition and results of other laboratory tests, including sequential hemoglobin or hematocrit measurements, reticulocyte counts, bilirubin, haptoglobin, and lactate dehydrogenase values (LDH$_1$:LDH$_2$).

Additional information on the laboratory and clinical management of patients with autoantibodies may be found in the sources listed in Suggested Reading.

Positive DAT Samples—General Considerations

Appropriate Evaluation

1. It is appropriate to determine the cause of a positive DAT in an anemic patient with clinical signs and symptoms of hemolysis; such studies serve to determine if the hemolysis has an immune basis. Other laboratory data may be informative, including evidence of reticulocytosis, hemoglobinemia and hemoglobinuria, absence of haptoglobin, and elevated levels of unconjugated serum bilirubin or the LDH isoenzyme LDH$_1$. If there is no evidence for hemolysis, then no further studies to determine the cause of the positive DAT are warranted.

2. A positive DAT on a recipient of a recent transfusion may indicate an alloimmune response to the recently transfused RBCs. However, eluate studies need not be performed on all blood samples from recent transfusion recipients manifesting a positive DAT because alloantibody activity will almost always be present in the serum. Data from the University of Michigan indicate that meaningful data observed solely by elution are obtained only rarely.

3. Elution studies on positive DAT samples from patients receiving certain drugs (eg, α-methyldopa and related compounds) do not distinguish between pathological autoantibody formation and that induced by the drug. Between 15% and 20% of patients receiving α-methyldopa develop a positive DAT, but less than 1% of these manifest clinical signs and symptoms of immune hemolysis. Surveillance for hemolysis among patients with such a drug-induced positive DAT may be appropriate; however, the need for extensive serologic investigation is questionable unless clinical signs of immune hemolysis appear. Even then, the need to investigate positive DAT samples on these patients should be undertaken following collaboration with the attending physician and only if the data will be used to influence clinical and/or transfusion management.

4. Approximately 3% of patients receiving high-dose intravenous penicillin develop a positive DAT. Eluates react specifically with RBCs coated with the drug or related compounds. Again, surveillance for hemolysis among patients with a penicillin-induced positive DAT may be appropriate, but until clinical symptoms appear, the need for extensive serologic investigation is questionable.

Recommended Testing

1. Elution studies performed as part of the evaluation of a positive DAT found during pretransfusion testing should focus on the detection of clinically significant alloantibodies made in response to recent transfusions. Because the most common specificities seen have Rh, Kell, or Kidd blood group specificity, and because these antibodies often exhibit dosage and give enhanced reactions with protease-treated RBCs, an ideal RBC test panel should include untreated RBCs as well as protease-treated RBCs of the following Rh phenotypes: R_1R_1, R_2R_2, and rr; of the enzyme-treated samples, at least one should be Jk(a+b−), one Jk(a−b+), and another K+.

2. A panel of RBCs similar to that described above is also ideal for the evaluation of blood samples with a positive DAT due to warm-reactive autoantibodies. Use of protease-treated RBCs of selected Rh phenotypes affords optimal detection of autoanti-Rh specificities.

References

1. Garatty G, Arndt PA. An update on drug-induced immune hemolytic anemia. Immunohematology 2007;23:105-19.

2. Judd WJ. Antibody elution from RBCs. In: Bell CA, ed. Seminar on antigen-antibody reactions revisited. Arlington, VA: AABB, 1985.

3. Roback J, Combs MR, Grossman B, Hillyer C, eds. Technical manual. 16th ed. Bethesda, MD: AABB (or current edition).

Suggested Reading

Beattie KM. Laboratory management of antibody specificities in warm autoimmune hemolytic anemia. In: Bell CA, ed. A seminar on laboratory management of hemolysis. Washington, DC: AABB, 1979:105-34.

Harmening D. Modern blood banking and transfusion practices. 5th ed. Philadelphia, PA: FA Davis, 2005.

Issitt, PD. Cold-reactive autoantibodies outside the I and P blood groups. In: Moulds JM, Woods LJ, eds. Blood groups: P, I, Sd^a and Pr. Arlington, VA: AABB, 1991:73-112.

Issitt PD, Anstee DJ. Applied blood group serology. 4th ed. Durham, NC: Montgomery Scientific Publications, 1998.

Judd WJ, Barnes BA, Steiner EA, et al. The evaluation of a positive direct antiglobulin test in pretransfusion testing revisited. Transfusion 1986;26:220-4.

Marsh WL. Aspects of cold-reactive autoantibodies. In: Bell CA, ed. A seminar on laboratory management of hemolysis. Washington, DC: AABB, 1979:87-103.

Mougey R. Cold autoimmune hemolytic anemia: A review of clinical and laboratory considerations. Immunohematology 1985;2:1-7.

Petz LD, Garratty G. Immune hemolytic anemias. 2nd ed. Philadelphia, PA: Churchill-Livingstone, 2004.

Roback J, Combs MR, Grossman B, Hillyer C, eds. Technical manual. 16th ed. Bethesda, MD: AABB, 2008 (or current edition).

Table XI-1.   Specificity of Cold-Reactive Autoantibodies: Comparison of Reactions with Untreated O, I+ RBCs

Anti-	RBCs				
	Oi_{adult}	Oi_{cord}	$A_1 I$	O, I FIC*	Auto
H*	→	(↓)	↓	↑	↓
HI*	↓	↓	↓	↑	↓
I^D	0	0	→	↑	→
I^F	↓	↓	→	(↑)	→
I^T	→	↑	→	↑	→
i	↑	↑	→	↑	→
Pr	→	→	→	0	→
Rx	→	→	→	↑	→

*In A_1 and A_1B individuals.

FIC = ficin-treated RBCs: When compared to group O, I+ RBCs, → = equally reactive; ↓ = markedly weaker; (↓) slightly weaker; ↑ = markedly stronger; (↑) slightly stronger.

0 = nonreactive.

Judd's Methods in Immunohematology
Investigation of Cases of Immune Hemolysis and/or a Positive DAT
Page 1 of 6

XI-A. Investigation of Cases of Immune Hemolysis and/or a Positive DAT

Purpose To provide a process for the management of patient samples with hemolysis and/or a positive DAT. (Also see Fig VIII-A-2.)

Before You Begin Through laboratory data system, phone, or requisition, obtain:

- Patient's transfusion, transplant, and pregnancy history.
- Medical diagnoses.
- Laboratory data indicative of hemolysis.
- Drug therapy history.

Operational Policy Samples with a strongly positive DAT caused by IgG coating may yield unwanted positive reactions with reagents formulated in a medium of high-protein content. Use low-protein content reagents when testing samples with a positive DAT.

Discuss the need for performing the Donath-Landsteiner test with the patient's clinicians.

Note: Serum, not plasma, collected as described in Procedure XI-L will be required.

Notify attending physician of significant findings.

Sample Requirements EDTA-anticoagulated blood, as a source of plasma and RBCs. Serum will be required for some studies indicated below.

Equipment/ Materials Results of DAT studies (Procedure XI-B).

Process   Consider the stages below in the management of samples with immune hemolysis and/or a positive DAT:

Stage	Description
1.	Evaluate the results of DAT studies in conjunction with the clinical and laboratory data according to the following criteria:

When the RBCs are ...	Then consider...

coated with C3 alone and there is evidence of gross hemolysis	• Cold agglutinin disease:
	  ○ Evaluate according to Process VIII-B.
	• PCH:
	  ○ Perform the Donath-Landsteiner test (Procedure XI-L).
	• Sepsis:
	  ○ Test for T and Tk activation (see Section XIV).
	• Drug-induced hemolysis:
	  ○ Test by Procedure XII-C, -D, -E, or -F, as indicated by drug history.

coated with C3, IgG, or IgG+C3, and the patient was reported to have a hemolytic transfusion reaction	• ABO incompatibility or hemolysis in units transfused:
	  ○ Inspect units and perform clerical check.
	  ○ Perform DAT and patient ABO type on pre- and posttransfusion samples.
	  ○ Examine pre- and posttransfusion samples for free hemoglobin.
	• Incompatibility due to alloantibodies:
	  ○ Perform IAT crossmatches, and test serum/plasma and eluate for alloantibodies.
	Note: Sensitive methods using serum, such as Procedures II-C and II-F, may be required to detect some alloantibodies.

		coated with IgG or IgG+C3, and there is a history of autoimmune disease, or history is unknown	warm autoimmune hemolytic anemia (WAIHA): • Test serum and eluate against a panel of phenotyped RBCs (see Section IV, Fig VIII-A-2, and Process VIII-A).
		coated with IgG or IgG+C3, and there is a relevant drug history	testing by Procedure XII-C, -D, -E, or -F, as indicated by drug history.
	2.	Evaluate the results of tests performed in Stage 1 according to the following criteria:	
		When…	**Then…**
		potent cold agglutinins are present	cold agglutinin disease is likely.
		the Donath-Landsteiner test result is positive	PCH is confirmed.
		tests for T- and/or Tk-activation are positive	the patient most likely has sepsis.
		tests for antibodies to drugs are positive	consider drug-induced immune hemolytic anemia.
		the unit is ABO incompatible or hemolyzed	investigate the cause and report as necessary to the FDA.
		alloantibodies were detected in pre- and/or posttransfusion samples	report as a DHTR and select antigen-negative units for future transfusion.

	IgG autoantibodies are present in the serum and/or eluate	• Consider WAIHA:
		Note: Many patients have IgG autoantibodies but do not hemolyze. Diagnosis of WAIHA is likely only if hemolysis is evident.
		  o Exclude underlying alloantibodies by adsorption. Select procedure from Section XI based on transfusion history.
		  o Proceed as described in Fig VIII-A-2.
		• Also consider drugs, especially α-methyl-dopa therapy.

	serum and elution studies are negative	• Consider passive antibody from non-ABO-type-specific blood components or transplants:
		  o Test serum and eluate against A_1 and B RBCs by an IAT (eg, Procedure II-I).
		• Consider drug-dependent antibody.
		  o Review medical records and discuss the need for further studies outlined above with the patient's clinician.

3.	Evaluate the patient's transfusion history in conjunction with the results of antibody identification, adsorption, and elution studies, when performed, according to the following criteria:	

When the patient...	Then...
has not been recently transfused and the serum displays an *Rh specificity* (eg, anti-e, but the patient's RBCs carry e antigen), and the antibody is adsorbed by the autologous RBCs	antibody is a relative Rh autoantibody: • Consider issuing e-negative units if transfusion with e-positive units do not produce the expected increase in hemoglobin/hematocrit. • Notify the patient's clinician that compatible units may be unobtainable.

	has not been recently transfused and the serum and eluate react equally with all RBC samples from a reagent RBC panel, and the antibody is adsorbed by the autologous RBCs	antibody is a panreactive autoantibody: • Issue least-reactive units when observed. • Notify the patient's clinician that compatible units may be unobtainable.
	has been recently transfused, and the serum (either unadsorbed or adsorbed with ZZAP-treated allogeneic RBCs) displays alloantibody specificity(ies)	consider an alloimmune response to transfusion: • Harvest the patient's autologous RBCs (see Section V and Fig VIII-A-2) and phenotype for the appropriate antigens or genotype. • Notify patient's clinician and issue a transfusion reaction report.
	has been recently transfused, the eluate is broadly reactive, and the serum adsorbed with allogeneic RBCs is nonreactive	harvest the patient's autologous RBCs (See Section V and Fig VIII-A-2) and test against the eluate: • If reactive, eluted antibody is an autoantibody. • If nonreactive, consider an alloantibody to a high-prevalence antigen. Perform tests with rare reagent RBCs and/or antibodies. • Notify the patient's clinician that compatible units may be unobtainable.

	has been recently transfused, the eluate is broadly reactive, and the serum adsorbed with allogeneic RBCs is reactive	• The adsorption is incomplete:
		  ○ Perform further adsorptions if possible.
		
		 • The antibody is directed toward an antigen destroyed by DTT or proteases:
		  ○ Perform adsorption with untreated, phenotypically matched RBCs, if available.

Section XI. Investigating Samples Containing Autoantibodies
Investigation of Cases of Immune Hemolysis and/or a Positive DAT

Page 6 of 6

**Effective
Date**

Approved by:	Printed Name	Signature	Date
Laboratory Management			
Medical Director			
Quality Officer			

XI-B. Antiglobulin Testing: Direct Tests with Anti-IgG and Anti-C3

Purpose

To provide instructions for the detection of in-vivo bound IgG and C3:

- In the investigation of immune hemolysis.

Background Information

Direct antiglobulin testing is used in the investigation of immune-mediated RBC destruction when IgG and/or complement (C3) may be bound to RBCs in vivo.

RBCs obtained directly from the patient are washed free of unbound globulins and tested against polyspecific (anti-IgG+C3) and/or monospecific AHG reagents (anti-IgG or -C3). Agglutination by a monospecific reagent suggests that the RBCs are coated with the corresponding globulin.

Operational Policy

Samples should be no more than 48 hours old.

Tests must be read immediately after centrifugation.

Note: Prepare fresh cell suspension just before washing.

Limitations

Unwanted Positive Reactions:

- Tests are overcentrifuged.
- Reagents are contaminated.

Unwanted Negative Reactions:

- RBCs are insufficiently washed.
- Tests were left to stand following centrifugation.
- RBCs left in suspension for an extended period and tested.

Sample Requirements

RBCs from an EDTA-anticoagulated blood sample: 0.1 mL.

Equipment/ Materials

Antihuman C3: containing anti-C3d.

Antihuman IgG: γ-chain specific.

Control RBCs: IgG-coated RBCs and C3d-coated RBCs; available commercially, or see Section VII.

Polyspecific antihuman globulin (PS-AHG): containing both anti-IgG and anti-C3.

Quality Control

1. On each day of use, test each AHG reagent against IgG- and C3d-coated RBCs:

   a) IgG-coated RBCs should react only with PS-AHG and anti-IgG.

   b) C3-coated RBCs should react only with PS-AHG and C3-coated RBCs.

2. On each occasion that this test is performed:

   a) Add IgG-coated RBCs to all negative tests with PS-AHG and anti-IgG.

   b) Centrifuge as for hemagglutination tests.

   c) Examine the RBCs macroscopically and grade and record the results.

   d) Agglutination of IgG-coated RBCs indicates that active AHG was added and that the RBCs were adequately washed before testing.

Procedure

Use the following steps to perform the procedure:

Step	Action
1.	Dispense 1 drop of 3%-5% sample RBCs (in saline or native plasma) into each of 4 appropriately labeled 12 × 75-mm test tubes.
2.	Wash the RBCs four times in saline and completely decant the final wash supernate.
3.	To 1 tube, add PS-AHG according to the manufacturer's directions.
4.	Similarly, set up tests with the anti-IgG and anti-C3 reagents.
5.	To the fourth tube, add 2 drops of saline.
6.	Gently agitate the contents of each tube.
7.	Centrifuge as for hemagglutination tests.
8.	Examine the RBCs macroscopically; grade and record the results.
9.	When test results with anti-C3 are negative, and if the manufacturer's directions so indicate, incubate tubes containing anti-C3 and saline at RT for 5 minutes. Repeat Steps 7 and 8.

10.	Add IgG-coated RBCs to all negative tests with anti-IgG or polyspecific AHG. Recentrifuge and examine the tests macroscopically for mixed-field agglutination. Repeat tests when IgG-coated RBCs are nonreactive.
11.	Interpret the reactions as follows:

If PS-AHG reacts…	And anti-IgG reacts…	And anti-C3 reacts…	And saline reacts…	Then coating proteins are…
+	+	+	0	IgG+C3.
+	+	0	0	IgG.
+	0	+	0	C3.
+	+	+	+	undetermined. Reactions: • Are indicative of spontaneous agglutination. • May be caused by IgM coating.
0	0	0	0	not present.

12.	If DAT is negative but clinical signs of hemolysis are indicated, the test may be repeated, substituting ice-cold saline or LISS in the washing step.

Reference   Garratty G. Immune hemolytic anemia associated with negative routine serology. Semin Hematol 2005 Jul;42:156-64.

Section XI. Investigating Samples Containing Autoantibodies
Antiglobulin Testing: Direct Tests with Anti-IgG and Anti-C3

Page 4 of 4

**Effective
Date**

Approved by:	Printed Name	Signature	Date
Laboratory Management			
Medical Director			
Quality Officer			

XI-C. Antiglobulin Testing: Direct Tests with Anti-IgM and Anti-IgA

Purpose

To provide instructions for the detection of in-vivo bound IgM and IgA:

- In the investigation of immune hemolysis.

Background Information

In rare cases of immune-mediated RBC destruction, globulins other than IgG or C3 may be bound to RBCs in vivo. This procedure facilitates recognition of RBCs coated with IgA or IgM.

Operational Policy

Samples should be no more than 48 hours old.

Tests must be read immediately after centrifugation.

Fresh RBC suspension must be prepared immediately before washing.

Limitations

Unwanted Positive Reactions:

- Tests are overcentrifuged.
- Reagents are contaminated.

Unwanted Negative Reactions:

- RBCs are insufficiently washed.
- Tests were left to stand following centrifugation.

Sample Requirements

RBCs from an EDTA-anticoagulated blood sample: 0.1 mL.

Equipment/ Materials

Antihuman IgM: goat or monoclonal anti-IgM (eg, Jackson ImmunoResearch Laboratories, West Grove, PA, or Sanquin Reagents, Amsterdam, the Netherlands); 1 mL. Use as recommended by the manufacturer, or titrate vs IgM-coated RBCs to determine optimal working dilution.

Antihuman IgA: goat or monoclonal anti-IgA (eg, Jackson ImmunoResearch Laboratories, West Grove, PA, or Sanquin Reagents, Amsterdam, the Netherlands); 1 mL. Use as recommended by the manufacturer, or titrate vs IgA-coated RBCs to determine optimal working dilution.

IgM-coated and IgA-coated RBCs: see Section VII.

Normal group A₁B (or groups A₁ and B) RBCs: for use as negative controls; washed four times and diluted to a 3%-5% suspension with saline.

pH 7.3 PBS.

Quality Control

On each day of use, show that IgM- and IgA-coated RBCs, and control A₁B (or A₁ and B) RBCs, give the expected reactions with anti-IgM and anti-IgA.

For each lot of anti-IgA and anti-IgM, show that there is no reactivity with IgG- or C3-coated RBCs.

Procedure

Use the following steps to perform the procedure:

Step	Action
1.	Dispense 1 drop of 3%-5% test RBCs (in saline or native plasma) into each of 3 appropriately labeled labeled 12 × 75-mm test tubes.
2.	Wash the RBCs four times in saline and completely decant the final wash supernate.
3.	To 1 tube, add 2 drops of the optimal dilution of anti-IgM.
4.	To another tube, add 2 drops of the optimal dilution of anti-IgA.
5.	To the third tube, add 2 drops of pH 7.3 PBS.
6.	Gently agitate the contents of each tube.
7.	Centrifuge as for hemagglutination tests.
8.	Examine the RBCs macroscopically; grade and record the results.
9.	Incubate negative tests for 5 minutes at RT. Repeat Steps 7 and 8.

10.	Interpret the reactions as follows:			
	If anti-IgA reacts…	**And anti-IgM reacts…**	**And PBS reacts…**	**Then coating proteins are…**
	+	0	0	IgA.
	0	+	0	IgM.
	+	+	+	undetermined: • Reactions are indicative of spontaneous agglutination.
	0	0	0	not present.
11.	If DAT is negative but clinical signs of hemolysis are indicated, the test may be repeated, substituting ice-cold saline or LISS in the washing step.			

**Effective
Date**

Approved by:	**Printed Name**	**Signature**	**Date**
Laboratory Management			
Medical Director			
Quality Officer			

XI-D. Antiglobulin Testing: Direct Tests with Polybrene

Purpose

To provide instructions for the detection of in-vivo bound IgG:

- In the investigation of DAT-negative autoimmune hemolytic anemia.

Background Information

In rare cases of warm autoimmune hemolytic anemia, IgG may be present on RBCs at levels so low that the conventional DAT (as performed in Procedure XI-B) is nonreactive. This procedure uses the cationic polymer, Polybrene, which causes aggregation of normal RBCs that can be dispersed with sodium citrate. However, sodium citrate does not disperse Polybrene-induced aggregation of IgG-coated RBCs.

Operational Policy

This procedure should be performed on freshly prepared suspensions of washed RBCs.

Limitations

Unwanted Positive Reactions:

- Tests are overcentrifuged.

- Polybrene is insufficiently dispersed.

Unwanted Negative Reactions:

- RBCs are insufficiently washed.

- Tests are shaken too vigorously.

Sample Requirements

Autologous serum or plasma: 0.1 mL.

RBCs: from an EDTA-anticoagulated sample, washed three times and diluted to a 3%-5% suspension in saline; 0.2 mL.

Equipment/ Materials

AHG: anti-IgG; need not be heavy-chain specific.

Control anti-D serum: 1 in 10,000 dilution (in AB serum) of commercially available high-protein (polyclonal, not chemically modified) anti-D serum.

Note: This yields a negative test result with Rh+ RBCs in LISS-antiglobulin tests; see Section II.

Control RhD+ RBCs: washed three times and diluted to a 3%-5% suspension with saline.

Pipettors with disposable tips to deliver 100 µL and 1 mL (eg, VWR, Batavia, IL).

Group AB serum.

IgG-coated RBCs: available commercially, or see Section VII.

Low-ionic medium.

Neutralizing reagent.

Polybrene aggregating solution.

Quality Control

The method includes positive and negative controls.

Confirm all negative reactions with IgG-coated RBCs.

Procedure

Use the following steps to perform the procedure:

Step	Action
1.	Wash 1 drop of each RBC sample with normal saline in appropriately labeled 10 or 12 × 75-mm test tubes. **Note**: Include 2 tubes containing Rh+ RBCs for control tests.
2.	Prepare 1% RBC suspensions by gently decanting the supernate and shaking the contents of the tubes lightly to resuspend the RBCs, then decanting the tubes forcefully to leave 1 drop of 1% RBCs.
3.	First add 100 µL of autologous serum or plasma, then 1 mL of low-ionic medium to appropriate tubes. Mix and incubate at RT for 1 minute.
4.	Similarly, set up positive and negative controls with Rh+ RBCs and dilute anti-D or AB serum, respectively. Mix and incubate at RT for 1 minute.
5.	Add 100 µL of aggregating solution to each tube and mix.
6.	Centrifuge at 1000 × g for 10 seconds (or equivalent) and decant the supernate. DO NOT RESUSPEND THE RBCs.
7.	Add 100 µL of neutralizing solution.
8.	Gently shake the tubes (shake rack gently at 45-degree angle for 10 seconds) and observe for persistent agglutination. Grade and record the results.

9.	Interpret the reactions as follows:	
	If agglutination is…	**Then the RBCs are…**
	present	coated with globulins.
	absent	DAT negative.
10.	Wash the RBCs four times with saline and completely decant the final wash supernate.	
11.	To the dry RBC buttons thus obtained, add anti-IgG according to the manufacturer's directions.	
12.	Centrifuge as for hemagglutination tests.	
13.	Examine the RBCs macroscopically; grade and record the results.	
14.	Interpret the reactions as follows:	
	If agglutination is…	**Then the RBCs are…**
	present	coated with IgG.
	absent	DAT negative.
15.	Add IgG-coated RBCs to all negative tests. Recentrifuge and examine the tests macroscopically for mixed-field agglutination. Repeat antibody detection tests when tests with IgG-coated RBCs are nonreactive.	

References   Garratty G, Postoway N, Nance S, Brunt D. The detection of IgG on RBCs of "Coombs negative" autoimmune hemolytic anemias. Transfusion 1982;22:430.

Lalezari P, Jiang AF. The manual Polybrene test: A simple and rapid procedure for detection of RBC antibodies. Transfusion 1980;20:206-11.

**Effective
Date**

Approved by:	Printed Name	Signature	Date
Laboratory Management			
Medical Director			
Quality Officer			

XI-E. Antiglobulin Testing: Enzyme-Linked DAT

Purpose   To provide instructions for the detection of in-vivo bound IgG:

- In the investigation of DAT-negative autoimmune hemolytic anemia.

Background Information   In the enzyme-linked direct antiglobulin test (ELDAT), RBCs from patients with suspected autoimmune hemolysis but with a negative conventional DAT are washed and incubated with anti-IgG plus alkaline phosphatase conjugate (IgG-AP). Unbound anti-IgG-AP is removed by washing, and a substrate is added that interacts with AP to produce a yellow color, the intensity of which is measured at 405 nm. Because this assay is exquisitely sensitive, it may demonstrate clinically significant autoimmune IgG coating at levels not detectable by the conventional DAT.

Operational Policy   Accuracy is essential when preparing RBC suspensions for use in the ELDAT. Dilute RBCs to approximately 2%. Determine actual suspension using an electronic particle counter and adjust to 2×10^8 RBCs/mL.

Limitations   Unwanted Positive Reactions:

- Unbound IgG-AP is not effectively removed.

Unwanted Negative Reactions:

- RBCs are insufficiently washed.

Sample Requirements   RBCs: from an EDTA-anticoagulated blood sample, washed six times and diluted to a 2% suspension with BSA-PBS. Determine actual suspension using an electronic particle counter and adjust to 2×10^8 RBCs/mL; a minimum of 1.5 mL is required.

**Equipment/
Materials**

Anti-D: RhIG; available commercially; obtain μg/mL content from manufacturer; dilute from 1:1000 to 1:128,000 with BSA-PBS.

Anti-IgG conjugate: ovine (sheep) antihuman IgG conjugated with AP (eg, MP Biomedicals, Irvine, CA). Determine the appropriate dilution for the anti-IgG-AP from titration studies (using serial twofold dilutions in BSA-PBS) with Rh+ RBCs precoated with a 1000× dilution of commercially prepared modified-tube (high-protein) anti-D. Plot the OD values against anti-IgG-AP dilution on linear graph paper. Choose a dilution of anti-IgG-AP that gives an OD value with Rh+ RBCs on the straight part of the curve, yet gives a low OD with Rh– RBCs.

BSA-PBS.

BSA-NS.

Laboratory film (eg, Parafilm, VWR, Batavia, IL).

ρ-nitrophenol phosphate (PNP) substrate: PNP (eg, Sigma-Aldrich, St Louis, MO), diluted to 2 mg/mL with 0.05 M carbonate buffer just before use.

Pippettors: to deliver 200-1000 μL (eg, VWR, Batavia, IL).

1 N NaOH.

Spectrophotometer (eg, Spectronic 200, VWR, Batavia, IL or equivalent): at wavelength of 405 nm.

Test tubes: glass, 12 × 75 mm. Prepare for EDAT by filling with BSA-PBS, discarding BSA-PBS after a few minutes, and inverting to drain.

Negative control RBC samples: six normal donor RBC samples, washed six times and diluted to a 2% suspension with BSA-PBS.

Positive control RBC samples: R_1R_1 or R_2R_2 RBCs precoated with dilutions of anti-D as follows:

1. Wash RBCs three times in BSA-PBS, and then wash once and dilute to a 2% suspension with BSA-LISS, as described above.

2. Dispense 1 mL of 2% R_1R_1 or R_2R_2 RBCs into 8 precoated 12 × 75-mm test tubes.

3. To 1 tube of each set, add 1 mL of a 1:1000 dilution of anti-D in BSA-LISS.

4. Similarly, set up tests with the other anti-D dilutions.

5. Incubate all tubes at 37 C for 15 minutes.

6. Wash the RBCs three times with pH 7.3 PBS and aspirate the final wash supernate.

7. Dilute the RBCs to a 2% suspension with BSA-PBS, as described above.

Quality Control

The procedure includes positive and negative controls.

Procedure

Use the following steps to perform the procedure:

Step	Action
1.	For each RBC sample (test, normal, and positive controls) dispense 0.5 mL of 2% RBCs into 3 precoated, appropriately labeled 12 × 75-mm glass test tubes.
2.	Wash the RBCs once with BSA-PBS and aspirate the final supernate.
3.	To duplicate tubes of each sample, add 0.2 mL anti-IgG-AP.
4.	To the third tube of each sample, add 0.2 mL BSA-PBS to serve as a "hemolysis control" tube.
5.	Cover the tubes with Parafilm and incubate at 37 C for 1 hour; mix periodically by gentle agitation during this time.
6.	Wash the RBCs three times with BSA-PBS and aspirate the final supernate.
7.	Dilute the RBCs in 0.5 mL BSA-NS and transfer to clean, appropriately labeled 12 × 75-mm test tubes.
8.	Centrifuge to pack the RBCs, and aspirate the supernate.
9.	Add 0.2 mL BSA-NS and 0.2 mL PNP to the RBC buttons.
10.	Mix well, cover the tubes with Parafilm, and incubate at 37 C for 60 minutes.
11.	Remove Parafilm and centrifuge to pack the RBCs.
12.	Transfer the supernates into clean test tubes and add 0.5 mL of 1 N NaOH (to stop the enzyme reaction).
13.	Read the OD of each supernate at 405 nm. **Note:** Read against a reagent blank consisting of PNP, 0.2 mL; BSA-NS, 0.2 mL; and 1 N NaOH, 0.5 mL.
14.	To evaluate the results for each sample, calculate the corrected OD by subtracting OD C from OD T, where T = test; C = hemolysis control.

15.	Take the average of the 2 corrected OD values for each test and control sample.
16.	Calculate the number of IgG molecules bound per RBC as follows: $$\frac{4 \times 10^{11} \times \text{RhIG anti-D content}}{\text{RhIG dilution} \times 2 \times 10^{8}}$$ Using the following assumptions: • 1 µg of anti-D contains 4×10^{11} molecules. • All anti-D molecules were bound in Step 3 of the Equipment Materials section.
17.	Plot the number of molecules bound per RBC at each anti-D dilution and plot against corrected OD values. Use the curve obtained to calculate the number of IgG molecules bound to the test RBCs.

References

Leikola J, Perkins HA. Enzyme-linked antiglobulin test: An accurate and simple method to quantitate RBC antibodies. Transfusion 1980;20:138-44.

Postoway N, Nance SJ, Garratty G. Variables affecting the enzyme-linked antiglobulin test when detecting and quantitating IgG RBC antibodies. Med Lab Sci 1985;42:11-19.

Wilson L, Wren MR, Issitt PD. Enzyme linked antiglobulin test: Variables affecting the test when measuring levels of RBC antigens. Med Lab Sci 1985;42:20-5.

Effective Date

Approved by:	Printed Name	Signature	Date
Laboratory Management			
Medical Director			
Quality Officer			

XI-F. Dispersing Autoagglutination

Purpose

To provide instructions for dispersing strongly agglutinated RBCs:

- Phenotyping and DAT studies on RBC samples that spontaneously agglutinate.

Background Information

IgM molecules consist of 5 radially arranged subunits linked by intersubunit disulphide (S-S) bonds that are susceptible to cleavage by thiol reagents such as 2-mercaptoethanol (2-ME) and dithiothreitol (DTT). The addition of 2-ME or DTT to RBCs that are spontaneously agglutinated by IgM autoantibodies in vitro results in unagglutinated RBC samples for use in blood grouping tests.

Operational Policy

Either DTT or 2-ME may be used for this procedure. The reagent should be used in a fume hood or in accordance with the institution's chemicals policy.

Limitations

Residual weak agglutination may be present following treatment of heavily coated RBCs.

Antigens that are susceptible to reducing agents (eg, Kell antigens) may be destroyed.

Sample Requirements

RBCs: from an EDTA-anticoagulated sample, washed three times with saline and diluted to a 50% suspension with PBS.

Equipment/ Materials

6% BSA.

Working Solution: dithiothreitol, 0.01 M (0.01 M DTT), or 2-ME, 0.1 M (0.1 M 2-ME).

pH 7.3 PBS.

Quality Control

Test treated and untreated RBCs with 6% BSA by immediate-spin technique.

Treat a control RBC sample carrying antigens for which the test RBCs are to be tested (eg, AB cells when treating to determine ABO type), in parallel with the test sample.

Procedure   Use the following steps to perform the procedure:

Step	Action
1.	To 1 volume of 50% patient and control RBCs in PBS, add an equal volume of 0.01 M DTT or 0.1 M 2-ME to each tube.
2.	Incubate at 37 C for 15 minutes (10 minutes for 2-ME).
3.	Wash RBCs three times with saline.
4.	Dilute the treated RBCs to a 3%-5% suspension with saline before use in blood typing tests (see Sections I and XIII).

Reference   Reid ME. Autoagglutination dispersal utilizing sulphydryl compounds. Transfusion 1978;18:353-5.

**Effective
Date**

Approved by:	**Printed Name**	**Signature**	**Date**
Laboratory Management			
Medical Director			
Quality Officer			

XI-G. Testing the Thermal Amplitude of a Cold-Reactive Autoantibody

Purpose

To provide instructions for determining the thermal amplitude of a cold-reactive IgG autoantibody:

- In the investigation of samples containing cold-reactive autoantibodies.

Background Information

Thermal amplitude tests may be used to assess the clinical significance of autoantibodies. Antibodies preferentially reactive in vitro at body temperatures are likely to cause significant RBC destruction in vivo, in contrast to RBCs that react preferentially below body temperature in vitro. The higher the thermal amplitude of the autoantibody, the greater the potential for immune hemolysis. Note that some IgM warm-reactive autoantibodies may react preferentially at 22 C.

Operational Policy

Samples should be collected, maintained, and separated at 37 C.

Limitations

Not applicable.

Sample Requirements

Serum: separated at 37 C from clotted blood samples maintained at 37 C: 0.3 mL.

Equipment/ Materials

Reagent RBCs: 2 samples of group O, adult I+, washed three times and diluted to a 3%-5% suspension with saline.

Water baths: 37 C, 30 C, and 22 C.

Quality Control

Check waterbaths before, once during, and at the end of each incubation phase. Acceptable temperature variation is ±1 C.

Procedure   Use the following steps to perform the procedure:

Step	Action
1.	Warm RBCs, serum, and 10 or 12 × 75-mm test tubes to 37 C.
2.	For each RBC sample to be tested, mix 3 drops of serum and 1 drop of 3%-5% RBCs in the prewarmed test tubes.
3.	Incubate at 37 C for 1 hour.
4.	Centrifuge as for hemagglutination tests and return tubes to 37 C for 5 minutes before reading.
5.	Examine the RBCs macroscopically; grade and record the results.
6.	Transfer the tubes to 30 C and incubate at this temperature for 1 hour.
7.	Centrifuge as for hemagglutination tests and return tubes to 30 C for 5 minutes before reading.
8.	Examine the RBCs macroscopically; grade and record the results.
9.	Transfer the tubes to 22 C and incubate at this temperature for 1 hour.
10.	Centrifuge as for hemagglutination tests.
11.	Interpret the results as follows:

If agglutination is present at…	Then the antibody…
22 C but not 30 C	has a limited thermal amplitude.
30 C but not 37 C	has potential clinical significance, depending, in part, on the strength of reactivity.
37 C	should be considered potentially clinically significant.

Reference   Judd WJ. Investigation and management of immune hemolysis: Autoantibodies and drugs. In: Wallace ME, Levitt JS, eds. Current applications and interpretation of the direct antiglobulin test. Arlington, VA: AABB, 1988:47-103.

**Effective
Date**

Approved by:	Printed Name	Signature	Date
Laboratory Management			
Medical Director			
Quality Officer			

Judd's Methods in Immunohematology
Diagnostic Testing of a Cold-Reactive Autoantibody by Titration
Page 1 of 3

XI-H. Diagnostic Testing of a Cold-Reactive Autoantibody by Titration

Purpose

To provide instructions for titration of a cold-reactive autoantibody:

- In the investigation of samples containing cold-reactive autoantibodies.

- To evaluate the antibody for clinical significance.

Background Information

Immune hemolysis by cold-reactive autoantibodies (particularly anti-I) may be related to autoantibody titer; the higher the titer the greater the hemolytic potential (clinical significance) of the autoantibody. This procedure may be used to determine the titer of cold-reactive autoanti-I.

Operational Policy

Samples should be collected, maintained, and separated at 37 C.

Calibrated pipettes should be used for preparing dilutions of serum.

Use a clean pipette tip for each tube to prevent carryover.

Limitations

Unwanted Positive Reactions:

- Carryover when preparing dilutions.

Sample Requirements

Serum: separated at 37 C from clotted blood samples maintained at 37 C; 0.3 mL.

Equipment/ Materials

Pipettors with disposable tips to deliver 100-500 µL (eg, VWR, Batavia, IL).

pH 7.3 PBS.

RBCs: 1% suspension of group O, I+ RBCs in pH 7.3 PBS. Prepare fresh daily from ACD or CPD anticoagulated blood collected within the previous 7 days. Wash three times with saline before dilution with PBS.

Quality Control

Not applicable.

Procedure   Use the following steps to perform the procedure:

Step	Action
1.	Dilute 0.2 mL of serum with 0.8 mL of pH 7.3 PBS.
2.	Using 12 × 75-mm test tubes, prepare 0.5-mL volumes of serial twofold dilutions of this 1 in 5 dilution with pH 7.3 PBS. The final dilution range should be from 1 in 10 to 1 in 20,480 (12 tubes).
3.	Add 0.5 mL of 1% RBCs to each dilution.
4.	Mix and incubate overnight at 4 C.
5.	DO NOT CENTRIFUGE: carefully place tubes in bath of melting ice and (1 tube at a time) examine the RBCs macroscopically for agglutination, starting with the highest dilution of serum. Grade and record the results.
6.	Report the titer as the reciprocal of the highest dilution of serum at which agglutination is observed.
7.	Interpret the results as follows:

If the titer is...	Then the antibody...
>40	is clinically significant.
>640 **Note:** Titers <640 may be obtained with autoanti-i; in such a situation, i_{cord} or i_{adult} RBCs may used instead of or in addition to I+ RBCs.	is likely to cause immune hemolysis.
<40	is not clinically significant.

Reference   Henry JB. Clinical diagnosis and management by laboratory methods. 16th ed. Philadelphia, PA: WB Saunders, 1979.

Effective Date

Approved by:	Printed Name	Signature	Date
Laboratory Management			
Medical Director			
Quality Officer			

Section XI. Investigating Samples Containing Autoantibodies
Determining Specificity of a Cold-Reactive Autoantibody by Titration

Page 1 of 3

XI-I. Determining Specificity of a Cold-Reactive Autoantibody by Titration

Purpose

To provide instructions for determining the specificity of a cold-reactive autoantibody:

- In the investigation of samples containing cold-reactive autoantibodies.

Background Information

Cold-reactive autoantibodies often do not display specificity except at dilution. For example, undiluted, potent anti-I will agglutinate I+, i_{cord}, and i_{adult} RBCs to the same degree (score); however, in titration studies, it can be shown that adult I+ RBCs are the strongest-reacting RBCs.

The following procedure may be used to determine specificity of autoantibodies associated with cold agglutinin syndrome (CAS). Such testing, in and of itself, is not diagnostic of CAS. However, autoantibody specificity may correlate with etiology; anti-I has been associated with *Mycoplasma pneumonia* infection, and anti-i with infectious mononucleosis and other disorders of the reticuloendothelial system.

Operational Policy

Samples should be collected, maintained, and separated at 37 C.

Calibrated pipettes should be used for preparing dilutions of serum.

Use a clean pipette tip for each tube to prevent carryover.

Limitations

Unwanted Positive Reactions:

- Carryover when preparing dilutions.

Sample Requirements

Serum: separated at 37 C from clotted blood samples maintained at 37 C; 2-3 mL.

Autologous RBCs: from anticoagulated sample.

Equipment/ Materials

Pipettors with disposable tips to deliver 100-1000 μL (eg, VWR, Batavia, IL).

pH 7.3 PBS.

Reagent RBCs: group O, I+, 2 samples; pooled group O RBCs pretreated with ficin or papain as described in Section III; RBCs of the same ABO type as the autologous RBCs (if other than group O); group O, i_{cord} or i_{adult} RBCs.

Quality Control

Not applicable.

Procedure

Use the following steps to perform the procedure:

Step	Action
1.	Wash reagent and autologous RBCs three times with saline and dilute to a 3%-5% suspension with pH 7.3 PBS.
2.	Prepare serial twofold dilutions of serum in pH 7.3 PBS; the dilution range should be from 1 in 2 to 1 in 4096 (12 tubes), and the volumes prepared should not be less than 0.5 mL.
3.	For each RBC sample to be tested, place 3 drops of each dilution into appropriately labeled 10 or 12 × 75-mm test tubes.
4.	Add 1 drop of a 3%-5% suspension of a selected RBC sample to 1 tube of each serum dilution. Similarly, set up tests with the other selected RBCs.
5.	Gently agitate the contents of each tube and incubate at RT for 15 minutes.
6.	Centrifuge as for hemagglutination tests.
7.	Examine the RBCs macroscopically; grade and record the results, starting with the highest dilution of serum.
8.	Transfer the tubes to 4 C and incubate at this temperature for 1 hour.
9.	Centrifuge as for hemagglutination tests.
10.	Examine the RBCs macroscopically; grade and record the results.
11.	Interpret the results according to Table XI-1.

Reference

Judd WJ. Investigation and management of immune hemolysis: Autoantibodies and drugs. In: Wallace ME, Levitt JS, eds. Current applications and interpretation of the direct antiglobulin test. Arlington, VA: AABB, 1988:47-103.

Section XI. Investigating Samples Containing Autoantibodies
Determining Specificity of a Cold-Reactive Autoantibody by Titration

Page 3 of 3

**Effective
Date**

Approved by:	Printed Name	Signature	Date
Laboratory Management			
Medical Director			
Quality Officer			

XI-J. Adsorbing Cold-Reactive Autoantibodies with Autologous RBCs

Purpose

To provide instructions for cold autologous adsorption:

- In the investigation of samples containing cold-reactive autoantibodies.

Background Information

Cold-reactive autoantibodies may mask the presence of underlying (concomitant) clinically significant alloantibodies. In this procedure, autoantibodies are removed from serum by adsorption with autologous RBCs that have been pretreated with a proteolytic enzyme. Treating RBCs with proteolytic enzymes enhances their adsorptive capacity by removing RBC membrane structures that otherwise hinder antigen-antibody association.

Note: Autoantibodies specific for protease-sensitive antigens (eg, Pr) will not be removed by this method.

Operational Policy

Autoadsorptions should not be used when the patient has been transfused within the previous 120 days.

Usually, 2-3 adsorptions are sufficient to remove the autoantibody; in rare instances, additional adsorptions may be required.

Limitations

Incorrect Results:

- Dilution of the plasma or serum may occur if care is not taken to remove all saline following RBC washes.

Sample Requirements

Plasma/serum for adsorption: 2 mL

Autologous RBCs: washed three times; 3 mL.

Equipment/ Materials

Ficin or papain: 1% wt/vol.

Glycine max (syn. *soja*) lectin (eg, Immucor, Norcross, GA, or see Section XIV).

Protein refractometer (eg, #47752-872, VWR, Batavia, IL).

Reagent RBCs: 3%-5% suspensions of group O, R_1R_1 and R_2R_2 RBCs.

5-mL graduated pipettes (eg, VWR, Batavia, IL).

Quality Control

Before use, confirm that the RBCs for adsorption have been treated with proteolytic enzyme. Untreated RBCs should be nonreactive with *G. max,* whereas complete agglutination should be observed with protease-treated RBCs.

Using a refractometer, measure the protein content of the adsorbed and unadsorbed serum. The adsorption process should not have lowered the protein content by more than 20% of the total protein in the unadsorbed sample.

Procedure

Use the following steps to perform the procedure:

Step	Action
1.	Mix 3 mL of RBCs with 1.5 mL of 1% papain or 1% ficin in a 16 × 100-mm test tube.
2.	Incubate at 37 C for 15 minutes.
3.	Wash the RBCs three times in saline and dispense 1-mL aliquots into each of 3 appropriately labeled 10 × 75-mm test tubes.
4.	Fill the tubes with saline and centrifuge to pack the RBCs ($\geq$1000 × g for at least 5 minutes). Remove as much of the supernate as possible.
5.	Mix 1 mL of enzyme-treated RBCs with 2 mL of autologous serum.
6.	Incubate at 4 C for 15-40 minutes.
7.	Centrifuge to pack the RBCs. Transfer the serum to another tube of enzyme-treated RBCs and mix well.
8.	Incubate at 4 C for 15-40 minutes.
9.	Centrifuge to pack the RBCs. Transfer the serum to the third tube of enzyme-treated RBCs and mix well.
10.	Incubate at 4 C for 30-40 minutes.
11.	Centrifuge to pack the RBCs. Transfer the adsorbed serum to a clean test tube. Test with group O reagent RBCs and 2-ME/DTT-treated autologous RBCs (see Procedure XI-F).

12.	Interpret the results as follows:			
	If the serum reacts with R₁R₁…	**And R₂R₂…**	**And Auto…**	**Then the autoantibody…**
	0	0	0 to ++	has been adsorbed, and the serum most likely does not contain alloantibodies.
	+/0*	+/0	0 to ++	has been adsorbed, and the serum may contain alloantibodies.
	++	++	+ to ++++	has not been fully adsorbed: • Repeat adsorption once more.
	*If alloantibodies are present, reactivity with the reagent RBCs may be variable in strength and may react with one reagent RBC sample and not the other.			
13.	Once the autoantibody has been adsorbed, test the serum in parallel with the unadsorbed serum by saline agglutination and antiglobulin techniques described in Section II.			

Effective Date

Approved by:	Printed Name	Signature	Date
Laboratory Management			
Medical Director			
Quality Officer			

XI-K. Adsorbing Cold Autoantibodies with Heterologous (Rabbit) RBCs

Purpose	To provide instructions for adsorption of strongly reactive cold autoantibodies with rabbit RBCs: • In the investigation of samples containing cold-reactive autoantibodies.
Background Information	Cold-reactive autoantibodies may mask the presence of underlying (concomitant) clinically significant alloantibodies. In the following procedure, autoantibodies are removed from serum by adsorption with rabbit RBCs, which readily adsorb IgM antibodies. Fixation with formalin permits extended storage of the RBCs for use in heterologous adsorption studies.
Operational Policy	Antibodies must be identified before adsorption because adsorption is not specific.
Limitations	<u>Unwanted Negative Reactions:</u> • Rabbit RBCs may adsorb alloantibodies of potential clinical significance if they are IgM.
Sample Requirements	Plasma/serum for adsorption: 2 mL.
Equipment/ Materials	Buffered formalin: 20% wt/vol. *Glycine max* (syn. *soja*) lectin (eg, Immucor, Norcross, GA, or see Section XIV). Magnetic stirrer and small stirring bar. pH 7.3 PBS. Rabbit RBCs: from 100 mL blood collected aseptically in Alsever's solution (eg, Pel-Freez Biologicals, Rogers, AR), washed three times with saline. Reagent RBCs: 3%-5% suspensions of group O, R_1R_1 and R_2R_2 RBCs. Protein refractometer (eg, #47752-872, VWR, Batavia, IL). 1-L beaker (eg, VWR, Batavia, IL). Pipettors with disposable tips to deliver 1 mL (eg, VWR, Batavia, IL).

**Quality
Control**

Using a refractometer, measure the protein content of the adsorbed and unadsorbed serum. The adsorption process should not have lowered the protein content by more than 20% of the total protein in the unadsorbed sample.

Procedure

Use the following steps to perform the procedure:

Step	Action
1.	Pack RBCs and add drop-wise into 1 L of 20% buffered formalin, mixing continuously during this process with a magnetic stirrer.
2.	Incubate overnight at RT.
3.	Wash the RBCs four times and dilute with an equal volume of pH 7.3 PBS. Store at 4 C indefinitely.
4.	Before use, dispense 1-mL aliquots of formalin-fixed rabbit RBCs into each of 2 appropriately labeled 10 × 75-mm test tubes.
5.	Fill the tubes with saline and centrifuge to pack the RBCs (≥1000 × g for at least 5 minutes). Remove as much of the supernate as possible.
6.	Mix 1 aliquot of formalin-fixed RBCs with 2 mL of autologous serum.
7.	Incubate at 4 C for 30-40 minutes.
8.	Centrifuge to pack the RBCs. Transfer the serum to another tube of formalin-fixed RBCs and mix well.
9.	Incubate at 4 C for 30-40 minutes.
10.	Centrifuge to pack the RBCs. Transfer the adsorbed serum to a clean test tube. Test with routine group O RBCs and 2-ME/DTT-treated autologous RBCs (see Procedure XI-F). Grade and record the results.

11.	Interpret the reactions as follows:			
	If the serum reacts with R_1R_1...	**And R_2R_2...**	**And Auto...**	**Then the autoantibody...**
	0	0	0 to ++	has been adsorbed, and the serum most likely does not contain alloantibodies.
	+/0*	+/0	0 to ++	has been adsorbed, and the serum may contain alloantibodies.
	++	++	+ to ++	has not been fully adsorbed: • Repeat adsorption once more.
	*If alloantibodies are present, the reactivity with the group O RBCs may be variable in strength and may react with one RBC sample and not the other.			
12.	Once adsorbed, test the serum in parallel with the unadsorbed serum by saline agglutination and antiglobulin techniques described in Section II.			

References

Dzik W, Yang R, Blank J. Rabbit erythrocyte stroma treatment of serum interferes with recognition of delayed hemolytic transfusion reactions (letter). Transfusion 1986;26:303-4.

Marks MR, Reid R, Ellisor SS. Adsorption of unwanted cold autoagglutinins by formaldehyde-treated rabbit red blood cells (abstract). Transfusion 1980;20:629.

Storry JR, Olsson ML, Moulds JJ. Rabbit red blood cell stroma bind immunoglobulin M antibodies regardless of blood group specificity (letter). Transfusion 2006;46:1260-1.

**Effective
Date**

Approved by:	Printed Name	Signature	Date
Laboratory Management			
Medical Director			
Quality Officer			

XI-L. Testing for PCH Using the Donath-Landsteiner Test

Purpose

To provide instructions for the detection of biphasic hemolysins as an aid to the diagnosis of paroxysmal cold hemoglobinuria (PCH):

- In the investigation of immune hemolysis.

- When there is evidence of acute hemolysis in the absence of positive test results for unexpected antibodies.

Background Information

PCH is a rare form of autoimmune hemolytic anemia. Characteristically, PCH is caused by IgG autoantibodies that act as biphasic hemolysins in vitro; ie, the IgG autoantibody binds complement components to RBCs at cold temperatures, and lysis of the coated RBCs occurs when the reactants are warmed to 37 C. This is the basis for the Donath-Landsteiner test. Most examples of the Donath-Landsteiner antibody manifest anti-P specificity; ie, they fail to react in Donath-Landsteiner tests with the very rare p and P^k RBCs. There are isolated reports of PCH caused by anti-i, -IH, and -Pr.

This procedure should be considered for patients with clinical signs and symptoms of hemolysis in the following situations:

- Cold agglutinins are not detected in the serum.

- C3 alone is present on the RBCs.

- The DAT is negative, the eluate is nonreactive, and the patient has hemoglobinemia and/or hemoglobinuria.

Note: PCH should not be confused with paroxysmal nocturnal hemoglobinuria (PNH), which is associated with absence of RBC membrane glycosylphosphatidylinositol-linked (GPI-linked) proteins.

Operational Policy

Blood samples must be drawn and maintained at 37 C before testing.

Fresh normal serum is included as a source of complement (patients with PCH often have low complement levels).

Limitations

Unwanted Positive Reactions:

- Samples were allowed to cool before testing.

Unwanted Negative Reactions:

- Hemolysis may be misinterpreted as a negative reaction.

Judd's Methods in Immunohematology
Testing for PCH Using the Donath-Landsteiner Test
Page 2 of 3

**Sample
Requirements**

Serum: 2-3 mL; separated at 37 C from clotted blood samples maintained at 37 C.

**Equipment/
Materials**

Human complement: freshly collected (within 6 hours of use) normal human serum (from a healthy volunteer) known to lack unexpected antibodies; 2-3 mL. May be stored frozen in 1-mL aliquots. Do not refreeze.

pH 7.3 PBS.

RBCs: 50% suspension of group O reagent RBCs in pH 7.3 PBS. Prepare fresh daily from ACD- or CPD-anticoagulated blood collected within the previous 7 days and washed three times with saline before dilution with PBS.

Sheep RBCs: available in most clinical immunology laboratories, or obtain commercially (eg, Pel-Freez Biologicals, Rogers, AR).

**Quality
Control**

This procedure includes control tests for lysis by mechanisms other than that produced by a biphasic hemolysin.

Before use, each batch of human complement should be shown to lyse sheep RBCs: use 1 drop of 3%-5% washed sheep RBCs in saline, 3 drops of human complement, and 15 minutes incubation at 37 C; centrifuge as for hemagglutination tests and examine the supernate for hemolysis.

Procedure

Use the following steps to perform the procedure:

Step	Action
1.	Prepare 10 or 12 × 75-mm test tubes as follows: a) 3 tubes each containing 10 drops of test serum. b) 3 tubes each containing 5 drops of test serum and 5 drops of human complement. c) 3 tubes each containing 10 drops of human complement.
2.	Add 1 drop of 50% RBCs to each tube and mix.
3.	Place 1 tube from each set at 37 C for 90 minutes.
4.	Place 2 tubes from each set in melting ice (0 C). After 30 minutes, remove 1 tube from each set and incubate at 37 C for 60 minutes. Leave remaining tubes at 0 C.

5.	Centrifuge all tubes to pack the RBCs. Examine the supernates for hemolysis; grade and record the results.
6.	Interpret the reactions as follows:

If the RBCs at 37 C react...	And RBCs at 0→37 C react...	And RBCs at 0 C react...	Then the Donath-Landsteiner test result is....
0	+/H	0	positive.
0	+/H	+/H	negative: • Probable cold-reactive antibody.
+/H	+/H	0	negative: • Probable warm-reactive antibody.
0	0	0	negative.

H = hemolysis.

Note: If no hemolysis is observed, take the RBCs from each tube, wash four times, and test a 3%-5% suspension with anti-C3, as described earlier in Process XI-A. If reactivity is observed, interpret agglutination as for hemolysis in the above table.

Reference Dacie JV, Lewis SM. Practical haematology. 4th ed. London: Churchill, 1968.

Effective Date

Approved by:

	Printed Name	Signature	Date
Laboratory Management			
Medical Director			
Quality Officer			

XI-M. Determining the Specificity of Warm-Reactive Autoantibodies by Titration

Purpose

To provide instructions for evaluating the relative specificity of a warm-reactive autoantibody:

- In the investigation of samples containing warm-reactive autoantibodies.

Background Information

Warm-reactive autoantibodies often exhibit relative Rh specificity—eg, autoanti-e that reacts strongly with e-positive RBCs but weakly with e-negative RBCs. Other warm-reactive autoantibodies display relative Rh specificity upon dilution. In hemolyzing patients with autoantibodies that display clear-cut Rh specificity with undiluted serum or eluate, there is some evidence that antigen-negative blood will survive better than the patient's RBCs. If relative Rh specificity can be demonstrated only by titration studies, the use of antigen-negative blood is debatable. However, limited data suggest that such blood may survive longer than the patient's RBCs. In the absence of hemolysis, the selection of antigen-negative blood is not required.

This procedure may also demonstrate underlying alloantibodies in sera containing warm-reactive autoantibodies, but it is not the optimal method to demonstrate concomitant alloantibodies, and it will be informative only if the alloantibody titer is greater than that of the autoantibody. Instead, adsorption studies are recommended (see Procedures XI-N and XI-O). Also see Procedures II-H, II-I, and Section VIII).

Operational Policy

Calibrated pipettes should be used for preparing dilutions of serum.

Use a clean pipette tip for each tube to prevent carryover.

Limitations

Unwanted Positive Reactions:

- Carryover when preparing dilutions.

Sample Requirements

Serum or eluate: 2 mL. See Section IV for elution techniques.

**Equipment/
Materials**

AHG: anti-IgG.

Pipettors with disposable tips to deliver 100-500 µL (eg, VWR, Batavia, IL).

Reagent RBCs: 3%-5% suspensions of group O, R_1R_1; O, R_2R_2; and O, rr RBCs.

**Quality
Control**

Not applicable.

Procedure

Use the following steps to perform the procedure:

Step	Action
1.	Prepare serial twofold dilutions of serum or eluate in saline. The dilution range should be from 1 in 2 to 1 in 1024 (10 tubes), and the volumes prepared should not be less than 0.5 mL.
2.	Place 3 drops of each dilution into each of 3 appropriately labeled 10 or 12 × 75-mm test tubes.
3.	To 1 tube of each dilution, add 1 drop of R_1R_1 RBCs. Similarly, test the R_2R_2 and rr RBCs.
4.	Gently agitate the contents of each tube. Incubate at 37 C for 30-60 minutes.
5.	Wash the RBCs four times with saline and completely decant the final wash supernate.
6.	To the dry RBC buttons thus obtained, add anti-IgG according to the manufacturer's directions.
7.	Centrifuge as for hemagglutination tests.
8.	Examine the RBCs macroscopically; grade and record the results, starting with the highest dilution of serum or eluate.
9.	On the basis of the results obtained, select the highest dilution of serum or eluate that gives a 2+ reaction with the most strongly reactive RBC sample.
10.	Prepare a sufficient volume of this dilution and test against a panel of reagent RBCs by saline antiglobulin technique (see Section II).

Judd's Methods in Immunohematology
Determining the Specificity of Warm-Reactive Autoantibodies by Titration
Page 3 of 3

11.	Interpret the results as follows:	
	If the diluted serum or eluate…	**Then…**
	is nonreactive with all RBC samples	the dilution was too high.
	reacts with some but not all RBC samples	check for blood group specificity.
	reacts equally with all RBC samples	no specificity is apparent.

Reference

Judd WJ. Investigation and management of immune hemolysis: Autoantibodies and drugs. In: Wallace ME, Levitt JS, eds. Current applications and interpretation of the direct antiglobulin test. Arlington, VA: AABB, 1988:47-103.

Effective Date

Approved by:	Printed Name	Signature	Date
Laboratory Management			
Medical Director			
Quality Officer			

XI-N. Adsorbing Warm-Reactive Autoantibodies with Enzyme-Treated Autologous RBCs

Purpose

To provide instructions for autoadsorption of warm-reactive autoantibodies:

- In the investigation of immune hemolysis and samples containing autoantibodies.

Background Information

Warm-reactive autoantibodies may mask the concomitant presence of alloantibodies in a serum. Recognition of alloantibodies is facilitated by removing serum autoantibodies by adsorption with autologous RBCs.

Autologous adsorption of warm-reactive autoantibodies can be achieved most effectively when coating antibody is first removed from the RBCs, and when the RBCs are pretreated with a proteolytic enzyme. Removal of coating antibody exposes antigen sites previously covered by autoantibody. Such sites are then available for binding to free autoantibody. Enzyme treatment enhances the adsorption process by removing RBC membrane structures that otherwise hinder antigen-antibody association.

Note: Because of the presence of donor RBCs carrying antigens to which the serum contains alloantibodies, reliable results may not be obtained with patients transfused within the preceding 120 days.

Operational Policy

This procedure is not suitable for patients transfused within the preceding 120 days.

Note: Two to three adsorptions are usually sufficient to remove the autoantibody; however, in rare instances additional adsorptions may be required.

Limitations

Unwanted Positive Reactions:

- Autoantibodies specific for papain-sensitive antigens will not be removed by this method.

Unwanted Negative Reactions:

- Dilution of the plasma or serum may occur if care is not taken to remove all saline following RBC washes.

Sample Requirements

Serum/plasma for adsorption: 2 mL.

Autologous RBCs: washed three times with saline; 3 mL.

Equipment/ Materials

5-mL graduated pipettes (eg, VWR, Batavia, IL).

6% BSA.

Ficin or papain: 1% wt/vol (see Section III).

Glycine max (syn. *soja*) lectin (eg, Immucor, Norcross, GA, or see Section XIV).

Reagent RBCs: 3%-5% suspensions of group O, R_1R_1; O, R_2R_2; and O, rr RBCs.

Protein refractometer (eg, #47752-872, VWR, Batavia, IL).

Quality Control

Before use, confirm that the RBCs for adsorption have been treated with proteolytic enzyme. Untreated RBCs should be nonreactive with *G. max,* whereas complete agglutination should be observed with protease-treated RBCs.

Using a refractometer, measure the protein content of the adsorbed and unadsorbed serum. The adsorption process should not have lowered the protein content by more than 20% of the total protein in the unadsorbed sample.

Procedure

Use the following steps to perform the procedure:

Step	Action
1.	Mix 3 mL of autologous RBCs with 1.5 mL of 1% papain or 1% ficin. Incubate at 37 C for 15 minutes.
2.	Wash the RBCs three times with saline and dispense 1-mL aliquots into each of 3 appropriately labeled 10 × 75-mm test tubes.
3.	Fill the tubes with saline and centrifuge to pack the RBCs (≥1000 × *g* for at least 5 minutes). Remove as much of the supernate as possible.
4.	Mix 1 aliquot of enzyme-treated RBCs with 2 mL of serum/plasma.
5.	Incubate at 37 C for 10-60 minutes.
6.	Centrifuge to pack the RBCs. Transfer the serum to the second tube of enzyme-treated RBCs and mix well.

7.	Incubate at 37 C for 10-60 minutes.
8.	Centrifuge to pack the RBCs. Transfer the serum to the third tube of enzyme-treated RBCs and mix well. **Note:** If the autoantibody is 2+ or less, then two adsorptions should be sufficient. Test the adsorbed serum as in Step 11.
9.	Incubate at 37 C for 10-60 minutes.
10.	Centrifuge to pack the RBCs. Transfer the adsorbed serum to a clean test tube.
11.	Test with group O reagent RBCs. Include autologous RBCs treated with chloroquine diphosphate or citric acid (see Section IV).
12.	Interpret the reactions as follows:

If the serum reacts with R_1R_1…	And R_2R_2…	And Auto…	Then the autoantibody…
0	0	0	has been adsorbed, and the serum most likely does not contain alloantibodies.
+/0*	+/0	0	has been adsorbed, and the serum may contain alloantibodies.
++	++	+ to ++++	has not been fully adsorbed: • Repeat adsorption once more.

*If alloantibodies are present, the reactivity with the reagent RBCs may be variable in strength and may react with one reagent RBC sample and not the other.

13.	Test the adsorbed serum in parallel with the unadsorbed serum using a saline indirect antiglobulin technique with an antibody identification panel (see Section II).

Reference   Morel PA, Bergren MO, Frank BA. A simple method for the detection of allo-antibody in the presence of autoantibody. Transfusion 1978;18:358.

**Effective
Date**

Approved by:	Printed Name	Signature	Date
Laboratory Management			
Medical Director			
Quality Officer			

XI-O. Adsorbing Autoantibodies with ZZAP-Treated Autologous RBCs

Purpose

To provide instructions for the adsorption of autoantibodies using autologous RBCs modified with a reagent mix of papain or ficin and DTT:

- In the investigation of immune hemolysis and samples containing autoantibodies.

Background Information

Autoantibodies may mask the concomitant presence of alloantibodies in a serum. Recognition of alloantibodies is facilitated by removing serum autoantibodies through adsorption with autologous RBCs.

ZZAP removes autoantibody coating the autologous RBCs by disrupting membrane-bound IgG through the combined action of a protease and a thiol reagent (see Section III for details). Furthermore, the use of a proteolytic enzyme enhances the adsorption process by removing RBC membrane structures that otherwise hinder antigen-antibody association. While this technique was initially developed to remove warm-reactive autoantibodies, it may be modified for adsorption of cold-reactive autoantibodies.

Note: Because of the presence of donor RBCs carrying antigens to which the serum contains alloantibodies, reliable results may not be obtained with patients transfused within the preceding 120 days.

Operational Policy

This procedure is not suitable for patients transfused within the preceding 120 days.

Note: Two adsorptions are usually sufficient to remove the autoantibody; however, in rare instances additional adsorptions may be required.

Limitations

Unwanted Positive Reactions:

- Autoantibodies specific for papain-sensitive (eg, En^a FS, Ge2) or thiol-sensitive antigens (eg, Kell antigens) will not be removed by this method.

Unwanted Negative Reactions:

- Dilution of the plasma or serum may occur if care is not taken to remove all saline following RBC washes.

Sample Requirements

Serum/plasma for adsorption: 2 mL.

Autologous RBCs: treated with ZZAP reagent as described in Section III; 2 mL.

Equipment/ Materials

Pipettors with disposable tips to deliver 1 mL (eg, VWR, Batavia, IL).

Glycine max (syn. *soja*) lectin (eg, Immucor, Norcross, GA, or see Section XIV).

Protein refractometer (eg, #47752-872, VWR, Batavia, IL).

Reagent RBCs: 3%-5% suspensions of group O, R_1R_1 and O, R_2R_2 RBCs.

ZZAP reagent.

Quality Control

Before use, confirm that the RBCs for adsorption have been treated with ZZAP. Treated RBCs should be nonreactive with *G. max,* whereas complete agglutination should be observed with protease-treated RBCs. RBCs should also be nonreactive with anti-k or other antibody to high-prevalence Kell antigen.

Using a refractometer, measure the protein content of the adsorbed and unadsorbed serum. The adsorption process should not have lowered the protein content by more than 20% of the total protein in the unadsorbed sample.

Procedure

Use the following steps to perform the procedure:

Step	Action
1.	Dispense 1-mL aliquots of washed, ZZAP-treated RBCs into each of 2 appropriately labeled 10 × 75-mm test tubes.
	Note: Remove a drop of ZZAP-treated RBCs, or salvage residual RBCs from test tubes or pipettes, and save for testing the efficacy of the adsorption process, as described in Step 8.
2.	Fill the tubes with saline and centrifuge to pack the RBCs (≥1000 × *g* for at least 5 minutes). Remove as much of the supernate as possible.
3.	Mix 1 aliquot of ZZAP-treated RBCs with 2 mL of test serum.
4.	Incubate at 37 C for 10-60 minutes (or at 4 C for removal of cold-reactive autoantibodies).

5.	Centrifuge to pack the RBCs. Transfer the serum to the second tube of ZZAP-treated RBCs and mix well.
6.	Incubate at 37 C for 10-60 minutes (or at 4 C for removal of cold-reactive autoantibodies).
7.	Centrifuge to pack the RBCs. Transfer the adsorbed serum to a clean test tube. Test with routine group O reagent RBCs and ZZAP-treated autologous RBCs.

8.	Interpret the reactions as follows:

If the serum reacts with R_1R_1...	And R_2R_2...	And Auto...	Then the autoantibody...
0	0	0	has been adsorbed, and the serum most likely does not contain alloantibodies.
+/0*	+/0	0	has been adsorbed, and the serum may contain alloantibodies.
++	++	+ to ++++	has not been fully adsorbed: • Repeat adsorption once more.

*If alloantibodies are present, the reactivity with the reagent RBCs may be variable in strength and may react with one reagent RBC sample and not the other.

9.	Test the adsorbed serum in parallel with the unadsorbed serum using a saline indirect antiglobulin technique with an antibody identification panel (see Section II).

Reference   Branch DR, Petz LD. A new reagent (ZZAP) having multiple applications in immunohematology. Am J Clin Path 1982;78:161-7.

**Effective
Date**

Approved by:	Printed Name	Signature	Date
Laboratory Management			
Medical Director			
Quality Officer			

XI-P. Adsorbing Autoantibodies with ZZAP-Treated Autologous RBCs (Micromethod)

Purpose

To provide instructions for adsorption of autoantibodies using autologous RBCs harvested from a patient sample containing transfused RBCs:

- When sample volumes are small.

- In the investigation of immune hemolysis and samples containing autoantibodies.

Background Information

This procedure may permit detection of concomitant alloantibodies in recently transfused patients with warm-reactive autoantibodies.

When serum from a recently transfused patient (ie, transfused within the preceding 120 days) is suspected of containing autoantibodies, a true "autologous" adsorption cannot be performed unless the patient's own RBCs are separated from the transfused population. In this procedure, autologous RBCs are separated from transfused RBCs and then treated with ZZAP reagent.

ZZAP removes autoantibody coating the autologous RBCs by disrupting membrane-bound IgG through the combined action of a protease and a thiol reagent (see Section III for details). Furthermore, the use of a proteolytic enzyme enhances the adsorption process by removing RBC membrane structures.

Operational Policy

Use an appropriate micromethod (capillary or column agglutination) to identify potential alloantibodies.

Note: Two adsorptions are usually sufficient to remove the autoantibody; however, in rare instances additional adsorptions may be required.

Limitations

Unwanted Positive Reactions:

- Autoantibodies specific for papain-sensitive (eg, En^a FS, Ge2) or thiol-sensitive antigens (eg, Kell antigens) will not be removed by this method.

Unwanted Negative Reactions:

- Dilution of the plasma or serum may occur if care is not taken to remove all saline following RBC washes.

Sample Requirements

Serum/plasma for adsorption: 0.4 mL.

Autologous RBCs: harvested by microhematocrit centrifugation, phthalate esters, or Percoll-Renografin procedures described in Section V; 0.2 mL.

Equipment/ Materials

Pipettors with disposable tips to deliver 100-500 µL (eg, VWR, Batavia, IL).

Glycine max (syn. *soja*) lectin (eg, Immucor, Norcross, GA, or see Section XIV).

Protein refractometer (eg, #47752-872, VWR, Batavia, IL).

Test tubes: 6 × 50-mm glass culture tubes (eg, VWR, Batavia, IL).

ZZAP reagent.

Quality Control

Before use, confirm that the RBCs for adsorption have been treated with proteolytic enzyme. Untreated RBCs should be nonreactive with *G. max,* whereas complete agglutination should be observed with protease-treated RBCs.

Using a refractometer, measure the protein content of the adsorbed and unadsorbed serum. The adsorption process should not have lowered the protein content by more than 20% of the total protein in the unadsorbed sample.

Procedure

Use the following steps to perform the procedure:

Step	Action
1.	Mix 0.2 mL of autologous RBCs with 0.4 mL of ZZAP reagent.
2.	Incubate at 37 C for 30 minutes.
3.	Dispense 0.1 mL of ZZAP-treated RBCs into each of 2 appropriately labeled 6 × 50-mm test tubes.
4.	Fill the tubes with saline and place inside a 10 or 12 × 75-mm test tube containing 0.5 mL of saline.
5.	Centrifuge to pack the RBCs ($\geq 1000 \times g$ for at least 5 minutes). Remove as much of the supernate as possible using a fine-bore Pasteur pipette.
6.	Add 0.2 mL of serum to 1 aliquot of ZZAP-treated RBCs and mix by aspiration through a fine-bore Pasteur pipette.
7.	Incubate at 37 C for 10-60 minutes.

8.	Centrifuge to pack the RBCs. Transfer the serum to the other tube of ZZAP-treated RBCs and mix well.
9.	Incubate at 37 C for 10-60 minutes.
10.	Centrifuge to pack the RBCs. Transfer the adsorbed serum to a clean test tube and use for reagent tests for unexpected antibodies in parallel with the unadsorbed serum, using Procedures VI-E or VI-F).
11.	Interpret the reactions for each aliquot of adsorbed serum as follows:

If the serum reacts with R_1R_1...	And R_2R_2...	And Auto...	Then the autoantibody...
0	0	0	has been adsorbed, and the serum most likely does not contain alloantibodies.
+/0*	+/0	0	has been adsorbed, and the serum may contain alloantibodies: • Proceed with Step 12.
++	++	+ to ++++	has not been fully adsorbed: • Repeat adsorption once more.

*If alloantibodies are present, the reactivity with the reagent RBCs may be variable in strength and may react with one reagent RBC sample and not the other.

12.	Test the adsorbed serum against a panel of reagent RBCs.

Reference   Mougey R. RBC separation methods and their applications. In: Myers M, Reynolds R, eds. Micromethods in blood group serology. Arlington, VA: AABB, 1983:19-36.

**Effective
Date**

Approved by:	Printed Name	Signature	Date
Laboratory Management			
Medical Director			
Quality Officer			

XI-Q. Adsorbing Warm-Reactive Autoantibodies with Allogeneic RBCs

Purpose

To provide instructions for the allogeneic adsorption of warm-reactive antibodies:

- In the investigation of immune hemolysis and samples containing autoantibodies.

Background Information

Warm-reactive autoantibodies may mask the presence of alloantibodies in a serum. When serum from a recently transfused patient (ie, transfused within the preceding 120 days) is suspected of containing autoantibodies, an autologous adsorption cannot be performed reliably because the transfused RBCs may adsorb alloantibodies. Recognition of alloantibodies may be facilitated by removal of autoantibodies through adsorption with allogeneic RBCs. The selection of such RBCs is influenced by what is known of the phenotype of the autologous RBCs. However, the number of allogeneic samples required for adsorption can be reduced because the ZZAP procedure destroys most antigens of the major blood groups, with the exception of ABO, Rh, and Kidd antigens (see Section III).

Operational Policy

Use RBCs matched for the patient's Rh and Jk type, if known.

If the phenotype is unknown, use RBCs of the following three Rh phenotypes: R_1R_1, R_2R_2, and rr. At least one sample should be Jk(a+b−), and one, Jk(a−b+).

Note: Two adsorptions are usually sufficient to remove the autoantibody; however, in rare instances additional adsorptions may be required.

Limitations

Unwanted Positive Reactions:

- Autoantibodies specific for papain-sensitive antigens will not be removed by this method.

Unwanted Negative Reactions:

- If the patient's serum contains a concomitant alloantibody to a high-prevalence antigen, it will also be adsorbed.

- Dilution of the plasma or serum may occur if care is not taken to remove all saline following RBC washes.

Sample Requirements Serum/plasma: from a recently transfused patient suspected to contain warm-reactive autoantibodies; 2-6 mL.

Equipment/ Materials Pipettors with disposable tips to deliver 1 mL (eg, VWR, Batavia, IL).

Glycine max (syn. *soja*) lectin (eg, Immucor, Norcross, GA, or see Section XIV).

Allogeneic RBCs treated with ZZAP reagent as described in Section III; 2 mL.

Reagent RBCs: 3%-5% suspensions of group O, R_1R_1 and O, R_2R_2 RBCs.

Protein refractometer (eg, #47752-872, VWR, Batavia, IL).

Quality Control Before use, confirm that the RBCs for adsorption have been treated with proteolytic enzyme. Untreated RBCs should be nonreactive with *G. max,* whereas complete agglutination should be observed with protease-treated RBCs.

Using a refractometer, measure the protein content of the adsorbed and unadsorbed serum. The adsorption process should not have lowered the protein content by more than 20% of the total protein in the unadsorbed sample.

Procedure Use the following steps to perform the procedure:

Step	Action
1.	Dispense 1 mL of each sample of ZZAP-treated RBCs into each of 2 appropriately labeled 10 × 75-mm test tubes.
2.	Fill the tubes with saline and centrifuge to pack the RBCs ($\geq$1000 × g for at least 5 minutes). Remove as much of the supernate as possible.
3.	Mix 1 aliquot of each ZZAP-treated RBC sample with 2 mL of test serum.
4.	Incubate at 37 C for 10-60 minutes
5.	Centrifuge to pack the RBCs. Transfer the serum to the other tube of ZZAP-treated RBCs of the same phenotype as used in Step 3 and mix well.
6.	Incubate at 37 C for 10-60 minutes.

7.	Centrifuge to pack the RBCs. Transfer the aliquots of adsorbed serum to clean test tubes.
8.	Test with group O reagent RBCs.
9.	Interpret the reactions for each aliquot of adsorbed serum as follows:

If the serum reacts with R_1R_1...	And R_2R_2...	And Auto...	Then the autoantibody...
0	0	0	has been adsorbed, and the serum most likely does not contain alloantibodies.
+/0*	+/0	0	has been adsorbed, and the serum may contain alloantibodies: • Proceed with Step 10.
++	++	+ to ++++	has not been fully adsorbed: • Repeat adsorption once more.

*If alloantibodies are present, the reactivity with the reagent RBCs may be variable in strength and may react with one reagent RBC sample and not the other.

10.	Test the adsorbed serum in parallel with the unadsorbed serum using a saline indirect antiglobulin technique with an antibody identification panel (see Section II).

Reference

Judd WJ. Investigation and management of immune hemolysis: Autoantibodies and drugs. In: Wallace ME, Levitt JS, eds. Current applications and interpretation of the direct antiglobulin test. Arlington, VA: AABB, 1988:47-103.

**Effective
Date**

Approved by:	Printed Name	Signature	Date
Laboratory Management			
Medical Director			
Quality Officer			

Section XII. Investigating Drug-Induced Hemolysis

This section contains procedures used in the investigation of suspected drug-induced immune hemolytic anemia (DIIHA).

General Considerations

When evaluating a case of suspected DIIHA, the following information should be obtained whenever possible:

- A drug history on the patient, including:

    o   Prescription drugs.

    o   Over-the-counter drugs.

    o   Alternative (herbal) medications.

- Timing and dosage of medication, including any medication received in the last 2 weeks or received at the time of acute hemolysis.

- History of any surgical procedures that may have required administration of antibiotics by a surgeon or an anesthesiologist.

This information will aid in determining the most likely causative drug because many patients receive more than one medication. Table XII-1 lists drugs reported to cause a positive direct antiglobulin test (DAT) and drug-induced hemolysis.

Indications that a drug study should be performed (and it has not been ordered) are a positive DAT, often strongly reactive (3+ to 4+), and a negative or disproportionately weak eluate as compared to the strength of the DAT. For example, if the DAT was 4+ because of IgG, one would expect the eluate to be 2+ to 4+ reactive with all cells tested. In the case of DIIHA, the eluate may be negative or weakly positive (weak to 1+). In addition to the serology, a clinical history of sudden hemolysis and drug ingestion at the time of hemolysis may indicate that drug studies should be performed.

Current Concepts in the Detection of Drug-Dependent Antibodies

Drug-dependent antibodies are known to cause immune hemolysis. Typical presenting serologic results include those often seen when evaluating a patient with warm autoimmune hemolytic anemia—a strong positive DAT (3+ to 4+) caused by IgG only, or IgG and C3 with broadly reactive serum antibody without the addition of drugs. In fewer cases, initial serologic tests appear like cold agglutinin syndrome, with a positive DAT (2+ to 3+) caused by C3 only and a cold-reactive antibody present in the serum. It is unusual to observe weak positive DATs caused by IgG or complement as have been historically reported for those drugs causing the so-called "immune complex" type of hemolysis, when the patient is actively experiencing hemolysis. DAT reactivity will decrease in strength rapidly after the patient is off the drug, often within a few weeks. Serum antibody reactivity in initial testing may occur if the drug is present in the patient's circulation and, thus, still present in the patient's serum. Alternatively, this reactivity may be the result of drug-independent autoantibody.

Classification

The mechanisms by which drugs induce immune hemolysis are not fully understood. For a review of the theories about these mechanisms, see the sources in Suggested Reading. Instead of referring to the detection of drug-dependent antibodies by the possible mechanism of hemolysis (induction of autoimmunity, drug adsorption, immune complex, membrane modification), the following classifications are used to describe how these antibodies are detected:

1. **Drug-independent autoantibody.** Classically, α-methyldopa, and now more commonly mefenamic acid and procainamide, may modify the immune system such that suppresser T-cells are no longer capable of controlling natural autoantibody production. Drugs are not necessary to detect the autoantibody. The serologic picture is indistinguishable from that seen in warm autoimmune hemolytic anemia with a strong positive (3+ to 4+) DAT and eluate reactive (2+ to 3+) with all reagent RBCs.

2. **Drugs that bind tightly to the RBC membrane.** Drugs such as the penicillins, traditionally, and second- and third-generation cephalosporins such as cefotetan more commonly today, bind effectively to RBC membranes. Antibodies primarily directed to the drug attach to the RBC-bound drug and result in a positive DAT. Hemolysis occurs infrequently and only when large daily doses are administered intravenously. IgG and sometimes C3 may be present on the RBCs. Drug-treated RBCs are required for serologic demonstration. Antibodies to the drug can be demonstrated in both the serum and eluate when tested against drug-treated RBCs. The drug-dependent antibody may be inhibited by pure drug (hapten inhibition).

3. **Drugs that do not bind to the RBC membrane.** Quinine or many nonsteroidal anti-inflammatory drugs (NSAIDs) may act as haptens and bind to proteins to form immunogens that evoke antibody production. Hemolysis is often acute and results from administration of only small quantities of the drug. IgG, in addition to C3, may be present on the RBCs. Eluates are usually nonreactive, and serum tests react only in the presence of the drug or one of its metabolites.

4. **Nonimmunologic adsorption of protein.** Cephalosporins and β-lactamase inhibitors (clavulanate, sulbactam, tazobactim) have also been involved. RBC membranes are modified by the drug such that all proteins (including albumin, immunoglobulins, and α and β globulins) are adsorbed nonimmunologically. Recent reports have indicated that hemolytic anemia may be caused by some β-lactamase inhibitors.

Additional Considerations

Certain biological materials may also account for a positive DAT, including allogeneic plasma products containing foreign antibody. Notable among these are non-ABO-type-specific blood components, and gamma globulin preparations containing Rh antibodies.

IgG-coating is seen with or without C3-coating and immune hemolysis. Specific antibody should be detected by elution. Furthermore, historically, anti-lymphocyte globulin (ALG) and anti-thymocyte globulin (ATG) preparations of equine (horse) origin had extremely high titers of anti-human species antibodies that caused passive acquisition of antibodies to result in a positive DAT.

Suggested Reading

Arndt PA, Garratty G The changing spectrum of drug-induced immune hemolytic anemia. Semin Hematol 2005;42:137-44.

Garratty G, Arndt PA. An update on drug-induced immune hemolytic anemia. Immunohematology 2007;3:105-19.

Johnson ST, Fueger JT, Gottschall JL. One center's experience: The serology and drugs associated with drug-induced immune hemolytic anemia—a new paradigm. Transfusion 2007;47:697-702.

Petz LD, Garratty G. Acquired hemolytic anemias. 2nd ed. Philadelphia, PA: Churchill-Livingstone, 2004.

Roback J, Combs MR, Grossman B, Hillyer C, eds. Technical manual. 16th ed. Bethesda, MD: AABB, 2008 (or current edition).

Table XII-1. Drugs Reported to Cause Immune Hemolysis and a Positive DAT*

Drug (Alternative Name)	Therapeutic Category	Method of Detecting Drug-Dependent Antibody[†]	Reported to be Reactive without Drug Added To Test?
Aceclofenac	NSAID	IPOD	No
Acetaminophen (Paracetamol)	NSAID	IPOD	No
Acyclovir	Antiviral	DTRC	No
Aminopyrine (Piramidone)	NSAID	DTRC	No
Amoxicillin	Antimicrobial	DTRC	No
Amphotericin B	Antimicrobial	IPOD	No
Ampicillin	Antimicrobial	DTRC/IPOD	No
Antazoline	Antihistamine	IPOD	No
Aspirin	Analgesic, antipyretic, anti-inflammatory	IPOD	No
Azapropazone (Apazone)	Anti-inflammatory, analgesic	DTRC	Yes
Buthiazide (Butizide)	Diuretic, Antihypertensive	IPOD	No
Carbimazole	Antithyroid	DTRC/IPOD	Yes
Carboplatin	Antineoplastic	DTRC/IPOD	Yes
Carbromal	Sedative, hypnotic	DTRC	No
Catechin [(+)-Cyanidanol-3; Cianidanol]	Antidiarrheal	DTRC/IPOD	Yes
Cefamandole	Antimicrobial	DTRC	No
Cefazolin	Antimicrobial	DTRC	No
Cefixime	Antimicrobial	DTRC/IPOD	No
Cefotaxime	Antimicrobial	DTRC/IPOD	Yes
Cefotetan[‡]	Antimicrobial	DTRC/IPOD	Yes
Cefoxitin	Antimicrobial	DTRC/IPOD	Yes
Cefpirome	Antibacterial	IPOD	No
Ceftazidime	Antimicrobial	DTRC/IPOD	Yes
Ceftizoxime	Antimicrobial	DTRC/IPOD	Yes
Ceftriaxone	Antimicrobial	IPOD	Yes
Cefuroxime	Antimicrobial	DTRC	No
Cephalexin	Antimicrobial	DTRC	No
Cephalothin[‡]	Antimicrobial	DTRC/DTRC	No
Chloramphenicol	Antimicrobial	DTRC	Yes
Chlorinated hydrocarbons	Insecticides	IPOD/DTRC	Yes
Chloropromazine	Antiemetic, antipsychotic	DTRC	Yes

Table XII-1. Drugs Reported to Cause Immune Hemolysis and a Positive DAT* (Cont.)

Drug (Alternative Name)	Therapeutic Category	Method of Detecting Drug-Dependent Antibody[†]	Reported to be Reactive without Drug Added To Test?
Chloropropamide	Antidiabetic	IPOD	Yes
Ciprofloxacin	Antibacterial	IPOD	Yes
Cisplatin[‡] (Cisdiaminodichloroplatinum)	Antineoplastic	IPOD/DTRC	No
Cladribine (2-chlorodeoxyadenosine)	Antineoplastic	IA	Yes
Clavulanate potassium (Clabulanic acid)	β-lactamase inhibitor	NIPA	No
Cloxacillin	Antibacterial	None	Yes
Cyclofenil	Gonad-stimulating principle	IPOD	Yes
Cyclosporin (Cyclosporine)	Immunosuppressant	DTRC	Yes
Dexchlorpheniramine maleate (Chlorpheniramine)	Antihistamine	IPOD	No
Diclofenac	NSAID	IPOD/DTRC	Yes
Diglycoaldehyde	Antineoplastic	NIPA	No
Diethylstillbestrol (Stillboestrol)	Estrogen	IPOD	No
Dipyrone	NSAID	IPOD/DTRC	No
Erythromycin	Antimicrobial	DTRC	No
Ethambutol	Antibacterial	IPOD/DTRC	No
Etodolac	NSAID	IPOD	No
Fenoprofen	NSAID	IPOD	Yes
Fluconazole	Antifungal	IPOD/DTRC	No
Fluorescein	Injectable dye	IPOD/DTRC	Yes
Fluorouracil	Antineoplastic	IPOD	No
Fludarabine	Antineoplastic	IA	Yes
Furosemide	Diuretic	IPOD	No
Glaphenine (Glaphenine)	Analgesic	None	Yes
Hydralazine	Antihypertensive	DTRC	No
Hydrochlorothiazide	Diuretic	IPOD/DTRC	Yes
9-Hydroxy-methyl-ellipticinium (Elliptinium acetate)	Antineoplastic	IPOD	No
Ibuprofen	NSAID	IPOD	Yes
Imatinib mesylate	Antineoplastic	DTRC	No
Insulin	Antidiabetic	DTRC	No
Isoniazid	Antimicrobial	IPOD/DTRC	No

Table XII-1. Drugs Reported to Cause Immune Hemolysis and a Positive DAT* (Cont.)

Drug (Alternative Name)	Therapeutic Category	Method of Detecting Drug-Dependent Antibody[†]	Reported to be Reactive without Drug Added To Test?
Latamoxef (Moxalactam)	Antimicrobial	None	Yes
Levofloxacin (Ofloxacin)	Antimicrobial	IPOD/DTRC	Yes
Levodopa (L-dopa)	Antiparkinsonian	IA	Yes
Mefenamic acid	NSAID	IA	Yes
Mefloquine	Antimicrobial	DTRC/IPOD	Yes
Melphalan	Antineoplastic	IPOD	No
6-Mercaptopurine	Antineoplastic	DTRC	No
Methadone	Analgesic	DTRC	No
Methotrexate	Antineoplastic, antirheumatic	DTRC/IPOD	Yes
Methyldopa	Antihypertensive	IA	Yes
Metrizoate-based radiographic contrast media	Used in x-rays	DTRC/IPOD	Yes
Minocycline	Antibacterial	IPOD	No
Nabumetone	Anti-inflammatory	IPOD	Yes
Nafcillin	Antimicrobial	DTRC	No
Naproxen	Anti-inflammatory, analgesic, antipyretic	IPOD	No
Nitrofurantoin	Antibacterial	IPOD	No
Nomifensine	Antidepressant	IPOD	Yes
Norfloxacin	Antimicrobial	DTRC	No
Oxaliplatin[‡]	Antineoplastic	DTRC/IPOD	Yes
p-Aminosalicylic acid (PAS)	Antimicrobial	IPOD	No
Penicillin G	Antimicrobial	DTRC/IPOD	No
Phenacetin (Acetophenetidin)	NSAID	IPOD	Yes
Phenytoin (Fenitoine)	Anticonvulsant, Anti-arrhythmic	DTRC	No
Piperacillin	Antimicrobial	IPOD/DTRC	Yes
Piperacillin and Tazobactam (Zosyn)	Antimicrobial	IPOD/DTRC	Yes
Probenecid	Uricosuric	IPOD	Yes
Procainamide	Anti-arrythmic	IA	Yes
Propyphenazone	NSAID	IPOD	No
Pyrazinamide	Antibacterial	DTRC/IPOD	No
Pyrimethamine (Pirimetamine)	Antimicrobial	DTRC	No
Quinidine	Antiarrhythmic, Antimicrobial	IPOD/DTRC	Yes

Table XII-1. Drugs Reported to Cause Immune Hemolysis and a Positive DAT* (Cont.)

Drug (Alternative Name)	Therapeutic Category	Method of Detecting Drug-Dependent Antibody[†]	Reported to be Reactive without Drug Added To Test?
Quinine	Antimicrobial	IPOD	Yes
Ranitidine	Antiulcerative	IPOD/DTRC	No
Rifabutin	Antibacterial	IPOD	No
Rifampin (Rifampicin)	Antibacterial	IPOD/DTRC	Yes
Stibophen	Antimicrobial	IPOD	No
Streptokinase	Thrombolytic	DTRC	Yes
Streptomycin	Antimicrobial	DTRC/IPOD	Yes
Sulbactam	β-lactamase Inhibitor	NIPA	No
Sulfasalazine	Anti-inflammatory	IPOD	No
Sulfisoxazole	Antibacterial	IPOD/DTRC	No
Sulindac	Anti-inflammatory	IPOD/DTRC	Yes
Suprofen	NSAID	IPOD	Yes
Tartrazine	Colorant	IPOD/DTRC	No
Tazobactam	β-lactamase Inhibitor	NIPA	No
Teicoplanin	Antimicrobial	IPOD	Yes
Temafloxacin	Antimicrobial	IPOD	No
Teniposide	Antineoplastic	IPOD	Yes
Tetracycline	Antimicrobial	DTRC	No
Thiopental sodium	Anesthetic	IPOD	No
Ticarcillin	Antimicrobial	DTRC	Yes
Tolbutamide	Antidiabetic	DTRC	No
Tolmetin	NSAID	IPOD	Yes
Triamterene	Diuretic	IPOD/DTRC	No
Trimellitic anhydride	Used in preparation of resins, dyes, adhesives, etc	DTRC	No
Trimothoprim and sulfamethoxazole (Bactrim)	Antibacterial	IPOD/DTRC	Yes
Vancomycin	Antibacterial	IPOD	No
Zomepirac	NSAID	IPOD	Yes

*Data drawn from Garratty G, Arndt PA. An update on drug-induced immune hemolytic anemia. Immunohematology 2007;3: 105-19.

[†]When two methods are listed, the first is more commonly reported to detect drug-dependent antibody; however, there are individuals whose drug-dependent antibody has been detected with the second method listed.

[‡]Nonimmunologic protein adsorption has been reported in some patients in whom drug-dependent antibody has been detected by other methods.

NSAID = nonsteroidal anti-inflammatory drug; IPOD = in presence of drug [patient serum + drug (1 mg/mL) + untreated RBCs]; DTRC = drug-treated RBCs (patient serum + drug-treated RBCs); IA = induction of autoimmunity (patient serum + untreated RBCs); NIPA = nonimmunologic protein adsorption (positive DAT).

XII-A. Dissolving Drugs in Solution

Purpose

To provide instructions for drug solutions for drug-dependent antibody testing:

- For dissolving drugs to be used for treating RBCs with penicillin, penicillin-derivatives, and cephalosporins.

- For dissolving drugs in 1-mg/mL solutions to be added to test mixtures.

Background Information

The solubility of the drug to be tested must be verified before attempting this procedure because drugs possess varying degrees of solubility in water. This information can be found in the *Physicians' Desk Reference* (PDR) or *The Merck Index*.

6% albumin may be used to solubilize drugs that are difficult to dissolve in PBS. It is particularly useful for testing insoluble or practically insoluble drugs such as probenecid in the presence of drug.

Note: Caution must be used when dissolving cephalosporins because the drug will bind covalently to albumin. This protein binding may reduce the concentration of the drug in solution; consequently, a weakly reactive drug-dependent antibody may not be detected.

Operational Policy

For best results, prepare the drug solution immediately before use. If drug solutions are stored, check the storage conditions particular to each drug. Appropriate controls must be run to verify the action of the drug after storage.

Limitations

Unwanted Positive Reactions:

- Nonspecific uptake of protein may result when RBCs are treated with some drugs (see Table XII-1).

- Some individuals have a drug-independent autoantibody. The patient serum will be positive when testing untreated normal RBCs, or in the absence of any drug in the test.

Unwanted Negative Reactions:

- If the drug binds covalently to albumin, and 6% albumin is used to dissolve the drug, the drug in solution may be lower than needed to detect the drug-dependent antibody.

- Drug prediluted by the pharmacy, particularly intravenous antibiotics, may not provide optimum drug concentration for drug-dependent antibody detection.

Sample Requirements

Not applicable.

Equipment/ Materials

Drug(s) in question: note dosage if drug is in tablet or capsule form.

Note: Request antibiotics in powder form for best results. Some drugs are available in the pure form through chemical companies. This is preferred to avoid fillers often added to tablets and capsules.

Any of the following diluents depending on the drug to be tested:

- pH 7.3 PBS.

- 1% albumin.

- 6% albumin.

- Barbital buffer: pH 9.6.

Quality Control

Test normal serum and appropriate diluents as negative controls.

Test a known serum from a patient with a drug-dependent antibody of the appropriate specificity, whenever possible, as a positive control.

Dissolving Procedure

Use the following steps to dissolve drugs into solution for Procedure XII-F (ie, to detect antibodies reacting in the presence of drug):

Step	Action
1.	Prepare drug according to the following conditions:
	If drug is in... **Then...**
	tablet form — crush tablet using mortar and pestle.
	capsule form — break seal and pour contents into weighing boat.
	powder form — proceed to Step 2.
	solution form — dilute to 1 mg/mL if possible.
2.	Weigh out drug according to the following conditions:
	If drug is in... **Then...**
	tablet or capsule form — use entire amount for dilution (eg, for a 250-mg tablet, dissolve in diluent).
	powder form — weigh out appropriate amount of drug [eg, 100 mg (0.1 g) of drug, or 10 mg (0.01 g) of drug].
	Note: Smaller amounts of drug can be weighed out to achieve the 1-mg/mL concentration.
3.	Add drug to an appropriate amount of diluent to obtain a 1-mg/mL concentration. **Example:** For 100 mg (0.1 g) of drug, dissolve in 100 mL of diluent; for 10 mg (0.01 g) of drug, dissolve in 10 mL of diluent.

4.	Dissolve drug and proceed as follows:	
	If drug...	**Then...**
	dissolves easily	proceed to Step 5.
	does not dissolve easily	incubate at 37 C with vigorous stirring, or check for solubility in *PDR*, *Merck Index*, or other literature, and dissolve in the appropriate solution. **Note:** Other diluents such as 1%-6% albumin, acetone, alcohol, or buffers of different pHs may be used. (See references for more information.)
	Note: Drugs in tablet form may have inert materials that do not dissolve. Drug may be present in the supernatant.	
5.	Centrifuge solution if precipitate is present, and use supernatant.	
6.	Check pH of drug solution: pH should be between 5.0 and 8.0. If so, drug solution is ready for testing in the presence of drug. Some drugs are light sensitive and need to be stored appropriately. Check *PDR* or *Merck Index* for more information on the stability of the drug.	
	If pH is...	**Then...**
	between 5.0 and 8.0	proceed to Procedure XII-F.
	below 5.0	adjust to desired pH.
	above 8.0	adjust to desired pH.

Penicillin Coating Procedure

Use the following steps when coating RBCs with drug (penicillin or penicillin derivatives) to be used in Procedure XII-C:

Note: If putative drug does not appear to coat cells (eg, cells are hemolyzed), check literature for alternative buffers, incubation temperature, and time.

Step	Action
1.	Prepare drug according to the following conditions:

If drug is in...	Then...
tablet form	crush tablet using mortar and pestle.
capsule form	break seal and pour contents into weighing boat.
powder form	proceed to Step 2.

Step	Action
2.	Weigh 300 mg of drug.
3.	Dissolve drug in 7.5 mL of pH 9.6 barbital buffer and proceed as follows:

If drug...	Then...
dissolves easily	proceed to Procedure XII-C.
does not dissolve easily	incubate at 37 C with vigorous stirring, or check for solubility in *PDR*, *Merck Index*, or other literature, and dissolve in the appropriate solution.

Note: The volume of drug-treated RBCs prepared can be reduced by preparing less drug solution as long as 40 mg/mL of drug concentration is maintained to coat the RBCs. For example, 150 mg of drug may be dissolved in 3.25 mL of pH 9.6 barbital buffer.

Note: Drugs in tablet form may have inert materials that do not dissolve.

Step	Action
4.	Centrifuge solution if necessary, and use supernatant. Drug solution is ready for treating RBCs.

Nonpenicillin Coating Procedure

Use the following steps when coating RBCs with drug (cephalosporins and other drugs for treating RBCs) to be used in procedure XII-C:

Note: If putative drug does not appear to coat cells (eg, cells are hemolyzed), check literature for alternative buffers, incubation temperature, and time.

Step	Action
1.	Prepare drug according to the following conditions:
	If drug is in... / **Then...**
	tablet form — crush tablet using mortar and pestle.
	capsule form — break seal and pour contents into weighing boat.
	powder form — proceed to Step 2.
2.	Weigh out 300 mg of drug.
3.	Dissolve drug in 7.5 mL of pH 7.3 PBS and proceed as follows:
	If drug... / **Then...**
	dissolves easily — proceed to Procedure XII-C.
	does not dissolve easily — incubate at 37 C with vigorous stirring, or check for solubility in *PDR*, *Merck Index*, or other literature, and dissolve in the appropriate solution.
	Note: The volume of drug-treated RBCs prepared can be reduced by preparing less drug solution as long as 40 mg/mL of drug concentration is maintained to coat the RBCs. For example, 150 mg of drug may be dissolved in 3.25 mL of pH 7.3 PBS.
	Note: Drugs in tablet form may have inert materials that do not dissolve.
4.	Centrifuge solution if necessary, and use supernatant. Drug solution is ready for treating RBCs.

References

O'Neil MJ, ed. The Merck index: An encyclopedia of chemicals, drugs, and biologicals. 14th ed. Whitehouse Station, NJ: Merck, 2006 (or current edition).

Petz LD, Garratty G. Acquired hemolytic anemias. 2nd ed. Philadelphia, PA: Churchill-Livingstone, 2004.

Physicians' desk reference. Montvale, NJ: Thomson Healthcare, 2008 (updated annually).

Effective Date

Approved by:	Printed Name	Signature	Date
Laboratory Management			
Medical Director			
Quality Officer			

XII-B. Preparing Urine for Detecting Metabolite-Dependent Antibodies

Purpose	To provide instructions for preparing urine to be used in detecting drug-dependent antibodies reacting in the presence of drug metabolites.
Background Information	Information on the pharmacokinetics of drugs can be found in the *PDR* or *Merck Index*. This information will provide the timeline for drug metabolism and aid in assessing when to collect specimens from an individual taking the drug.
	A first-morning urine collection may provide a high concentration of drug metabolite, particularly if the volunteer drug recipient is on a therapeutic dose of the drug.
	A fresh complement source has been noted to aid in the detection of some drug-dependent antibodies (see Petz and Garratty in the reference list), although in no instance has it been shown to be required to detect drug-dependent antibody.
	Some drug-dependent antibodies will show enhanced reactivity when tested against protease (ficin or papain)-treated RBCs.
Operational Policy	Urine from volunteers who have ingested therapeutic levels of the drug is required as a source of drug metabolites.
Limitations	Failure to adjust the pH of the urine to normal will result in hemolysis of the reagent RBCs.
Sample Requirements	Urine from a volunteer drug recipient.
Equipment/ Materials	Litmus paper: pH 7.0 range.

Quality Control

Test patient serum and normal RBCs with a known example of metabolite-dependent antibody, if available. Normal reagent RBCs in the presence of drug metabolite should react 2+ to 4+.

Note: In order to preserve rare control serum/plasma, it is not necessary to test the known metabolite-dependent antibody against untreated RBCs in the presence of diluent.

Procedure

Use the following steps to complete the procedure:

Step	Action
1.	Identify a volunteer drug recipient who is taking a therapeutic dose of the drug in question.
2.	Review the pharmacokinetics of the drug in *PDR* or *Merck Index* and obtain urine from the volunteer drug recipient at the appropriate intervals to collect the optimum amount of drug metabolite. **Note:** Different times may be required for different drugs. Alternatively, collect a first morning urine sample from the volunteer drug recipient.
3.	Centrifuge urine sample(s) for 3-5 minutes and remove supernatant.
4.	Check pH of urine: pH should be between 5.0 and 8.0. If so, urine is now ready for testing in the presence of drug.<table><tr><th>If pH is…</th><th>Then…</th></tr><tr><td>between 5.0 and 8.0</td><td>proceed to Procedure XII-G.</td></tr><tr><td>below 5.0</td><td>adjust to desired pH.</td></tr><tr><td>above 8.0</td><td>adjust to desired pH.</td></tr></table>
5.	Store at 1-6 C, or aliquot and store below –20 C until required.

References

O'Neil MJ, ed. The Merck index: An encyclopedia of chemicals, drugs, and biologicals. 14th ed. Whitehouse Station, NJ: Merck, 2006 (or current edition).

Petz LD, Garratty G. Acquired hemolytic anemias. 2nd ed. Philadelphia, PA: Churchill-Livingstone, 2004.

Physicians' desk reference. Montvale, NJ: Thomson Healthcare, 2008 (updated annually).

**Effective
Date**

Approved by:	Printed Name	Signature	Date
Laboratory Management			
Medical Director			
Quality Officer			

XII-C. Detecting Drug-Dependent Antibodies Reacting with Drug-Treated RBCs

Purpose   To provide instructions for detecting drug-dependent antibodies able to bind to drug-treated RBCs—in particular, penicillin and many cephalosporins.

Background Information   Penicillins and second- and third-generation cephalosporins may induce an IgG immune response (for example, penicillin-dependent antibody) that can be recognized in tests with RBCs treated with the drug. When testing native (undiluted) serum, a positive result is likely indicative of a drug-dependent antibody. Titration studies may need to be performed to ensure reactivity is the result of a pathologic drug-dependent antibody vs those often found in normal individuals. Considerations:

- IgM drug-dependent antibodies will agglutinate drug-treated RBCs, but not the same untreated RBCs at room temperature unless reactivity is due to low-titer preexisting antibodies.

- IgG drug-dependent antibodies will react by IAT against drug-treated RBCs, but not the same untreated RBCs unless reactivity occurs to low titer as indicated above.

- Many normal individuals have low-titer drug-dependent antibody, but the titer is usually <32.

When selecting RBCs for drug treating, e+ RBCs are preferred because it has been shown that many drug-dependent antibodies have relative Rh specificity. Using e+ RBCs may enhance detection of antibodies.

Note: Rare drug-dependent antibodies have been shown to have specificity to other blood group antigens.

Operational Policy   Untreated RBCs should not react with patient serum or eluate. If positive reactions are observed, reactivity may be the result of a non-drug-related antibody (a specific alloantibody), a drug-independent autoantibody, or a drug-dependent antibody resulting from the continued presence of the drug the patient is taking in the patient's plasma.

Note: Titration of patient serum and subsequent testing of the dilutions against untreated and drug-treated RBCs may be necessary. If drug-dependent antibody is present, the titer against the drug-treated RBCs will be greater than against untreated RBCs.

Limitations

Caution:

- Antibodies to cephalosporins may cross-react with RBCs treated with penicillin.

- See Procedure XII-D for an alternative method that also permits detection of antibodies to semisynthetic penicillins.

Incorrect Results:

- Incorrect technique has been used.

- Drug has been omitted.

- Wrong reagent has been used.

Note: Caution must be taken when testing cefotetan-coated RBCs because these cells are also effective at nonspecific protein uptake. In addition, some individuals have "naturally occurring" cefotetan-dependent antibody.

Unwanted Positive Reactions:

- Nonspecific uptake of protein may result when RBCs are coated with some drugs (see Table XII-1).

- Some individuals have a drug-independent autoantibody. The patient serum will be positive when testing untreated normal RBCs, or in the absence of any drug in the test.

Sample Requirements

Serum or eluate (see Section IV): 0.3 mL.

Equipment/ Materials

Alsever's solution.

Control serum or eluate: with known drug-dependent antibody to be tested, if available.

Drug solution (see Procedure XII-A).

Fresh RBCs: group O, rr, washed three times with saline; 1 mL.

Negative control: pooled normal serum (or plasma), or normal serum or plasma from a single donor.

AHG: polyspecific.

Quality Control

Test treated RBCs with a known example of drug-dependent antibody, if available. Treated (positive control) RBCs should react 3+ to 4+.

Note: In order to preserve rare control serum/plasma, it is not necessary to test the known drug-dependent antibody against untreated RBCs.

Test normal serum and appropriate diluents as negative controls.

Drug-Treating Procedure

Use the following steps to treat RBCs with drug:

Note: If alloantibodies are present in patient serum, antigen-negative cells must be used in testing.

Step	Action
1.	Wash group O, rr RBCs three times in saline. Save an aliquot of untreated RBCs to use as a normal control (untreated RBCs).
2.	Mix 0.5 mL of rr RBCs with 7.5 mL of drug solution. **Note:** Prepare drug solution immediately before adding to RBCs.
3.	Incubate at RT for 1 hour with occasional mixing.
4.	Wash three times with saline or until hemolysis is gone. Dilute to a 3%-5% suspension with 10 mL of Alsever's solution and store at 4 C. **Note:** If treated RBCs will not be stored, the cell suspension may be prepared with normal saline.
5.	Dilute the remaining (treated) 0.5 mL of RBCs to a 3%-5% suspension with 10 mL of Alsever's solution and store at 4 C. **Note:** Cell suspensions may be prepared using normal saline if RBCs will not be stored.

Detecting Antibodies Procedure

Use the following steps to detect drug-dependent antibodies using drug-treated RBCs:

Note: Test the patient's serum and eluate against drug-treated and untreated RBCs. Also test the appropriate positive and negative (normal) controls. If patient serum was positive in routine testing, titrate the patient serum.

Step	Action
1.	Add 2 drops each of patient serum or serum dilution, eluate, positive control, and negative control to the appropriately labeled tubes.
2.	Add 1 drop each of 3%-5% cell suspension of drug-treated RBCs and the untreated RBCs to the appropriate tubes.
3.	To detect IgM drug-dependent antibodies, incubate at RT for 15 minutes: • Centrifuge. • Dislodge the cell buttons gently. • Examine macroscopically for agglutination. • Grade and record the results. **Note:** This step may be omitted if desired. Proceed to Step 4.
4.	Mix and incubate at 37 C for 30-60 minutes: • Centrifuge. • Dislodge the cell buttons gently. • Examine macroscopically for agglutination. • Grade and record the results.
5.	Wash each tube three to four times with saline and completely decant the final wash supernate. To the dry cell buttons add 2 drops of AHG: • Mix and centrifuge. • Dislodge the cell buttons gently. • Examine macroscopically for agglutination. • Grade and record the results. **Note:** Polyspecific AHG is preferred to detect complement-dependent reactivity. Centrifuge and read for agglutination.

6.	Add 1 drop of IgG-coated RBCs to all tubes with negative antiglobulin results:		
	• Mix gently.		
	• Centrifuge.		
	• Examine macroscopically for agglutination.		
	• Grade and record the results.		
7.	Interpret the reactions as follows:		
	If...	**And...**	**Then...**
	• Patient serum + drug-treated RBCs are positive • Normal serum + drug-treated RBCs are negative	• Patient serum + normal RBCs are negative • Normal serum + normal RBCs are negative	patient has a drug-dependent antibody.
	• Patient serum + drug-treated RBCs are positive • Normal serum + drug-treated RBCs are negative	• Patient serum + normal RBCs are positive • Normal serum + normal RBCs are negative	patient has a drug-independent autoantibody: • Test dilution(s) of patient serum with drug-treated and normal RBCs, or adsorb serum and repeat drug antibody testing using adsorbed serum.
	• Patient serum + drug-treated RBCs are positive • Normal serum + drug-treated RBCs are positive	• Patient serum + normal RBCs are negative • Normal serum + normal RBCs are negative	positive reaction could be caused by nonspecific uptake of proteins onto the drug-treated RBCs: • Test dilution(s) of patient serum (1:20 or 1:100) and normal serum vs drug-treated RBCs. Pathologic drug-dependent antibody titer will be reactive at titer values >20 in most cases.

References   Petz LD, Garratty G. Acquired hemolytic anemias. 2nd ed. Philadelphia, PA: Churchill-Livingstone, 2004.

Roback J, Combs MR, Grossman B, Hillyer C, eds. Technical manual. 16th ed. Bethesda, MD: AABB, 2008 (or current edition).

Effective Date

Approved by:	Printed Name	Signature	Date
Laboratory Management			
Medical Director			
Quality Officer			

XII-D. Detecting Antibodies to Semisynthetic Penicillins

Purpose

To provide instructions for preparing iso-osmolar solutions of semisynthetic penicillins, in addition to penicillin and Keflin, for use in RBC coating:

- In the investigation of drug-induced positive DATs and immune hemolysis associated with semisynthetic penicillin therapy.

Background Information

Semisynthetic penicillins may induce an IgG immune response (anti-penicillin antibody) that can be recognized in tests with RBCs coated with the specific drug. Boric Acid Buffer (BAB) has an osmolarity of 200 mOsm/kg; addition of the given amount of drug to 15 mL of BAB will bring the osmolarity to 300 mOsm/kg. To attain a final osmolarity of 300 mOsm/kg, 0.75 mM of each drug must be added to 15 mL of BAB. The required mg amount of each drug is calculated by multiplying the molecular weight of the drug by 0.75.

Operational Policy

Not applicable.

Limitations

Incorrect Results:

- Incorrect technique has been used.

- Drug has been omitted.

- Wrong reagent has been used.

Unwanted Positive Reactions:

- Non-specific uptake of protein may result when RBCs are coated with some drugs (see Table XII-1).

- Some individuals have a drug-independent autoantibody. The patient serum will be positive when testing untreated normal RBCs, or in the absence of any drug in the test.

- Antibodies to cephalosporins may cross-react with RBCs treated with penicillin.

Unwanted Negative Reactions:

- Drug prediluted by the pharmacy, particularly intravenous antibiotics, may not provide optimum drug concentration for drug-dependent antibody detection.

Sample Requirements

Serum and/or eluate (see Section IV): 0.3 mL.

Note: Dilute the serum 1 in 20 with saline before testing with drug-treated RBCs.

Equipment/ Materials

Alsever's solution.

Boric acid buffer (BAB): pH 9.6-10.

Drug solutions: prepare by dissolving the following amounts in 15 mL of BAB:

- Disodium carbenicillin, 317 mg.

- Potassium penicillin G, 279 mg.

- Sodium ampicillin, 279 mg.

- Sodium cephalothin, 314 mg.

- Sodium methicillin, 302 mg.

- Sodium nafcillin, 327 mg.

- Sodium oxacillin, 318 mg.

Osmometer (eg, single-sample osmometer, model 3250, VWR, Batavia, IL).

RBCs: group O, rr; 1 mL per drug plus 1 mL for controls, washed three times with saline.

Negative control: pooled normal serum (or plasma), or normal serum or plasma from a single donor.

Quality Control

Check osmolarity of drug solutions. Osmolarity should be 300 ±20 mOsm/kg.

Test treated RBCs with a known example of drug-dependent antibody, if available. Treated (positive control) RBCs should react 3+ to 4+.

Note: In order to preserve rare control serum/plasma, it is not necessary to test the known drug-dependent antibody against untreated RBCs.

Test normal serum and appropriate diluents as negative controls.

Procedure   Use the following steps to perform the procedure:

Step	Action
1.	To 15 mL of each drug solution, add 1 mL of rr RBCs and mix well.
2.	Incubate at 37 C for 2 hours (1 hour for sodium cephalothin).
3.	Wash three times with saline. Dilute to a 3%-5% suspension with Alsever's solution and store at 4 C. **Note:** Treated RBCs may be diluted in saline if cells will be used immediately.
4.	Dilute 1 mL of untreated RBCs to a 3%-5% suspension with Alsever's solution and store at 4 C.
5.	Test eluate or serum against drug-treated and untreated RBCs by saline agglutination tests at RT and by saline IATs (see Section II).
6.	Examine the RBCs macroscopically; grade and record the results.
7.	Interpret the reactions as follows:

If...	And...	Then...
• Patient serum + drug-treated RBCs are positive • Normal serum + drug-treated RBCs are negative	• Patient serum + normal RBCs are negative • Normal serum + normal RBCs are negative	patient has a drug-dependent antibody.
• Patient serum + drug-treated RBCs are positive • Normal serum + drug-treated RBCs are negative	• Patient serum + normal RBCs are positive • Normal serum + normal RBCs are negative	patient has a drug-independent autoantibody: • Test dilution(s) of patient serum with drug-treated and normal RBCs, or adsorb serum and repeat drug antibody testing using adsorbed serum.

• Patient serum + drug-treated RBCs are positive • Normal serum + drug-treated RBCs are positive	• Patient serum + normal RBCs are negative • Normal serum + normal RBCs are negative	positive reaction could be caused by nonspecific uptake of proteins onto the drug-treated RBCs: • Test dilution(s) of patient serum (1:100) and normal serum vs drug-treated RBCs. Pathologic drug-dependent antibody titer will be reactive at titer values >20 in most cases.
patient serum + untreated RBCs are negative	known control drug-dependent antibody is positive	patient does not have drug-dependent antibody.
patient serum + untreated RBCs are negative	known control drug-dependent antibody is not available	interpretation of test for drug-dependent antibody cannot be reliably made.

Reference   Judd WJ. Investigation and management of immune hemolysis: Autoanti-bodies and drugs. In: Wallace ME, Levitt JS, eds. Current applications and interpretation of the direct antiglobulin test. Arlington, VA: AABB, 1988:47-103.

Effective Date

Approved by:	**Printed Name**	**Signature**	**Date**
Laboratory Management			
Medical Director			
Quality Officer			

XII-E. Detecting Cephalothin-Dependent Antibodies

Purpose
To provide instructions for detecting cephalothin-dependent antibodies that bind effectively to drug-coated RBCs.

Note: There have been reported cases of cephalothin-dependent antibodies reacting in the presence of drug.

Background Information
Cephalothin has been reported to induce an IgG immune response (cephalothin-dependent antibody) that can be recognized in tests with RBCs treated with the drugs..

Operational Policy
Not applicable.

Limitations

Caution:

- Antibodies to penicillin may cross-react with RBCs coated with cephalosporin.

- Normal sera will react with cephalothin (Keflin)-coated RBCs because such RBCs adsorb all proteins nonimmunologically. This reactivity does not occur with incubation times as short as 15 minutes, or if the serum is diluted 1 in 20 with PBS before testing.

- Eluates do not contain sufficient protein to account for nonimmunologic adsorption of globulins by Keflin-treated RBCs. Thus, reactivity of an eluate with cephalosporin-coated RBCs is indicative of antibody to cephalosporins or cross-reacting antibodies to penicillin.

- Some cephalothin-dependent antibodies may react only in the presence of drug.

Note: See Procedure XII-D for an alternative method that also permits detection of antibodies to semisynthetic penicillins.

Incorrect Results:

- Incorrect technique has been used.

- Drug has been omitted.

- Wrong reagent has been used.

Sample Requirements

Serum and/or eluate (see Section IV): 0.3 mL.

Note: Serum may be diluted 1 in 20 with saline before testing with cephalothin-coated RBCs because many normal individuals will have cephalothin-dependent antibody.

Equipment/ Materials

Alsever's solution.

Cephalosporin solution: sodium cephalothin (Keflin), 0.3 g; pH 6.0 PBS, 10 mL.

Note: If cephalosporin other than cephalothin (Keflin) is implicated, use Procedure XII-A.

Control serum: with cephalothin-dependent antibody, if available.

RBCs: group O, rr, 1 mL, washed three times with saline.

Negative control: pooled normal serum (or plasma), or normal serum or plasma from a single donor.

Quality Control

Test treated RBCs by saline-IAT with a known example of cephalothin-dependent antibody, if available. Treated RBCs should react 3+ to 4+; untreated (control) RBCs should be nonreactive.

Procedure

Use the following steps to complete the procedure:

Step	Action
1.	Mix 0.5 mL of RBCs with 5 mL of cephalothin solution.
2.	Incubate at 37 C for 30-60 minutes. Mix occasionally during incubation.
3.	Wash three times with saline or PBS. Dilute to a 3%-5% suspension with Alsever's solution and store at 4 C.
4.	Dilute the remaining (uncoated) 0.5 mL of RBCs to a 3%-5% suspension with 10 mL of Alsever's solution and store at 4 C.
5.	Test eluate or diluted serum against both drug-treated and untreated RBCs by saline agglutination tests at RT and by saline IATs as described in Section II.
6.	Examine the RBCs macroscopically; grade and record the results.

7.	Interpret the reactions as follows:		
	If...	**And...**	**Then...**
	patient eluate and/or serum + drug-treated RBCs are positive	no reactivity is seen with untreated RBCs	cephalothin-dependent antibody is present.
	known cephalothin-dependent antibody control is positive and drug-treated RBCs are positive	no reactivity is seen with untreated RBCs	test is valid.
	known cephalothin-dependent antibody control is not available	patient testing is negative	interpretation of test for drug-dependent antibody cannot be reliably made.

References   Petz LD, Garratty G. Acquired hemolytic anemias. 2nd ed. Philadelphia, PA: Churchill-Livingstone, 2004.

Effective Date

Approved by:	Printed Name	Signature	Date
Laboratory Management			
Medical Director			
Quality Officer			

XII-F. Detecting Drug-Dependent Antibodies Reacting in the Presence of Drug

Purpose

To provide instructions for detecting drug-dependent antibodies reacting in the presence of drug:

- For the detection of drug-dependent antibodies specific for drugs that do not bind effectively to the RBC membrane.

Background Information

When testing native (undiluted) serum, a positive result is likely indicative of a drug-dependent antibody. Titration studies may need to be performed to ensure reactivity is caused by a pathologic drug-dependent antibody vs those often found in normal individuals. Considerations:

- IgM drug-dependent antibodies will agglutinate normal RBCs in the presence of drug, but not the same untreated RBCs without added drug at room temperature unless preexisting low-titer antibodies are present.

- IgG drug-dependent antibodies will react by IAT against normal RBCs in the presence of drug, but not the same untreated RBCs without added drug unless preexisting low-titer antibodies are present.

When selecting RBCs for testing in the presence of drug metabolite, e+ RBCs are preferred because it has been shown that many drug-dependent antibodies have relative Rh specificity. Using e+ RBCs may enhance detection of antibodies.

Note: Rare drug-dependent antibodies have been shown to have specificity to other blood group antigens.

A fresh complement source has been noted to aid in the detection of some drug-dependent antibodies (see Petz and Garratty in the reference list), although in no instance has it been shown to be required to detect drug-dependent antibody.

Some drug-dependent antibodies will show enhanced reactivity when tested against protease (ficin or papain)-treated RBCs.

Operational Policy

Untreated RBCs should not react with patient serum or eluate. If positive reactions are observed, reactivity may be the result of a non-drug-related antibody (a specific alloantibody), a drug-independent autoantibody, or a drug-dependent antibody resulting from the continued presence of the drug the patient is taking in the patient's plasma.

Note: Titration of the patient serum and subsequent testing of the dilutions with normal RBCs in the presence of drug may be necessary. If drug-dependent antibody is present, the titer in the presence of drug will be greater than against normal RBCs without drug added to the test.

Limitations

Incorrect Results:

- Incorrect technique has been used.

- Drug has been omitted.

- Drug could not be dissolved in solution.

- Wrong reagent has been used.

Note: Caution must be taken when testing cefotetan-coated RBCs because these cells are also effective at nonspecific protein uptake. In addition, some individuals have "naturally occurring" cefotetan-dependent antibody.

Unwanted Positive Reactions:

- Some individuals have a drug-independent autoantibody. The patient serum will be positive when testing untreated normal RBCs, or in the absence of any drug in the test.

Unwanted Negative Reactions:

- Rare complement-binding drug-dependent antibodies may not agglutinate in the presence of drug if fresh normal serum as a source of complement is not added.

- Some drug-dependent antibodies will be detected only when testing enzyme-treated RBCs in the presence of drug.

Sample Requirements	Serum or plasma.

Equipment/ Materials	Drug(s) in question: in the form administered (tablet, solution, capsule), dissolved in pH 7.3 PBS, 1% albumin, or 6% albumin (see Procedure XII-A).

Negative control: pooled normal serum (or plasma), or normal serum or plasma from a single donor.

Positive control: known drug-dependent antibody serum, if available.

AHG: polyspecific preferred.

IgG-coated RBCs (see Section VIII, or obtain commercially).

Litmus paper: pH 7.0 range.

Diluent without drug: pH 7.3 PBS, 1% albumin, or 6% albumin.

RBCs: group O, rr reagent RBCs, washed three times with saline and diluted to a 3%-5% suspension.

Note: If alloantibodies are present, appropriate antigen-negative cells should be used.

Ficin- or papain-treated RBCs: group O, rr reagent RBCs; 3%-5% suspensions, prepared as described in Section III

Quality Control	Test patient serum and normal RBCs with a known example of drug-dependent antibody, if available. Normal reagent RBCs in the presence of drug should react 3+ to 4+.

Note: In order to preserve rare control serum/plasma, it is not necessary to test the known drug-dependent antibody against untreated RBCs in the presence of diluent.

Test normal serum and appropriate diluent as negative controls.

Confirm all negative antiglobulin test results with IgG-coated RBCs.

Procedure   Use the following steps to detect antibodies to perform the procedure:

Step	Action
1.	Using 0.1 mL (2 drops) of each reactant, prepare 1 or 2 sets (if testing enzyme-treated RBCs) of the following mixtures: • Patient serum + drug. • Patient serum + diluent (PBS or 1% or 6% albumin). • Normal serum + drug. • Normal serum + diluent (PBS or 1% or 6% albumin). • Diluent (PBS or 1% or 6% albumin) + drug.
2.	To 1 set of test mixtures, add 1 drop of untreated RBCs.
3.	To the other set, add 1 drop of enzyme-treated RBCs. **Note:** This step may be omitted in initial testing. See Limitations.
4.	To detect IgM drug-dependent antibodies, incubate at RT for 30 minutes. Then: • Centrifuge. • Dislodge the cell buttons gently. • Examine macroscopically for agglutination. • Grade and record the results. **Note:** This step may be omitted if desired. Proceed to Step 5.
5.	Mix the contents of each tube and incubate at 37 C for 1 hour, mixing the contents of each tube periodically. Then: • Centrifuge. • Dislodge the cell buttons gently. • Examine macroscopically for agglutination. • Grade and record the results.
6.	Wash each tube three to four times with saline and completely decant the final wash supernate. To the dry cell buttons, add 2 drops of AHG: • Mix and centrifuge. • Dislodge the cell buttons gently. • Examine macroscopically for agglutination. • Grade and record the results. **Note:** Polyspecific AHG is preferred to detect complement-dependent reactivity. Centrifuge and read for agglutination.

7.	Add 1 drop of IgG-coated RBCs to all tubes with negative antiglobulin test results: • Mix gently. • Centrifuge. • Examine macroscopically for agglutination. • Grade and record the results.
8.	Interpret the reactions as follows:

If hemolysis or agglutination is observed in ...	Then...
• Patient serum + drug and • All other tubes are negative	• Drug-dependent antibody is present. • Eluate + drug may or may not be positive.
• Patient serum + drug and • Patient serum + diluent	prepare serial dilutions (1:2, 1:4, etc) and retest.
• Other than those above normal serum + drug or • Diluent + drug	test is invalid: • Investigate cause and retest if appropriate.
none of the tests	drug-dependent antibody may be prozoning. Prepare serial dilutions (1:2, 1:4, etc) and retest: • Perform additional testing using enzyme-treated RBCs (Step 3) and/or • Retest adding a fresh complement source or • Retest using serum or urine metabolites of the drug.

Judd's Methods in Immunohematology
Detecting Drug-Dependent Antibodies Reacting in the Presence of Drug
Page 6 of 6

References

Garratty G. Laboratory investigation of drug-induced immune hemolytic anemia. In: Bell CA, ed. A seminar on laboratory management of hemolysis (supplement). Washington, DC: AABB, 1979.

Petz LD, Branch DR. Drug-induced hemolytic anemia. In: Chaplin H, ed. Methods in hematology: Immune hemolytic anemias. New York: Churchill-Livingstone, 1985:47-94.

Petz LD, Garratty G. Acquired hemolytic anemias. 2nd ed. Philadelphia, PA: Churchill-Livingstone, 2004.

Roback J, Combs MR, Grossman B, Hillyer C, eds. Technical manual. 16th ed. Bethesda, MD: AABB, 2008 (or current edition).

Effective Date

Approved by:

	Printed Name	Signature	Date
Laboratory Management			
Medical Director			
Quality Officer			

XII-G. Detecting Metabolite-Dependent Antibodies Reacting in the Presence of Drug

Purpose

To provide instructions for detecting drug-dependent antibodies reacting in the presence of drug metabolites.

Background Information

Some drugs (notably diclofenac and etodolac) elicit antibody formation against metabolites of the drug rather than epitopes on the native drug. Serum and/or urine from volunteers who have ingested therapeutic levels of the drug are required as a source of these metabolites. Information on the pharmacokinetics of drugs can be found in the *PDR* or *Merck Index*. This information will provide the timeline for drug metabolism and aid in assessing when to collect specimens from an individual taking the drug. Considerations:

- IgM metabolite-dependent antibodies will agglutinate RBCs in the presence of drug metabolite, but not the same RBCs without added drug metabolite at room temperature.

- IgG metabolite-dependent antibodies will react by IAT in the presence of drug, but not the same RBCs without added drug metabolite.

When selecting RBCs for testing in the presence of drug metabolite, e+ RBCs are preferred because it has been shown that many drug-dependent antibodies have relative Rh specificity. Using e+ RBCs may enhance the detection of antibodies.

Note: Rare drug-dependent antibodies have been shown to have specificity to other blood group antigens.

A fresh complement source has been noted to aid in the detection of some drug-dependent antibodies, although in no instance has it shown to be required to detect drug-dependent antibody.

Some drug-dependent antibodies will show enhanced reactivity when tested against protease (ficin or papain)-treated RBCs.

Operational Policy

This procedure should be considered when the drug is known to be rapidly metabolized. It is useful when use of other methods for detecting antibody have been uninformative.

Limitations

Incorrect Results:

- Incorrect technique has been used.

- Drug has been omitted.

- Inactive complement has been used.

- Wrong reagent has been used.

Unwanted Positive Reactions:

- Some individuals have a drug-independent autoantibody. The patient serum will be positive when testing untreated normal RBCs, or in the absence of any drug in the test.

Unwanted Negative Reactions:

- Rare complement-binding drug-dependent antibodies may not agglutinate in the presence of drug if fresh normal serum as a source of complement is not added.

- Some drug-dependent antibodies will be detected only when testing enzyme-treated RBCs in the presence of drug.

Sample Requirements

Serum: 3 mL.

Equipment/ Materials

AHG: polyspecific preferred.

Serum metabolites: serum samples from volunteer drug recipients collected at the appropriate time interval as determined and separated; 1 mL serum per sample. Keep at 1-6 C, or aliquot and store below −20 C until required.

Urine metabolite (see Procedure XII-B).

Human complement: freshly collected, normal human serum known to lack unexpected antibodies; 1 mL.

IgG-coated RBCs (see Section VIII, or obtain commercially).

pH 7.3 PBS.

RBCs: group O, rr reagent RBCs, washed three times with saline and diluted to a 3%-5% suspension with PBS.

Ficin- or papain-treated RBCs: group O, rr reagent RBCs; 3%-5% suspensions, prepared as described in Section III.

Sheep RBCs: available in most clinical immunology laboratories, or obtain commercially (eg, Pel-Freez Biologicals, Rogers, AR).

Quality Control

Test patient serum and normal RBCs with a known example of metabolite-dependent antibody, if available. Normal reagent RBCs in the presence of drug should react 3+ to 4+.

Note: In order to preserve rare control serum/plasma, it is not necessary to test the known metabolite-dependent antibody against untreated RBCs in the presence of diluent.

Test normal serum and appropriate diluent as negative controls.

Before use, each batch of human complement should be shown to lyse sheep RBCs. Use 1 drop of 3%-5% washed sheep RBCs in saline and 3 drops of human complement, with 15 minutes incubation at 37 C. Centrifuge as for hemagglutination tests and examine the supernate for hemolysis.

Confirm all negative antiglobulin test results with IgG-coated RBCs.

Procedure

Use the following steps to perform the procedure:

Step	Action
1.	Using 0.1 mL (2 drops) of each reactant, prepare 1 or 2 sets (if testing enzyme-treated RBCs) of the following mixtures: • Patient serum + drug-metabolite (urine or serum). • Patient serum + diluent (PBS or 1% or 6% albumin). • Normal serum + drug-metabolite (urine or serum). • Normal serum + diluent (PBS or 1% or 6% albumin). • Diluent (PBS or 1% or 6% albumin) + drug-metabolite (urine or serum).
2.	To 1 set of test mixtures, add 1 drop of untreated RBCs.

3.	To the other set, add 1 drop of ficin-treated RBCs.
	Note: This step may be omitted in initial testing. See Limitations.
4.	To detect IgM drug-dependent antibodies, incubate at RT for 30 minutes. Then:
	• Centrifuge.
	• Dislodge the cell buttons gently.
	• Examine macroscopically for agglutination.
	• Grade and record the results.
	Note: This step may be omitted if desired. Proceed to Step 5.
5.	Mix the contents of each tube and incubate at 37 C for 1 hour, mixing the contents of each tube periodically. Then:
	• Centrifuge.
	• Dislodge the cell buttons gently.
	• Examine macroscopically for agglutination.
	• Grade and record the results.
6.	Wash each tube three to four times with saline and completely decant the final wash supernate. To the dry cell buttons, add 2 drops of AHG:
	• Mix and centrifuge.
	• Dislodge the cell buttons gently.
	• Examine macroscopically for agglutination.
	• Grade and record the results.
	Note: Polyspecific AHG is preferred to detect complement-dependent reactivity. Centrifuge and read for agglutination.
7.	Add 1 drop of IgG-coated RBCs to all tubes with negative antiglobulin test results:
	• Mix gently.
	• Centrifuge.
	• Examine macroscopically for agglutination.
	• Grade and record the results.

8.	Interpret the reactions as follows:	
	If hemolysis or agglutination is observed in...	**Then...**
	• Patient serum + serum or urine metabolite and • All other tubes are negative	metabolite-dependent antibody is present. **Note:** Eluate + serum or urine metabolite may or may not be positive.
	• Patient serum + serum or urine metabolite and • Patient serum + diluent	prepare serial dilutions (1:2, 1:4, etc) and retest.
	• Other than those above normal serum + serum or urine metabolite or • Diluent + serum or urine metabolite	test is invalid: • Investigate cause and retest if appropriate.
	none of the tests	• Perform additional testing using enzyme-treated RBCs and/or • Retest with the addition of complement if not performed in initial testing.

References   Bougie D, Johnson ST, Weitekamp LA, Aster RH. Sensitivity to a metabolite of diclofenac as a cause of acute immune hemolytic anemia. Blood 1997;90:407-13.

Cuhha PD, Lord RS, Johnson ST, et al. Immune hemolytic anemia caused by sensitivity to a metabolite of etodolac, a nonsteroidal anti-inflammatory drug. Transfusion 2000;40:663-8.

O'Neil MJ, ed. The Merck index: An encyclopedia of chemicals, drugs, and biologicals. 14th ed. Whitehouse Station, NJ: Merck, 2006 (or current edition).

Physicians' desk reference. Montvale, NJ: Thomson Healthcare, 2008 (updated annually).

Salama A, Mueller-Eckhardt C. The role of metabolite-specific antibodies in nomifensine-dependent immune hemolytic anemia. N Engl J Med 1985;313:469-74.

**Effective
Date**

Approved by:	Printed Name	Signature	Date
Laboratory Management			
Medical Director			
Quality Officer			

Section XIII. Investigating ABO Typing Problems

Problems encountered in ABO typing are often associated with apparent absence of expected anti-A and/or anti-B, such as occurs with samples from newborns or from patients with immune deficiency disorders. Rarely, apparent absence of expected anti-A or anti-B may be caused by prozoning, excessive amounts of blood group substances, or a subgroup in which the presence of A or B RBC antigens cannot be detected by conventional agglutination tests but may be demonstrated by adsorption/elution studies. Some subgroups give mixed-field reactions with anti-A and/or anti-B; other causes of mixed-field reactions include recent transfusion, marrow transplantation, polyagglutination, and rare genetic mosaics. In other instances, discrepant ABO typing results may be caused by the presence of contaminants in reagent antisera or unexpected antibodies in test sera, including autoantibodies and antibodies to reagent RBC constituents. These causes of ABO typing results are discussed more fully below and are also summarized in Table XIII-1; Table XIII-2 summarizes the reactions of rare ABO phenotypes.

One of the major changes since the first edition (and continuing past the second edition) of this book has been the almost complete switch from polyclonal ABO reagents to monoclonal reagents. Some ABO discrepancies such as polyagglutination are only rarely detected because the naturally occurring anti-T and -Tn found in human polyclonal sera are not present in monoclonal reagents. However, monoclonal reagents are not without their quirks, and discrepancies are still regularly encountered.

Included in this section are specific serologic procedures used in the resolution of problems that may be encountered in routine ABO typing tests. Additional tests that may be required are described in Sections IX and XIV. Some guidelines have been included to assist in the selection of these procedures. If no conclusion can be drawn from the serologic tests, referral of the sample to a molecular testing laboratory can be valuable because the molecular basis of many subgroups of A and B antigens have been defined.

Causes of ABO Typing Discrepancies

Technical Factors

There are many technical factors that may contribute to erroneous ABO typing results. These include improper storage of reagents; use of incorrect technique; use of the wrong reagent; omission of antisera; use of antisera contaminated with bacteria, foreign matter, or the contents of other reagent vials; and incorrect centrifugation of tests.

IgM Autoantibodies

RBCs from patients with autoimmune hemolytic anemia caused by cold-reactive antibodies (cold agglutinin syndrome, or CAS) may agglutinate spontaneously at temperatures below 37 C. The IgM-mediated auto-agglutination can be obviated by incubating the RBCs with thiol reagents such as dithiothreitol (DTT) or 2-mercaptoethanol (2-ME). Also, potent

IgM agglutinins may mask the presence of anti-A and/or anti-B in the sera of these individuals; serum ABO typing can be performed at 37 C using group O RBCs as a control for auto-agglutination in addition to A_1 and B RBCs.

Weak or Absent Antigen Expression

A and B antigen expression may be depressed in leukemia, or weakly expressed because of inheritance of rare alleles at the ABO locus or inheritance of a variant H gene. The latter controls the development of H substance from which A and B antigens develop. Weakened A antigen expression is also occasionally observed in pregnancy, with a return to normal antigen strength after delivery.

In some rare phenotypes, the expression of A or B may be so weak that direct tests with anti-A or anti-B are nonreactive. That the RBCs carry weak A or B antigens is indicated by absence of the corresponding antibody from the serum. In phenotypes such as A_2 and A_2B, anti-A_1 may be present in the serum and cause an apparent exception to Landsteiner's Law (see Procedure XIII-C) inasmuch as A antigen is present on the RBCs, and anti-A is apparent in the serum. A_2 and A_2B phenotypes arise from inheritance of a variant gene (A^2) at the ABO locus, or from gene interaction in which the B gene suppresses the expression of the A gene. The A antigen in A_2 and A_2B phenotypes is probably both quantitatively and qualitatively different from A antigen in the more common A_1 phenotype. Thus Landsteiner's Law is not violated; the anti-A_1 that is formed is not an antibody against a self-antigen (autoantibody).

Very rarely, apparent weak or absent antigen may be seen in women with ovarian cysts that contain high concentrations of soluble blood group substances. The soluble blood group substance may spill over into the blood stream and neutralize tests with anti-A or anti-B when unwashed RBCs are used for ABO typing,

Mixed-Field Reactions

Mixed-field reactions are generally seen when testing RBCs from patients recently transfused with non-ABO-type-specific RBCs (eg, group O to group A/B) or shortly after marrow transplantation. Rarely are mixed-field reactions caused by leukemic changes or true genetic mosaicism (chimerism or dispermy). Mixed-field agglutination with anti-A and anti-A,B is also characteristic of Tn and A_3 RBCs.

Missing or Weak Anti-A and Anti-B

As discussed previously, anti-A and anti-B are absent in the sera of newborns, and reliance must be placed on the results of RBC typing when interpreting the results of ABO typing tests on blood from neonates. There are also congenital and acquired immune deficiency disorders in which the expected anti-A and/or anti-B may be absent. Of particular note is the weak or missing anti-A and/or anti-B seen in elderly patients. Incubation of tests and studies with enzyme-pretreated A, B, and O RBCs may be helpful in resolving discrepancies caused by absent agglutinins. The defect may not always be in the serum; apparent absence of anti-A or anti-B is associated with RBC mosaicism and is seen when A and/or B are weakly expressed on RBCs.

Anti-A and/or Anti-B Prozones

Sera with high-titer (ie, >5000) IgG anti-A and/or anti-B may be nonreactive with A_1 and/or B RBCs by immediate-spin technique. This prozone phenomenon is the result of steric hindrance of agglutination by C1, the first component of human complement, which is bound to the RBCs by IgG antibody before agglutination can occur. This phenomenon can be obviated by 1) use of EDTA-anticoagulated plasma, which lacks calcium ions essential for the integrity of the C1 molecule, 2) use of reagent RBCs suspended in preservative containing EDTA, 3) inactivation of complement by incubating sera at 56 C, or 4) dilution of the serum, 1 in 10 with saline. Hemolysis of A and/or B RBCs will occur if serum/RBC mixtures are incubated in the presence of active complement.

B(A) Phenotype

RBCs from group B individuals with high levels of galactosyltransferase are agglutinated by selected potent monoclonal anti-A reagents (eg, clones MHO4 or ES15). The B gene-specified transferase synthesizes trace amounts of A antigen that can be recognized through the use of reagents formulated from these antibodies.

Polyagglutination

Polyagglutinable RBCs have abnormal membrane structures such that they are agglutinated by normal adult human sera. Causes include membrane modifications by microbial enzymes (T, Th, Tk, and Tx) and acquired-B polyagglutination as well as incomplete membrane carbohydrate biosynthesis resulting from somatic mutation (Tn syndrome). Occasionally, polyagglutinability can be an inherited characteristic [hereditary erythroblastic multinuclearity associated with positive acidified serum (HEMPAS), NOR, or Cad]. Polyagglutinable RBCs are classified through the use of lectins, which are agglutinins derived primarily from plant seeds.

Naturally occurring agglutinins in human serum react with unique surface structures present on polyagglutinable RBCs. Anomalous reactions sometimes are seen in ABO typing tests with human source reagents, particularly with Tn and acquired-B RBCs. Tn RBCs carry A-like antigens and, therefore, are agglutinated by anti-A, whereas acquired-B RBCs carry a B-like antigen that cross-reacts with human anti-B.

Monoclonal reagents vary in their ability to react with Tn and acquired-B antigens. Current Food and Drug Administration (FDA)-licensed monoclonal anti-A and -A,B do not react with Tn RBCs. An increased incidence in the detection of acquired-B RBCs was observed through the use of some FDA-licensed monoclonal anti-B blood grouping reagents formulated from the anti-B clone ES4. Reactivity with acquired-B cells has been shown to be dependent on the pH of the final reaction milieu, with strongest reactivity associated with reagents having higher pH values (ML Beck and WJ Judd, unpublished observations). Since recognition of this phenomenon, reagent manufacturers have reformulated their reagents in an acid-buffered diluent. However, these modified reagents may react with serum-suspended acquired-B RBCs because the acid diluent may not have the buffering capacity to lower the pH of serum (ML Beck and WJ Judd, unpublished observations).

Abnormal Serum Proteins

Sera with reversed albumin-to-globulin ratios cause RBCs to form rouleaux, which may be mistaken for agglutination. See Procedure VIII-K for management of samples manifesting rouleaux.

Antibodies to Reagent Constituents

Antibody in the serum of a test sample against a reagent constituent may account for ABO typing discrepancies. Antibodies to polycarboxyl groups on EDTA and to yellow tartrazine #5 have been implicated. With antibodies to polycarboxyl groups, reagent A_1 and B RBCs suspended in a preservative containing EDTA (to prevent lysis by complement-binding anti-A or anti-B) are agglutinated. This reactivity can be abolished by washing the RBCs with saline before testing. With blood samples containing antibodies to yellow tartrazine #5 (used to color anti-B), unwanted reactions will be seen if serum suspended RBCs are used for blood typing.

Guidelines for Resolving ABO Typing Discrepancies

For the results of ABO typing tests (when performed by Procedure I-A) to be valid, there must always be, for each ABO type, 1) two positive and two negative test results and 2) concordance between RBC and serum results (ie, Landsteiner's Law must not be violated). Moreover, a valid positive test result is considered to be a reaction ≥2+; when weaker reactions are observed, additional testing is necessary.

Table XIII-1 summarizes reaction patterns that violate the first two rules stated above and lists the possible causes. The flow chart (Fig XIII-1) shows a suggested pathway for the investigation of ABO discrepancies.

The following are some suggested guidelines for problem-solving based on these reaction patterns.

Apparent Absent or Weak Antigen

1. Wash the RBCs and repeat the tests with extended incubation. See Procedure XIII-C. Consider inhibition with soluble blood group substance if marked enhancement is obtained by immediate-spin technique using washed RBCs. Also, see Procedure XIII-D.

2. Treat the RBCs with enzyme and retest (employ adequate controls). See Procedure XIII-D.

3. Adsorb/elute with anti-A and/or anti-B. See Procedure XIII-E.

4. Determine transfusion history (especially O RBC transfusions).

5. Determine diagnosis (especially leukemia and pregnancy).

6. Determine if patient is a marrow transplant recipient.

7. Determine if there is evidence for twinning at birth.

8. Perform ABH secretor studies. See Procedure XIII-G.

9. Perform rosetting tests (Procedure XIII-F) to detect minor RBC populations, or RBC separation techniques (Procedure XIII-I) if two populations of RBCs are grossly present.

10. If weak A or B appears to be an inherited characteristic, determine the RBC H antigen expression. See Procedure XIII-H.

Apparent Absent or Weak Agglutinin

1. Incubate the tests. See Procedure XIII-C.

2. Test the serum at room temperature and 4 C with two examples each of A_1, B, and O RBCs, and the autologous RBCs. Use Procedure II-H.

3. Test the serum at room temperature and 4 C with two examples each of enzyme-treated A_1, B, and O, and the autologous RBCs (use Procedure II-H). A cold autoadsorption (to remove enzyme-enhanced autoantibodies or enzyme-dependent panagglutinins) may be necessary before testing (see Procedures XI-J and XI-K).

4. Determine the age and diagnosis of the patient (eg, newborn, impaired immunity).

5. Determine the transfusion history of the patient (eg, whether non-ABO-type-specific plasma infusions were given).

Apparent Extra Antigens

1. Wash the RBCs and repeat the tests. If the tests are nonreactive, consider antibody in the patient or donor serum to an ingredient of the ABO typing reagent (eg, antibody to reagent dye).

2. Test the patient or donor serum at room temperature with two examples of group O RBCs and the autologous RBCs using Procedure II-H. If the serum contains cold-reactive autoagglutinins, consider spontaneous agglutination of RBCs. Treat the patient or donor RBCs with 2-ME or DTT and repeat the tests (see Procedure XI-F).

3.   Test the washed RBCs with a different manufacturer's reagents using Procedure I-A:

    a.   Use other polyspecific reagents if the primary reagent is of human origin.

    b.   Use monoclonal reagents of different origin if the aberrant primary reagent is monoclonal.

4.   Determine the diagnosis of the patient (eg, septicemia, gastrointestinal lesion).

5.   If acquired-B is suspected from Steps 3 and 4 above, repeat the tests with acidified anti-B. See Procedure XIV-G.

6.   Perform ABH secretor studies. See Procedure XIII-G.

7.   If polyclonal anti-A demonstrates a mixed-field reaction, treat RBCs with papain or ficin and retest (see Procedure XIII-D). Consider Tn-polyagglutination (see Section XIV) if repeat tests are nonreactive.

Apparent Extra Agglutinin(s)

1.   Test the serum at room temperature and 4 C with 2 examples each of A_1, A_2, B, O, and O, I– (cord and/or adult) RBCs as well as the autologous RBCs using Procedure II-H. Evaluate reactions for the presence of coldreactive auto- or alloantibodies (eg, anti-I, anti-M). When autoantibodies are present, autoadsorb the serum and repeat the tests, or perform the tests with A_1 and B RBCs by a low-ionic-strength saline in-direct antiglobulin test (LISS-IAT). If a specific alloagglutinin is present, repeat the tests with A_1 and B RBCs lacking the relevant antigen(s).

2.   Wash the reagent RBCs and repeat the tests. If the discrepancy is resolved with washed RBCs, consider antibody to an ingredient in the reagent RBC preservative.

3.   Test the serum with fresh A_1 and B RBCs. If the discrepancy is resolved, consider antibody to stored RBCs.

Mixed-Field Agglutination

1.   Determine if patient was/is recently/currently pregnant (indicating possible massive fetomaternal hemorrhage) or transfused (especially O RBCs to a group A/B patient).

2.   Determine the diagnosis of the patient (leukemia or pregnancy is especially important).

3.   Determine if patient is a marrow transplant recipient.

4.   Determine if there is evidence for twinning at birth.

5.   If responses in Steps 1-3 are negative, treat RBCs with enzyme and retest (employ adequate controls). See Procedure XIII-D.

6.   Perform RBC separation techniques (Procedure XIII-I) if two populations of RBCs are present. Phenotype separated RBC populations.

7.   Perform ABH secretor studies. See Procedure XIII-G.

Suggested Reading

Beattie KM. Discrepancies in ABO typing. In: Walker RH, ed. A seminar on problems encountered in pretransfusion tests. Washington, DC: AABB, 1972:129-65.

Beattie KM. Perspectives on some usual and some unusual ABO phenotypes. In: Bell CA, ed. A seminar on antigens on blood cells and body fluids. Washington, DC: AABB, 1980:97-149.

Khan F, Khan RH, Sherwani A, et al. Lectins as markers for blood grouping. Med Sci Monit 2002;8:RA293-300.

Olsson ML, Irshaid NM, Hosseini-Maaf B, et al. Genomic analysis of clinical samples with serologic ABO blood grouping discrepancies: Identification of 15 novel A and B subgroup alleles. Blood 2001;98:1585-93.

Pierce SR. Anomalous blood bank results. In: Dawson RB, ed. Trouble-shooting the crossmatch. Washington, DC: AABB, 1977:85-114.

Roback J, Combs MR, Grossman B, Hillyer C, eds. Technical manual. 16th ed. Bethesda, MD: AABB, 2008 (or current edition).

Judd's Methods in Immunohematology

Table XIII-1. Causes of ABO Typing Discrepancies

Cause of Apparent Absent Antigen	Missing Reactivity				Cause of Apparent Absent Agglutinin
	Anti-A	Anti-B	A₁	B	
	0	0	0	+	Non-ABO-type-specific plasma infusions/inheritance of a weak A/B subgroup
	0	0	+	0	Prozone of anti-A,B/newborn/impaired immune response
Leukemia/excess blood group substance*	+	0	0	0	Newborn/impaired immune response/inheritance of a weak A/B subgroup
	0	+	0	0	

Cause of Apparent Extra Antigen	Additional Reactivity				Cause of Apparent Extra Agglutinin
	Anti-A	Anti-B	A₁	B	
Antibody to a reagent component in anti-A* Antibody to low-prevalance antigen in anti-A Tn-polyagglutination	+	0	+	+	Anti-A₁ Antibody to a reagent component/stored RBCs Cold-reactive auto/alloantibody
Antibody to a reagent component in anti-B* Antibody to low-prevalance antigen in anti-B	0	+	+	+	Antibody to a reagent component/stored RBCs Cold-reactive auto/alloantibody
Spontaneous agglutination of RBCs	+	+	+	+	Cold-reactive auto/alloantibody
Spontaneous agglutination of RBCs Antibody to a reagent component in anti-B* Antibody to low-prevalance antigen in anti-B Acquired-B phenomenon/polyagglutination	+	+	0	+	Passive anti-B Cold-reactive alloantibody
Spontaneous agglutinination of RBCs Antibody to a reagent component in anti-A* Antibody to low-prevalance antigen in anti-A B(A) phenomenon/polyagglutination	+	+	+	0	Anti-A₁ Passive anti-A Cold-reactive alloantibody

*Potential problem when using serum-suspended RBCs for ABO typing.
+ = reactive; 0 = nonreactive.

Table XIII-2. Some Anomalous or Uncommon ABO Typing Results*

RBCs + Anti-					Serum/Plasma + RBCs					Secretor Status‡	Probable Phenotype
A	A₁	B	A,B	H†	A₁	A₂	B	0	Auto		
+	0	0	+	s	+	0	+	0	0	A and H	A_2 with anti-A_1
(+)	0	+	+	w	+	0	0	0	0	A, B, and H	A_2B with anti-A_1
mf	0	0	mf	w	0	0	+	0	0	A and H	A_3
0	0	0	(+)	s	+	0	+	0	0	H	A_x with anti-A_1
e	0	0	e	s	0	0	+	0	0	H	A_{el}
w	0	0	w	s	0	0	+	0	0	A and H	A_{weak}
w	0	0	w	0	(+)	+	+	+	0	—	A_h
0	0	w	w	0	+	+	+	+	0	—	B_h
0	0	0	0	0	+	+	+	+	0	—	O_h
mf	+	0	mf	s	+	+	+	0	0	H	O, Tn
(+)	0	+	+	+	+	+	0	0	+	B and H	B(A)
+	(+)	(+)	+	w	0	0	+	0	0	A and H	Acquired-B

***Note:** Unless otherwise stated, reactions shown are those obtained with polyclonal anti-A, -B, and -AB; different reactions may be obtained using monoclonal reagents.

†*Ulex europaeus* lectin.

‡Antigens in the saliva of *Se* individuals.

mf = mixed-field; s = strong; w = weak; e = reactions seen only by adsorption/elution tests; ( ) = reactions may be less than the normal 3+ or 4+.

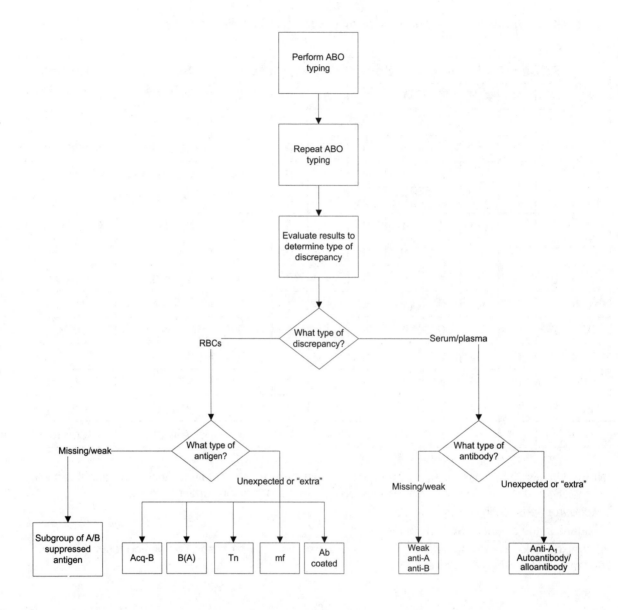

Figure XIII-1. Flow chart for the investigation of ABO discrepancies. Acq-B = acquired-B; Ab = antibody.

XIII-A. Investigation of Mixed-Field Reactions

Purpose

To provide a process for investigating mixed-field reactions observed during ABO typing.

Before You Begin

From hospital and laboratory data systems, phone, or requisition, obtain the patient's:

- Transfusion/transplantation history.
- Medical diagnoses.
- Birth records (evidence of twinning).
- Raw data (reactions) from initial ABO typing.

Operational Policy

Wash RBCs three times with pH 7.3 PBS before testing to prevent erroneous results caused by extraneous antibodies.

Sample Requirements

Patient RBCs treated with papain or ficin, as described in Section III.

Equipment/ Materials

Monoclonal anti-A known to lack activity for B(A) RBCs.

Monoclonal anti-B known to lack activity for acquired-B RBCs.

Process

Consider the factors outlined in the stages below when investigating mixed-field reactions observed during ABO typing:

Stage	Description	
1.	Evaluate anti-A and anti-B results as follows...	
	When mixed field reactions...	**Then consider...**
	occur in tests with anti-A and/or anti-B	• Weak antigen expression. • Recent transfusions. • Marrow or stem cell transplantation. • Genetic chimera.

2.	Repeat RBC ABO tests with protease-treated RBCs and evaluate the reaction pattern as follows:	
	When protease treatment ...	**Then consider...**
	enhances reactions	• A weak A or B subgroup. • Weak antigen expression caused by leukemic change.
	does not enhance reactions	• A3 phenotype. • A mixed cell population.
3.	Evaluate the history of the donor/patient and proceed as follows:	
	When there is a history ...	**Then consider...**
	of a blood transfusion or hematopoietic transplant	an artificial chimera—ie, mixed populations of donor and recipient RBCs.
	twinning in utero	true chimera.

Effective Date

Approved by:	Printed Name	Signature	Date
Laboratory Management			
Medical Director			
Quality Officer			

XIII-B. Investigation of Nonconcordant ABO Typing Reactions

Purpose To provide a process for investigating nonconcordant reactions observed during ABO typing.

Background For any valid reaction pattern observed in ABO typing tests using anti-A and anti-B on RBCs and A_1 and B RBCs on serum/plasma, there should be two positive test results and two negative test results, and the RBC reactions should not conflict with the serum/plasma reactions. When fewer than two positive test results are observed, antigens and/or expected antibodies will appear to be absent. When more than two positive test results are observed, extra antigens or antibodies will appear to be present.

The use of washed test and reagent RBCs in this procedure eliminates typing discrepancies caused by rare antibodies to reagent constituents. Selection of specific monoclonal reagents eliminates discrepancies caused by acquired-B and the B(A) phenotype.

Note: Polyagglutination should not be a cause of ABO typing discrepancies using currently available monoclonal antibody reagents.

Before You Begin From hospital and laboratory data systems, phone, or requisition, obtain the patient's:

- Transfusion/transplantation history.
- Medical diagnoses.
- Birth records (evidence of twinning).
- Raw data (reactions) from initial ABO typing.

Operational Policy Wash test and reagent A_1 and B RBCs three times with pH 7.3 PBS before testing.

Sample Requirements EDTA-anticoagulated or clotted whole blood.

Equipment/
Materials

Monoclonal anti-A known to lack activity for B(A) RBCs.

Monoclonal anti-B known to lack activity for acquired-B RBCs.

A_1 and B reagent RBCs.

Process

Consider the factors outlined in the stages below when investigating apparent absent antigens/antibodies and apparent extra antigens/antibodies observed during ABO typing:

Stage	Description				
1.	Repeat tests with washed patient and reagent RBCs and evaluate the reaction pattern as follows:				
	When the reaction pattern is...				**Then consider...**
	Anti-A	**Anti-B**	**A_1**	**B**	
	0	0	0	0	newborn/impaired immune response, prozone, marrow transplant, para-Bombay.
	0	0	0	+	leukemia, chimera, marrow transplant, para-Bombay, non-ABO-type-specific plasma infusions.
	0	0	+	0	
	+	0	0	0	newborn/impaired immune response.
	0	+	0	0	
	+	+	+	+	spontaneous RBC agglutination, cold-reactive non-ABO antibody.
	+	0	+	+	anti-A_1, cold-reactive non-ABO antibody, passive anti-A.
	0	+	+	+	cold-reactive non-ABO antibody, passive anti-B.
	+	+	+	0	anti-A_1, passive anti-A, cold-reactive non-ABO antibody.

2.	Evaluate the above considerations in light of the patient's history as follows:	
	When there is...	**Then consider ...**
	spontaneous RBC agglutination	treating patient's RBCs wirh DTT/2-ME and repeating ABO/Rh type.
	massive RBC transfusion or hematopoietic transplant	blood type change in vivo (eg, group O to group A or group B).
	twinning in utero	true chimera: • Submit sample for cytogenetic analysis.
	large-volume plasma transfusion	use of non-ABO-type-specific plasma.
	immune deficiency (disease state, newborn, elderly)	that low levels of anti-A/-B may be present: • Incubate serum/plasma ABO tests at cold temperatures (include group O RBCs to confirm specificity).
	leukemia	loss of antigen due to disease: • Enhance reactivity by repeating RBC ABO typing with papain- or ficin-treated RBCs.
	no informative history	para-Bombay phenotype: • Test RBCs with *Ulex europaeus* lectin. • Submit sample for molecular analysis.

Effective Date

Approved by:	Printed Name	Signature	Date
Laboratory Management			
Medical Director			
Quality Officer			

XIII-C. Evaluating an ABO Discrepancy

Purpose

To provide instructions for the initial evaluation of an ABO testing discrepancy between the results of the antigen testing and results of tests for naturally occurring antibodies in the plasma/serum.

Background Information

The basic rule in ABO typing is that of Lansteiner's Law, that there should be concordance between RBC and serum results: where an antigen is lacking on the RBCs, there should be an antibody present in the plasma/serum. Most of the major causes of such discrepancies have been summarized in the introduction to this section. The procedure that follows should assist in identifying the nature of the problem; additional testing may be required to confirm suspicions, depending on the result obtained.

Operational Policy

Because this procedure is for the purpose of evaluating apparent unwanted positive or negative reactions, the Quality Control section should be strictly adhered to, and the validity of the test results should be based on these results.

When agglutination occurs, reactions greater than 2+ are expected; observation of weaker reactions necessitates further study before valid conclusions can be made.

Limitations

Not applicable.

Sample Requirements

Clotted or anticoagulated whole blood: separate serum/plasma; 1 mL.

RBCs: washed three times and diluted to a 3%-5% suspension with saline.

Equipment/ Materials

Anti-A_1 (optional): *Dolichos biflorus* lectin, available commercially or prepared as described in Section XIV.

Anti-H (optional): *Ulex europaeus* lectin, available commercially or prepared as described in Section XIV.

Anti-A, -B, and -A,B: the reactivity described in Quality Control is based on polyclonal reagents. Slightly different findings than those presented may be encountered with monoclonal reagents.

Reagent RBCs: 3%-5% suspensions of A_1, A_2, B, and O RBCs.

Quality Control

Daily, for each lot of reagents in use, demonstrate that:

1. Anti-A agglutinates (4+) groups A_1 and A_2 RBCs but not groups B and O RBCs.

2. Anti-B agglutinates (4+) group B RBCs but not groups A_1, A_2, and O RBCs.

3. Anti-A_1 agglutinates (3+ to 4+) group A_1 RBCs but not group A_2 RBCs.

4. Anti-H agglutinates (3+ to 4+) group O and/or A_2 RBCs and reacts weakly (1+) or not at all with A_1 RBCs.

Procedure

Use the following steps to perform the procedure:

Step	Action
1.	Dispense 2-3 drops of serum/plasma into 5 appropriately labeled 10 or 12 × 75-mm test tubes.
2.	To 1 tube, add 1 drop of A_1 RBCs. Similarly, set up tests with A_2, B, O, and the test RBCs. Gently mix the contents within each tube.
3.	Dispense 1 drop of anti-A into an appropriately labeled 10 or 12 × 75-mm test tube. Set up similar tubes for anti-B, anti-A,B, and, if desired, anti-A_1 and anti-H.
4.	Add 1 drop of test RBCs to each tube containing reagent antiserum or lectin and gently mix the contents within each tube.
5.	Allow tests with lectins to stand at RT for the length of time stipulated by the reagent manufacturer, or for 5 minutes if reagents are prepared as described in Section XIV.
6.	Centrifuge as for hemagglutination tests.
7.	Examine the RBCs macroscopically; grade and record the results.
8.	Centrifuge all other tubes as for hemagglutination tests.
9.	Examine the RBCs macroscopically for agglutination and hemolysis; grade and record the results.

10.	Interpret the reactions as follows:	
	If the RBCs...	**Then...**
	agglutinate with anti-A or anti-B	antigen is present.
	agglutinate with anti-A,B only	the RBCs are weakly antigen-positive: • A subgroup (eg, A_x) is indicated.
	do not agglutinate with anti-A, anti-B, or anti-A,B	antigen is absent.
	If the serum/plasma...	**Then the serum/plasma contains...**
	agglutinates (or hemolyzes) A_1 and A_2 RBCs but not B or O RBCs	anti-A.
	agglutinates (or hemolyzes) B RBCs but not A or O RBCs	anti-B.
	agglutinates (or hemolyzes) A_1 RBCs but not A_2, B, or O RBCs	anti-A_1: • A subgroup of A is indicated.
	does not agglutinate or hemolyze reagent test RBCs	Weak ABO agglutinins or none at all.
11.	Repeat Steps 8 and 9 after 15 minutes incubation at RT. Interpret tests as in Step 10.	
12.	If additional anomalous reactions are encountered, refer to Process XIII-B.	

Reference   Walker RH, ed. A seminar on problems encountered in pretransfusion tests. Washington, DC: AABB, 1972:129-65.

**Effective
Date**

Approved by:	Printed Name	Signature	Date
Laboratory Management			
Medical Director			
Quality Officer			

XIII-D. Using Protease-Treated RBCs for ABO Typing Resolution

Purpose

To provide instructions for the evaluation of ABO typing using protease-treated RBCs.

Background Information

Mixed-field agglutination reactions in tests with ABO typing sera may be the result of 1) weak antigen expression (eg, A_3 RBCs), 2) a recent transfusion or marrow transplantation, 3) RBC mosaicism associated with chimerism or dispermy, or 4) polyagglutination (especially with Tn RBCs), if using polyclonal reagents. As shown in Step 5, results of tests with protease-treated RBCs serve to indicate the cause of mixed-field agglutination.

Operational Policy

Do not read tests microscopically because unwanted positive results may be encountered.

Do not refreeze enzyme solutions.

Limitations

Unwanted Positive Reactions:

- Incorrect concentration of enzyme was used.

Unwanted Negative Reactions:

- Enzyme is inactive.

- Incorrect technique was used.

- Enzyme preparation buffer is the wrong pH.

- A test component has been omitted.

Sample Requirements

RBCs from clotted or anticoagulated blood: 3%-5% suspensions of both untreated (washed three times) and ficin- or papain-pretreated RBCs (see Section III); 0.5 mL of each.

Equipment/ Materials

Anti-A, -B, and -A,B.

Reagent RBCs: 3%-5% suspensions of A_1, B, and O RBCs, both untreated and pretreated with ficin or papain.

Quality Control

The procedure includes both positive and negative controls for each typing reagent.

Procedure

Use the following steps to perform the procedure:

Step	Action
1.	To 1 drop of each RBC sample, add 2 drops of anti-A in appropriately labeled 10 or 12 × 75-mm test tubes.
2.	Set up similar tests with anti-B and -A,B reagents.
3.	Gently agitate the contents of each tube and incubate at RT for 15 minutes.
4.	Centrifuge as for hemagglutination tests.
5.	Examine the RBCs macroscopically and interpret the results as follows:

If reactivity of the protease-treated RBCs is…	Then…
enhanced	weak antigen (eg, an antigen subgroup) is present.
unaffected	two populations are mostly likely present.
abolished	Tn polyagglutination is likely.*

*Only with polyclonal anti-A and -A,B.

Effective Date

Approved by:	Printed Name	Signature	Date
Laboratory Management			
Medical Director			
Quality Officer			

XIII-E. Confirming Weak A Or B Antigen Expression by Adsorption and Elution

Purpose

To provide instructions for the detection of weak A or B antigen not detectable by routine blood grouping techniques.

Background Information

RBCs with a weak expression of A or B antigens may not be directly agglutinated by anti-A or anti-B, but may adsorb the specific antibody, which subsequently can be recovered by elution. The elution of anti-A from A_x RBCs is best demonstrated by the IgM component of anti-A,B, whereas the A antigen of the A_m phenotype is best demonstrated by the IgG components of anti-A and anti-A,B.

Operational Policy

Eluates must be tested directly after preparation.

Tests may be limited to adsorption/elution with a single reagent, as deemed appropriate.

Monoclonal antibodies are not suitable for this procedure because high unwanted positivity.

Limitations

Unwanted Positive Reactions:

- RBCs were washed insufficiently.

- Monoclonal antibodies were used.

Unwanted Negative Reactions:

- Elution temperature was incorrect.

- Eluate contains too much free hemoglobin.

Sample Requirements

RBCs from clotted or anticoagulated blood: 3 mL packed RBCs, washed six times with saline.

Judd's Methods in Immunohematology
Confirming Weak A Or B Antigen Expression by Adsorption and Elution
Page 2 of 4

Equipment/
Materials

AHG: anti-IgG or polyspecific reagent.

6% BSA.

Controls:

- Artificial mixture of 3%-5% A_1 or B RBCs in group O RBCs to serve as a positive control: 3 mL packed RBCs, washed six times with saline.

- 100% group O RBCs to serve as a negative control: 3 mL packed RBCs, washed six times with saline.

IgG-coated RBCs: see Section VIII, or obtain commercially.

Polyclonal anti-A, -B, and -A,B: either commercial reagents or high-titer donor plasma (see Procedure XIII-K).

Reagent RBCs: two examples each of A_1, B, and O RBCs, washed three times and diluted to a 3%-5% suspension with saline.

Note: Use papain- or ficin-treated RBCs, prepared by as described in Procedure III-D, in critical studies.

Saline: chilled to 4 C.

Water bath: at 56 C.

Pipettors with disposable tips to deliver 0.5-1 mL (eg, VWR, Batavia, IL).

Quality
Control

Perform the procedure with the positive control and negative control RBCs. Tests are valid when anti-A or anti-B is recovered from the artificial RBC mixture, but no antibody is eluted from the group O RBCs.

Procedure

Use the following steps to perform the procedure:

Step	Action
1.	Dispense 1 mL of each antiserum into appropriately labeled 13 × 100-mm test tubes.
2.	Add 0.5 mL of packed test RBCs to each tube.
3.	Similarly, set up tests with control samples.
4.	Mix and incubate at 37 C for 1 hour.
5.	Resuspend the RBCs and transfer tubes to 4 C for 2 hours.
6.	Wash the RBCs six times with 4 C saline. Save the final wash supernate for parallel testing with the eluate.
7.	Add 1 mL of 6% BSA to each tube of packed RBCs and mix well.

8.	Place the tubes at 56 C for 10 minutes and stir periodically with applicator sticks.
9.	Centrifuge to pack the intact RBCs and harvest the supernate (eluate).
10.	Test each eluate and final wash supernate against the reagent RBCs at RT and 4 C using the saline agglutination procedure described in Section II.
11.	Examine the RBCs macroscopically; grade and record the results.
12.	Interpret the reactions as follows:

If agglutination is...	Then...
present	weak antigen (eg, an antigen subgroup) is present.
absent	the test RBCs are antigen-negative.

13.	Transfer the tubes to 37 C for 1 hour.
14.	Centrifuge as for hemagglutination tests.
15.	Examine the RBCs macroscopically; grade and record the results.
16.	Interpret the reactions as follows:

If agglutination is...	Then...
present	weak antigen (eg, an antigen subgroup) is present.
absent	the test RBCs are antigen-negative.

17.	Wash the RBCs four times with saline and completely decant the final supernate.
18.	To the dry RBC buttons thus obtained, add AHG according to the manufacturer's directions.
19.	Centrifuge as for hemagglutination tests.
20.	Examine the RBCs macroscopically; grade and record the results.

21.	Interpret the reactions as follows:	
	If agglutination is...	**Then...**
	present	weak antigen (eg, an antigen subgroup) is present.
	absent	the test RBCs are antigen-negative.
22.	Add IgG-coated RBCs to all negative tests. Recentrifuge and examine the tests macroscopically for mixed-field agglutination. Repeat antibody detection tests when tests with IgG-coated RBCs are nonreactive.	

Reference

Beattie KM. Perspectives on some usual and some unusual ABO phenotypes. In: Bell CA, ed. A seminar on antigens on blood cells and body fluids. Washington, DC: AABB, 1980:97-149.

Effective Date

Approved by

	Printed Name	Signature	Date
Laboratory Management			
Medical Director			
Quality Officer			

XIII-F. Detecting Minor RBC Populations and ABO Mixtures

Purpose

To provide instructions for the detection of subpopulations of A or B antigen-positive RBCs where ABO typing discrepancies are apparent.

Background Information

Addition of anti-A (or -B) to a predominantly group O RBC sample containing a minor population of group A (or B) RBCs may not always cause observable agglutination of the minor RBC population. Insufficient A or B RBCs may be present such that antigen-antibody interactions involving multiple RBCs, necessary to form agglutinates, do not readily occur. The use of appropriate indicator RBCs to form rosettes around the minor RBC population precoated with anti-A (or -B) affords a sensitive method for detecting the minor population.

Operational Policy

Not applicable.

Limitations

Not applicable.

Sample Requirements

RBCs from clotted or anticoagulated blood: 0.1 mL.

Equipment/ Materials

Polyspecific anti-A or anti-B, as appropriate.

Controls:

- Artificial mixture of 3%-5% A_1 or B RBCs in group O RBCs to serve as a positive control.
- 100% group O RBCs to serve as a negative control.

Indicator RBCs: group A_1 and/or B (as appropriate).

Quality Control

The procedure includes tests with positive and negative control samples. Rosettes should be present in the positive control sample, but not in the negative control sample.

Procedure   Use the following steps to perform the procedure:

Step	Action
1.	Wash all RBC samples three times and dilute to a 3%-5% suspension with saline.
2.	Dispense 1 drop of anti-A (or -B) in a 10 or 12 × 75-mm test tube.
3.	Add 1 drop of test RBCs and mix well.
4.	Similarly, set up positive and negative control tests.
5.	Incubate at RT for 15 minutes.
6.	Wash the RBCs eight times with saline.
7.	Add 1 drop of A_1 or B RBCs (A_1 if anti-A used; B if anti-B used).
8.	Mix and incubate at RT for 5 minutes, gently agitating the contents of the tube during this time.
9.	Centrifuge as for hemagglutination tests and gently resuspend the RBCs.
10.	Centrifuge again as for hemagglutination tests.
11.	Examine the RBCs microscopically for the presence of RBC rosettes.
12.	Interpret the reactions as follows:

If rosettes are...	Then...
discrete, around a small population of RBCs	two populations of RBCs are present.
diffuse, throughout the whole field	the RBCs are likely a single population with weak antigen expression (eg, a subgroup).

**Effective
Date**

Approved by

	Printed Name	Signature	Date
Laboratory Management			
Medical Director			
Quality Officer			

XIII-G. Determining ABH Secretor Status

Purpose

To provide instructions for determining the presence or absence of soluble ABH blood group antigens in saliva.

Background Information

The *ABO* and *H* genes govern the expression of A, B, and H antigens on RBCs. In saliva and other body fluids, however, the presence of water-soluble A, B, and H antigens is determined by *ABO* and *Se* genes. When *Se* is present, those antigens whose expression is controlled by the *ABO* locus will also be found in the secretions. The presence of secreted antigens can be ascertained using a hemagglutination-inhibition assay.

Operational Policy

Polyclonal reagents should be used for this procedure, either commercially available or high-titer donor plasma (see Procedure XIII-K).

Limitations

Unwanted Positive Reactions:

- False inhibition has been reported with monoclonal anti-A and anti-B; hence, the stipulation that polyclonal reagents be used.

Unwanted Negative Reactions:

- Saliva has been improperly prepared.

Sample Requirements

Saliva under investigation: prepared as described in Section VIII; 0.5 mL.

Equipment/ Materials

Anti-A: polyclonal (human) reagent.

Anti-B: polyclonal (human) reagent.

Anti-H: *Ulex europaeus* lectin, commercially available or prepared as described in Section XIV.

pH 7.3 PBS.

RBCs: A_1, B, and O RBCs, washed three times and diluted to a 3%-5% suspension with saline.

Pipettors with disposable tips to deliver 0.1-1.0 mL (eg, VWR, Batavia, IL).

Quality Control

Test saliva samples from Le(a+b–) and Le(a–b+) individuals in parallel. Include a PBS control to verify that nonreactive tests are due to inhibition of antibody and not dilution.

Procedure

Use the following steps to perform the procedure:

Step	Action
1.	Dilute 0.1 mL of anti-A with 0.9 mL of PBS.
2.	Dilute 0.1 mL of anti-B with 0.9 mL of PBS.
3.	Dispense 0.1-mL volumes of dilute anti-A into 2 10 or 12 × 75-mm test tubes. Prepare similar tubes with dilute anti-B and with anti-H lectin.
4.	Add 0.1 mL of saliva to 1 tube of each reagent.
5.	Add 0.1 mL of PBS to the other tubes.
6.	Shake the contents of each tube and incubate at RT for 30 minutes.
7.	Add 1 drop of the appropriate indicator RBCs: A_1 to tubes containing anti-A, B to tubes containing anti-B, and O to tubes containing anti-H.
8.	Mix and incubate at RT for 15 minutes.
9.	Centrifuge as for hemagglutination tests.
10.	Examine the RBCs macroscopically; grade and record the results.

Step	Action			
11.	Interpret the reactions as follows:			
	If agglutination is...			**Then the test subject is a...**
	Anti-A	**Anti-B**	**Anti-H**	
	+	+	0	secretor of H antigen.
	0	+	0	secretor of A and H antigens.
	+	0	0	secretor of B and H antigens.
	0	0	0	secretor of A, B, and H antigens.
	+	+	+	nonsecretor.

**Effective
Date**

Approved by	Printed Name	Signature	Date
Laboratory Management			
Medical Director			
Quality Officer			

XIII-H. Determining H Antigen Expression

Purpose

To provide instructions for the detection of H antigen on RBCs.

Background Information

The expression of H antigen content on RBCs is related to ABO type. Because H antigen is the terminal antigen on group O RBCs, these RBCs are strongly H positive. The glycosyltransferases encoded by *A* and *B* genes use H as a substrate, and thus the sequence in decreasing order of H antigen expression is $O > A_2 > A_2B > B > A_1 > A_1B$. Some rare variant phenotypes are associated with a weakened expression or absence of H, and like A and B antigens, H may be depressed in certain disease states and on some polyagglutinable RBC types.

Determination of H expression can be useful when evaluating a potential A or B subgroup.

Operational Policy

Not applicable.

Limitations

Not applicable.

Sample Requirements

RBCs: washed three times and diluted to a 3%-5% suspension with saline; 1 mL.

Equipment/ Materials

Anti-H: *Ulex europaeus* lectin, available commercially, or a crude saline extract prepared as described in Section XIV.

BSA: 22% wt/vol; containing 0.1% (vol/vol) Tween 20 (Sigma-Aldrich, St Louis, MO) as a wetting agent.

pH 7.3 PBS.

RBCs: washed three times and diluted to a 3%-5% suspension with saline; include A_1, A_2, B, and O RBCs (controls) for comparative purposes.

Quality Control

The procedure includes tests with RBC samples carrying predictable expression of H.

Procedure   Use the following steps to perform the procedure:

Step	Action
1.	Prepare serial twofold dilutions of anti-H lectin in pH 7.3 PBS. The dilution range should be from 1 to 1:2048 (12 tubes), and the volumes prepared should not be less than 0.1 mL for each RBC sample to be tested.
2.	Mix 1 drop of test RBCs with 2 drops of each dilution in appropriately labeled 10 or 12 × 75-mm test tubes.
3.	Similarly, set up tests with control A_1, A_2, B, and O RBCs.
4.	Incubate at RT for 30 minutes.
5.	Add 2 drops of 22% BSA to each tube and mix well.
6.	Incubate at RT for 5 minutes.
7.	Centrifuge as for hemagglutination tests.
8.	Examine the RBCs macroscopically; grade and record the results.
9.	Add the reaction scores of individual tubes for each RBC sample. Compare the sum of scores obtained with the test RBCs with that obtained with each control sample to determine the relative H antigen content of the test RBCs.
10.	Compare the sum of scores obtained from the test RBCs with those from the controls:

If the sum of scores with the test sample…	Then report H content of test RBCs as…
matches that of one of the controls (±5)	comparable to that control sample.
is intermediate between two control samples	intermediate between those control samples.

**Effective
Date**

Approved by	Printed Name	Signature	Date
Laboratory Management			
Medical Director			
Quality Officer			

XIII-I. Separating A:O Mixtures

Purpose

To provide instructions for separating populations of A and O RBCs in a mixture.

Background Information

Agglutinated RBCs are heavier and, therefore, sediment quicker in suspension than do unagglutinated RBCs. This facilitates separation of RBC mixtures by differential agglutination. With lectin reagents to human A blood group antigen, dispersal of agglutinates is accomplished by the addition of soluble blood group A substance.

Operational Policy

The procedure may be modified for separating B:O mixtures using GS I lectin from *Griffonia simplicifolia*, available from E-Y Laboratories, San Mateo, CA.

Limitations

Unwanted Positive Reactions:

- RBCs are improperly washed.

- Rouleaux is present.

- RBCs are polyagglutinable.

Unwanted Negative Reactions:

- RBCs are not permitted enough time to agglutinate.

Sample Requirements

RBCs: washed three times and diluted to 3%-5% suspension with saline; 0.5 mL.

Equipment/ Materials

Anti-A blood typing reagent.

22% or 30% BSA.

Control sample: artificial mixture of A and O RBCs (1:1), washed three times and diluted to a 50% suspension with saline.

Human group A saliva: containing water-soluble blood group A substance (see Appendix A and Procedure XIII-G).

Lectin anti-A, *Phaseolus lunatus* (syn. *limensis*, or lima beans): prepared as described in Section XIV.

pH 7.3 PBS.

Petri dishes: as used routinely in microbiology laboratories.

Test RBCs: washed three times and diluted to 50% suspension with saline.

Quality Control

The procedure includes tests with an artificial mixture of A and O RBCs.

Procedure

Use the following steps to perform the procedure:

Step	Action
1.	Dispense 2 mL of lectin into a clean Petri dish.
2.	Add 0.5 mL of 50% test RBCs and rock the Petri dish until agglutinates no longer increase in size.
3.	Similarly, set up tests with artificial A:O mixture.
4.	Using a clean Pasteur pipette, transfer the agglutinates (group A RBCs) into clean 10 or 12 × 75-mm test tubes; then: a) Fill the tube with BSA and mix by inversion. b) Allow the agglutinates to settle and transfer the unagglutinated (group O) RBCs in the supernate to a clean 10 or 12 × 75-mm test tube.
5.	Repeat Steps 4a and 4b twice more. a) Wash the agglutinated RBCs three times with saline. b) Add 2 mL of A-secretor saliva and incubate at RT for 1 hour. c) Wash the group A RBCs three times with saline before testing with anti-A and PBS.
6.	Wash the unagglutinated group O RBCs three times with saline before testing with anti-A.

7.	Examine tests microscopically and interpret the reactions as follows:		
	If tests with anti-A and the A population show...	**And the tests with PBS are...**	**Then...**
	no free RBCs	negative	a pure group A population has been obtained: • Phenotype the group A RBCs.
	no free RBCs	positive	inhibition with saliva was not complete: • Repeat Step 5b.
	free RBCs	negative	separation is incomplete: • Repeat Steps 4a and 4b.
	If tests with anti-A and the O population show...		**Then...**
	no agglutinated RBCs		a pure group O population has been obtained: • Phenotype the group O RBCs.
	agglutinated RBCs		separation is incomplete: • Repeat Steps 4a and 4b.

References   Beattie KM. Discrepancies in ABO typing. In: Walker RH, ed. A seminar on problems encountered in pretransfusion tests. Washington, DC: AABB, 1972:129-65.

Booth PB, Plaut G, James JD, et al. Blood chimerism in a pair of twins. Brit Med J 1957;i:1456-8.

Effective Date

Approved by	Printed Name	Signature	Date
Laboratory Management			
Medical Director			
Quality Officer			

Judd's Methods in Immunohematology
Detecting A and B Transferases by Conversion of Group O RBCs
Page 1 of 3

XIII-J. Detecting A and B Transferases by Conversion of Group O RBCs

Purpose

To provide instructions for detecting active A and/or B glycosyltransferases in serum or plasma by adding A or B antigens to group O RBCs.

Background Information

In the presence of their substrate uridine diphosphate (UDP)-sugars, the A- and B-gene-specified transferases (3-α-N-acetylgalactoaminyltransferase and 3-α-galactosyltransferase) will cause group O RBCs to acquire A or B antigens in vitro that can be detected in direct tests with the appropriate antisera. Thus, indirectly, the presence of the ABO-gene-specific transferases in sera can be detected using this method.

Operational Policy

Plasma from EDTA samples is not suitable for use in this procedure because of the chelating properties of EDTA.

Limitations

Unwanted Positive Reactions:

- Too much $MnCl_2$ in the serum-to-RBC mixture.

Unwanted Negative Reactions:

- Too much $MnCl_2$ in the serum-to-RBC mixture.
- EDTA plasma used.

Sample Requirements

Test serum or ACD plasma: 1 mL.

Equipment/ Materials

Groups A, B, and O sera: 1 mL of each to serve as controls.

Group O RBCs: washed three times and diluted to a 50% suspension with saline.

Manganese chloride ($MnCl_2$).

Uridine 5'-diphosphogalactose: UDP-galactose (eg, Sigma-Aldrich, St Louis, MO).

Uridine 5'-diphospho-N-acetylgalactosamine: UDP-N-acetylgalactosamine (eg, Sigma-Aldrich, St Louis, MO).

Quality Control   This procedure includes positive and negative controls.

Procedure   Use the following steps to perform the procedure:

Step	Action
1.	Dispense 1 mL of the test and control samples into 2 sets of appropriately labeled 10 or 12 × 75-mm test tubes.
2.	Moisten the end of a small-circle applicator stick with saline and use to add a small amount (ie, that which will adhere to the end of the stick) of UDP-galactose to one set of tubes.
3.	Repeat Step 2 with UDP-N-acetylgalactosamine to the other set of tubes.
4.	Similarly, add a small amount of $MnCl_2$ to each tube.
5.	Add 1 drop of 50% O RBCs to each tube.
6.	Mix and incubate at 37 C for between 1 and 3.5 hours.
7.	Wash the RBCs three times with saline.
8.	Determine the presence of B antigens on the treated RBC samples (tests and controls) using anti-A, -B, and -A,B, as described in Procedure XIII-C.
9.	Interpret the reactions as follows:

If RBCs treated with the test serum and UDP-galactose...	And the RBCs treated with the control samples and UDP-galactose...	Then...
type as group B	type as expected	the test serum contains the B-gene-specified transferase.
type as group O	type as expected	the test serum lacks the B-gene-specified transferase.
type as group O	do not type as expected	the results are invalid: • Consider inactive substrate.

Judd's Methods in Immunohematology
Detecting A and B Transferases by Conversion of Group O RBCs
Page 3 of 3

	If RBCs treated with the test serum and UDP-*N*-acetyl-galactosamine...	And the RBCs treated with the control samples and UDP-*N*-acetyl-galactosamine...	Then...
	type as group A	type as expected	the test serum contains the A-gene-specified transferase.
	type as group O	type as expected	the test serum lacks the A-gene-specified transferase.
	type as group O	do not type as expected	the results are invalid: • Consider inactive substrate.

Reference   Valko DA, et al. A simple method for detection of the *B*-gene specified transferase (abstract). Transfusion 1981;21:624.

Effective Date

Approved by	**Printed Name**	**Signature**	**Date**
Laboratory Management			
Medical Director			
Quality Officer			

XIII-K. Selecting Plasma Containing High-Titer Anti-A and/or Anti-B

Purpose

To provide instructions for the selection of polyclonal anti-A and anti-B of high titer from donor plasma samples.

Background Information

Monoclonal anti-A and anti-B blood grouping reagents are now the reagents of choice, and there are very few polyclonal reagents available. Many monoclonal antibodies are more sensitive than their polyclonal counterparts, and more potent. However, they are not suitable for some procedures such as adsorption/elution because they may give unwanted positive reactions. Identification of high-titer donor plasma can provide a source of polyclonal anti-A and/or anti-B that may be used in these procedures.

Operational Policy

Plasma is suitable if the sample is to be used directly; otherwise conversion to serum is recommended (see Procedure XV-K).

Limitations

Not applicable.

Sample Requirements

Plasma or serum from group A and group B blood donors: 0.2 mL.

Equipment/ Materials

Reagent RBCs: 3%-5% suspensions of A_1, B, and O RBCs, untreated and papain (or ficin)-treated RBCs (see Procedure III-G).

6% BSA.

Quality Control

Not applicable.

Procedure   Use the following steps to perform the procedure:

Step	Action
1.	Prepare 1:100 dilutions of all donor plasma/serum samples by diluting a 5-µL sample in 495 µL of 6% BSA.
2.	Pipette 2 drops of each dilution into each of 2 tubes, 10 or 12 × 75 mm.
3.	For all group B samples, add 1 drop of untreated A_1 RBCs to 1 tube, and papain-treated A_1 RBCs to the other.
4.	For all group A samples, repeat with group B RBCs.
5.	Mix and incubate at RT for 15 minutes.
6.	Centrifuge and examine the RBCs macroscopically.
7.	Interpret the reactions as follows: <table><tr><th>If agglutination is…</th><th>Then the sample…</th></tr><tr><td>2+ or less</td><td>does not contain high-titer agglutinins.</td></tr><tr><td>>2+</td><td>contains high-titer agglutinins.</td></tr></table>
8.	Select plasma samples with high-titer agglutinins for adsorption/ elution studies (see Procedure XIII-E).
9.	Selected samples of the same ABO group may be pooled.

Effective Date

	Printed Name	Signature	Date
Approved by			
Laboratory Management			
Medical Director			
Quality Officer			

Section XIV. Investigating RBC Polyagglutination

Polyagglutination is a condition in which RBCs are agglutinated by ABO-compatible adult human sera but not by cord blood sera. The RBCs have abnormal membrane structures as a result of 1) microbial enzymes that modify cell surface carbohydrates, 2) incomplete bio-synthesis of the RBC membrane following somatic mutation, or 3) the inheritance of rare alleles. The abnormal membrane structures are recognized by specific naturally acquired polyagglutinins present in normal adult sera.

Although serologic problems caused by polyagglutination are uncommon, the abnormality should always be considered whenever discrepant ABO typing results are seen (especially with polyclonal antisera), and when intravascular hemolysis occurs in the absence of RBC transfusion or after transfusion with plasma-containing components. Furthermore, polyag-glutination may result in a positive direct antiglobulin test (DAT), due to C3 activation, or a positive serologic crossmatch when donor RBCs are polyagglutinable.

The techniques described in this section are used to identify polyagglutination, although some methods have much wider application—notably the use of lectins as alternatives to human sera for blood typing purposes. Some lectins are also useful for investigating variant MN phenotypes.

The serologic characteristics of the various forms of polyagglutination are summarized in Table XIV-1. The sources below provide detailed reviews of polyagglutination and describe the various applications of lectins in immunohematology.

Suggested Reading

Beck ML, Judd WJ, eds. Polyagglutination. Washington, DC: AABB, 1980.

Judd WJ. Polyagglutination. Immunohematology 1992;8:58-69.

Judd WJ. The role of lectins in blood group serology. CRC Crit Rev Clin Lab Sci 1980;12: 171-212.

Table XIV-1. Reactions of Polyagglutinable RBCs* with Lectins

Lectin	RBCs										
	T	Tk	Th	Tx	Tn	Cad	Nor	VA	HEMPAS	HbM~Hyde Park~	Acquired-B
Griffonia simplicifolia I	0	0	0	0	+	0	0	0	0	0	+
Griffonia simplicifolia II	0	+	0	0	0	0	0	0	0	+	0
Dolichos biflorus	0	0	0	0	+	+	0	0	0	0	w/0
Helix pomatia	+	0	/	/	+	+	0	+	+	+	+
Phaseolus limensis	0	0	0	0	0	0	0	0	0	/	+
Leonorus cardiaca	0	0	0	0	0	+	0	0	0	0	0
Arachis hypogaea	+	+	+	+	0	0	0	0	0	w	(+)
Glycine max	+	0	0	0	+	0	0	0	0	+	0
Salvia horminum	0	0	0	0	+	+	0	0	0	w	0
Salvia sclarea	0	0	0	0	+	0	0	0	0	0	0
Ulex europaeus[†]	>	≤	=	=	≥	≤	=	≤	≤	>	=
Vicia cretica	+	0	+	0	0	0	0	0	0	w	0

*All RBCs are group O except for acquired-B RBCs.

[†]Reactions with *U. europaeus* compared to reactivity of group O RBCs: > = stronger than; ≤ = equal to or weaker than; = = equal to; ≥ = equal to or stronger than.

0 = nonreactive; + = reactive; w/0 = often weakly reactive or nonreactive; / = not tested; (+) = often reactive due to T and/or Tk activiation; w = weakly reactive.

XIV-A. Detecting Polyagglutination with AB and Cord Blood Serum

Purpose

To provide instructions for testing RBCs with group AB and cord blood sera:

- Demonstration of polyagglutination.

Background Information

By definition, polyagglutinable RBCs are agglutinated by most adult sera, regardless of ABO type, but not by cord blood sera. This procedure serves to confirm the polyagglutinable status of RBCs.

Operational Policy

Because of the presence of cold agglutinins in normal sera, use AB sera prepared as described in Appendix A if 4-C studies are required.

Limitations

Incorrect Results:

- Incorrect technique.
- Improper storage of reagents.
- Use of sera contaminated with antibodies to RBC antigens.

Sample Requirements

Test RBCs: washed three times and diluted to a 3%-5% suspension with PBS.

Equipment/ Materials

A_1 and B RBCs: washed three times and diluted to a 3%-5% suspension with PBS.

AB serum from adults: four to six examples (see Appendix A) or use AB donor plasma.

Autologous serum: to serve as an autocontrol.

Cord blood sera: from two to three cord blood samples.

Neuraminidase-treated (T-activated) RBCs: prepared as described in Section III. Alternatively, use known Tn RBCs.

Quality Control

The method includes tests with positive and negative control samples.

Judd's Methods in Immunohematology
Detecting Polyagglutination with AB and Cord Blood Serum
Page 2 of 3

Procedure   Use the following steps to perform the procedure:

Step	Action
1.	Dispense 2-3 drops of each serum sample into each of 4 appropriately labeled 10 or 12 × 75-mm test tubes.
2.	To 1 tube of each sample, add 1 drop of test RBCs.
3.	Similarly, set up tests with the control (A, B, and T-activated) RBCs.
4.	Mix and incubate at RT for 15 minutes.
5.	Centrifuge as for hemagglutination tests.
6.	Examine the RBCs macroscopically; grade and record the results.
7.	Interpret the reactions with the test RBCs* as follows:

If AB sera are...	And cord blood sera are...	Then...
reactive	nonreactive	test RBCs are polyagglutinable.
nonreactive	nonreactive	test RBCs are not polyagglutinable.
reactive	reactive	consider spontaneous agglutination.

*When controls react as expected.

Reference   Moulds JJ. Polyagglutination: Overview and resolution. In: Beck ML, Judd WJ, eds. Polyagglutination. Washington, DC: AABB, 1980:1-22.

**Effective
Date**

Approved by:	Printed Name	Signature	Date
Laboratory Management			
Medical Director			
Quality Officer			

XIV-B. Preparing Crude Extracts of Lectins

Purpose
To provide instructions for preparing lectins from seeds and other sources:

- Studies of ABO typing problems.
- Investigation of polyagglutination.
- Determination of secretor status.

Background Information
Lectins are carbohydrate-binding proteins obtained primarily from seeds. Their biological reactivity can be inhibited by the addition of simple sugars. Many lectins agglutinate RBCs and, as such, they have been used as alternatives to human sera for blood typing purposes. They are also invaluable reagents in the investigation of RBC polyagglutination.

Operational Policy
Add Tween 20 (Sigma-Aldrich, St Louis, MO), a wetting agent, to prevent adhesion of lectin proteins to glass surfaces and facilitate the reading of agglutination. Tween 20 may not readily go into solution. Prepare a 10% vol/vol solution in pH 7.3 PBS and warm to 37 C before use. Add 100 μL of this to every 10 mL of lectin preparation.

Limitations
Incorrect Results:

- Improper storage of reagents.
- Use of incorrect technique.
- Use of wrong reagent.

Sample Requirements
Seeds: from health food stores or reputable seed suppliers (JL Hudson, La Honda, CA, or Park Seed Company, Greenwood, SC). The following seeds, given with the antibodies they agglutinate, are useful in investigating RBC surface markers (see also Table XIV-1):

- *Arachis hypogaea* (peanut), anti-T/Tk.
- *Dolichos biflorus*, anti-A_1/Tn/Cad (may give weak reactions with anti-A_2).
- *Glycine max* (soybean), anti-T/Tn/Cad and protease-treated RBCs.

- *Salvia horminum*, anti-Tn/Cad.

- *Salvia sclarea*, anti-Tn.

- *Ulex europaeus*, anti-H (agglutinates O RBCs > A_2 > B > A_2B > A_1 > A_1B).

- *Vicia graminea*, anti-N_{VG}.

Equipment/ Materials	Control RBCs: for each lectin, include examples of known positive and negative RBCs (see above), washed three times and diluted to a 3%-5% suspension in pH 7.3 PBS.
	pH 7.3 PBS.
	Pestle and mortar.
	10-mL test tubes.
	22% BSA.
	Tween 20.
Quality Control	Lectins are standardized against known reactive and nonreactive RBCs.
Procedure	Use the following steps to perform the procedure:

Step	Action
1.	For each 1 g of seeds, add 5-10 mL of PBS.
2.	Soak the seeds overnight in PBS at 4 C.
3.	Grind seeds with a pestle and mortar. Add an additional 5 mL of PBS and regrind the seeds.
4.	Remove the saline extract from the seed debris and centrifuge to remove particulate matter.
5.	Carefully transfer the supernate into a clean test tube, avoiding any fatty material. Recentrifuge and repeat this step until a clear supernate is obtained.
6.	Add an equal volume of 22% BSA, and add Tween 20 at a final concentration of 0.1% vol/vol.
7.	Prepare serial twofold doubling dilutions of lectin in 11% BSA + 0.1% Tween 20.

8.	Mix 2 drops of each lectin dilution with the appropriate control RBCs.
9.	Incubate at RT for 5 minutes: • Centrifuge. • Examine the RBCs macroscopically for agglutination. • Grade and record the results.
10.	Determine the titer of the lectin vs the positive control RBCs: the titer is the reciprocal of the highest dilution yielding a 1+ reaction.
11.	Proceed as follows:

If the titer is…	And the negative control RBCs are…	Then…
≥8	nonreactive	the lectin is suitable for use: • Store refrigerated.
≥8	reactive	dilute lectin to a point at which negative control RBCs are nonreactive and repeat the titration.
≤8	reactive or nonreactive	lectin is unsuitable for use.

Effective Date

Approved by:	Printed Name	Signature	Date
Laboratory Management			
Medical Director			
Quality Officer			

XIV-C. Preparing Solutions of Purified Lectins

Purpose

To provide instructions for preparing lectins from seeds and other sources:

- Studies of ABO typing problems.
- Investigation of polyagglutination.
- Determination of secretor status.

Background Information

Lectins are carbohydrate-binding proteins obtained primarily from seeds. Their biological reactivity can be inhibited by the addition of simple sugars. Many lectins agglutinate RBCs and, as such, they have been used as alternatives to human sera for blood typing purposes. They are also invaluable reagents in the investigation of RBC polyagglutination.

Operational Policy

Add Tween 20 (Sigma-Aldrich, St Louis, MO), a wetting agent, to prevent adhesion of lectin proteins to glass surfaces and facilitate the reading of agglutination. Tween 20 may not readily go into solution. Prepare a 10% vol/vol solution in pH 7.3 PBS and warm to 37 C before use. Add 100 µL of this to every 10 mL of lectin preparation.

Limitations

Incorrect Results:

- Improper storage of reagents.
- Use of incorrect technique.
- Use of wrong reagent.

Sample Requirements

Purified lectin proteins (eg, E-Y Laboratories, San Mateo, CA). See Table XIV-1.

Equipment/ Materials

Control RBCs: for each lectin, include examples of known positive and negative RBCs, washed three times and diluted to a 3%-5% suspension in pH 7.3 PBS.

Distilled water.

11% BSA + Tween 20.

Quality Control

Lectins are standardized against known reactive and nonreactive RBCs.

Procedure

Use the following steps to perform the procedure:

Step	Action
1.	Reconstitute the lyophilized lectin protein with pH 7.3 PBS, and label the vial with the protein concentration in mg/mL.
2.	Add an equal volume of 22% BSA, and add Tween 20 at a final concentration of 0.1% vol/vol.
3.	Prepare serial twofold doubling dilutions of lectin in 11% BSA + 0.1% Tween 20.
4.	Mix 2 drops of each lectin dilution with the appropriate control RBCs.
5.	Incubate at RT for 5 minutes: • Centrifuge. • Examine the RBCs macroscopically for agglutination. • Grade and record the results.
6.	Determine the titer of the lectin vs the positive control RBCs: the titer is the reciprocal of the highest dilution yielding a 1+ reaction.
7.	Proceed as follows: <table><tr><th>If the titer is...</th><th>And the negative control RBCs are...</th><th>Then...</th></tr><tr><td>≥8</td><td>nonreactive</td><td>the lectin is suitable for use: • Store refrigerated.</td></tr><tr><td>≥8</td><td>reactive</td><td>dilute lectin to a point at which negative control RBCs are nonreactive and repeat the titration.</td></tr><tr><td>≤8</td><td>reactive or nonreactive</td><td>lectin is unsuitable for use.</td></tr></table>

**Effective
Date**

	Printed Name	Signature	Date
Approved by			
Laboratory Management			
Medical Director			
Quality Officer			

XIV-D. Aggregating RBCs with Polybrene

Purpose

To provide instructions for performing the Polybrene (Sigma-Aldrich, St Louis, MO) aggregation test:

- Investigation of polyagglutination.

- Studies of MN-variant phenotypes.

- Recognition of sialic acid deficiency.

Background Information

N-acetylneuraminic acid (NeuAc), a sialic acid, carries a negatively charged carboxyl group. NeuAc residues are present on a number of RBC surface structures, notably sialoglycoproteins; as such, they account for approximately 95% of the total surface charge and likely prevent RBCs from spontaneously aggregating when in suspension.

Polybrene, a positively charged polymer, causes aggregation of negatively charged RBCs. A possible explanation for this that the RBC surface negative charge is neutralized, although the mechanism is probably more complex. In any event, this aggregation can be a crude indicator of RBC surface charge when investigating polyagglutinable blood or samples of a variant MN phenotype.

Treatment of RBCs with proteases (eg, ficin or papain) removes the majority of the sialic acid residues by cleaving the N-terminal regions of the sialoglycoproteins that carry them.

Operational Policy

Polybrene adheres to the surface of glass containers; thus, it is important to store the stock reagent in plastic containers to prevent weakening of the solution during storage.

Limitations

Incorrect Results:

- Improper storage of reagents.

- Use of incorrect technique.

- Use of wrong reagent.

Sample Requirements

Test RBCs: washed three times and diluted to a 3%-5% suspension with pH 7.3 PBS.

Equipment/ Materials	Negative control RBCs: 3%-5% suspension of ficin-pretreated RBCs in pH 7.3 PBS (see Section III).
	Positive control RBCs: 3%-5% suspension of untreated RBCs in pH 7.3 PBS.
	pH 7.3 PBS.
	Stock Polybrene solution: 10% wt/vol hexadimethrine bromide.

Quality Control	The procedure includes tests with positive and negative controls.

Procedure   Use the following steps to perform the procedure:

Step	Action
1.	Dilute the stock 10% Polybrene solution 1 in 250 with pH 7.3 PBS.
2.	In appropriately labeled 10 × 75-mm test tubes, mix 2 drops of RBCs with 2 drops of dilute Polybrene.
3.	Gently agitate the contents of each tube and observe for aggregation using an illuminated concave mirror. Note the time at which aggregation of the positive control commences.
4.	Continue to agitate the tubes for a further 2 minutes and examine all tubes macroscopically for aggregation; record the results.
5.	Interpret the reactions as follows:

If the RBCs...	Then the RBC sialic acid content is...
aggregate	normal.
do not aggregate	reduced.

References   Issitt PD. Polyagglutination. In: Walker RH, ed. A seminar on problems encountered in pretransfusion tests. Washington, DC: AABB, 1972:81-106.

Moulds JJ. Polyagglutination: Overview and resolution. In: Beck ML, Judd WJ, eds. Polyagglutination. Washington, DC: AABB, 1980:1-22.

Steane EA. Cited by: Issitt PD, Issitt CH. Applied blood group serology. 2nd ed. Oxnard, CA: Spectra Biologicals, 1975:262.

**Effective
Date**

Approved by	Printed Name	Signature	Date
Laboratory Management			
Medical Director			
Quality Officer			

XIV-E. Acetylating RBCs

Purpose

To provide instructions for treating RBCs with acetic anhydride:

- Studies on acquired-B phenomenon.
- Studies on glycophorins A and B.

Background Information

A_1 RBCs may acquire B-like antigens in vivo by the action of bacterial deacetylases that convert N-acetylgalactosamine (GalNAc, the blood group A immunodominant sugar) into galactosamine ($GalNH_2$). The latter is similar to galactose (blood group B immunodominant sugar) and cross-reacts with anti-B reagents. Acquired-B antigens are changed back to normal A_1 determinants following reacetylation with acetic anhydride.

Note: After acetic anhydride treatment, acquired-B RBCs react with *Dolichos biflorus* (anti-A_1) lectin in accordance with their genetically determined A_1 status.

Although the procedure is primarily used in studies on acquired-B RBCs, it was initially developed to study the interaction between MN antigens and *Vicia graminea* lectin. Acetylation of RBCs modifies carbohydrate residues in the N-terminal regions of glycophorin A (GPA; MN sialoglycoprotein) and glycophorin B (GPB; Ss sialoglycoprotein). Acetic-anhydride-treated M+N− RBCs react with anti-N_{VG} lectin; thus, acetylation of RBCs can be used to ascertain the presence of latent N_{VG} receptors on intact GPA, or on GPB of RBCs treated with purified trypsin, as described in Section III.

Operational Policy

Avoid contact between acetic anhydride vapors and water or air. Contact between acetic anhydride and water, alcohols, strong oxidizers, chromic acid, amines, or strong caustics may cause fires and explosions.

Exposure to acetic anhydride in either the liquid or vapor form causes severe irritation of the eyes, skin, and mucous membranes in humans. Avoid breathing vapors, and protect eyes and mouth from vapors. Perform this procedure under a chemical hood.

Avoid contact of acetic anhydride with skin; wear protective clothing when performing this procedure.

Acetic anhydride should be stored in a cool, dry, well-ventilated area in tightly sealed containers that are labeled in accordance with the Hazard Communication Standard of the Occupational Safety and Health Administration (29 CFR 1910.1200). Outside or detached storage is preferred. Inside storage must be in a standard flammable-liquids storage room or cabinet. Containers of acetic anhydride should be protected from physical damage and should be separated from water, alcohols, strong oxidizers, chromic acid, amines, strong caustics, heat, sparks, and open flame. Because containers that formerly contained acetic anhydride may still hold product residues, they should be handled appropriately.

Limitations

Incorrect Results:

- Improper storage of reagents.
- Use of incorrect technique.
- Use of wrong reagent.

Sample Requirements

Test RBCs: washed three times and packed.

Equipment/ Materials

Acetic anhydride, $(CH_3CO)_2O$ (eg, Sigma-Aldrich, St Louis, MO).

0.2 M PBS-glycerol: pH 8.5.

0.5 M phosphate buffer: pH 8.5.

10-mL volume measuring cylinder.

Chemical hood and protective clothing (see Operational Policy).

Control RBCs: acquired-B or M+N– RBCs, washed three times and packed.

Pipettors with disposable tips to deliver 50 μL and 250 μL (eg, VWR, Batavia, IL).

Magnetic stirrer and small stirring bar (eg, VWR, Batavia, IL).

Reactive reagent anti-B, human or formulated from ES4, or *V. graminea* lectin (anti-N_{VG}).

Small glass or plastic beaker/flask (eg, 25-mL capacity): one for each sample to be treated.

Quality Control   Save an aliquot of washed RBCs for control purposes.

Procedure   Use the following steps to perform the procedure:

Step	Action
1.	Dispense 0.25 mL of each packed RBC sample into an appropriately labeled glass or plastic beaker/flask.
2.	To each, add 7.5 mL of 0.2 M PBS-glycerol.
3.	With continued stirring (magnetic stirrer) under a chemical hood, slowly add 50 μL of acetic anhydride to each RBC suspension.
4.	Continue stirring at RT for 10 minutes.
5.	Neutralize the acetic anhydride by adding 5 mL of 0.5 M pH 8.5 phosphate buffer to each beaker/flask.
6.	Wash the RBCs four times with saline.
7.	Test in parallel with untreated/control RBCs.
8.	When testing reactivity between anti-B and acquired-B RBCs, interpret the reactions as follows:

If treated RBCs...	And untreated RBCs...	Then...
react with anti-B	react with anti-B	B antigen is normal.
do not react with anti-B	react with anti-B	B antigen is acquired.

When testing reactivity between anti-N_{VG} and M+N– RBCs, interpret the reactions as follows:

If treated RBCs...	And untreated RBCs...	Then...
react with anti-N_{VG}	do not react with anti-N_{VG}	GPB is normal.
do not react with anti-N_{VG}	do not react with anti-N_{VG}	a variant GPB may be present.

Reference   Lisowska E, Duk M. Effect of modification of amino groups of human erythrocyte M, N, and N_{VG} blood group specificities. Vox Sang 1975;28: 392-7.

**Effective
Date**

Approved by:	Printed Name	Signature	Date
Laboratory Management			
Medical Director			
Quality Officer			

XIV-F. Inhibiting Acquired-B Reactivity

Purpose

To provide instructions for inhibiting the acquired-B reactivity of mono-clonal anti-B:

- Studies on acquired-B RBCs.

Background Information

A_1 RBCs may acquire B-like antigens in vivo by the action of bacterial deacetylases that convert α-N-acetylgalactosamine (α-GalNAc, blood group A immunodominant sugar) into α-galactosamine (α-GalNH$_2$). The latter is similar in structure to α-galactose (α-Gal, blood group B immu-nodominant sugar) and cross-reacts with anti-B reagents.

Acquired-B antigens are readily detected by certain monoclonal (eg, ES4) anti-B formulated at a neutral or alkaline pH. Strong examples will even react with such monoclonal anti-B at an acid pH. This reactivity can be inhibited by the simple addition of GalNH$_2$-HCl, which does not inhibit the reactivity between these anti-B and RBCs with a normal expression of B antigen.

Operational Policy

Use 0.3 M GalNH$_2$-HCl when testing anti-B formulated at a neutral or alka-line pH.

Limitations

Incorrect Results:

- Improper storage of reagents.
- Use of incorrect technique.
- Use of wrong reagent.

Sample Requirements

Test RBCs: from clotted or anticoagulated blood samples, washed three times and diluted to a 3%-5% suspension with PBS.

Equipment/ Materials

Known acquired-B RBCs, if available.

0.1 M **D**-galactosamine HCl (GalNH$_2$-HCl).

Normal group B RBCs.

pH 7.3 PBS.

Reactive reagent anti-B (eg, formulated with ES4).

Procedure

Use the following steps to perform the procedure:

Step	Action
1.	For each RBC sample to be tested, mix 1 drop of monoclonal anti-B with 1 drop of 0.1 M GalNH$_2$-HCl in an appropriately labeled 10 or 12 × 75-mm test tube.
2.	Similarly, mix 1 drop of anti-B with 1 drop of pH 7.3 PBS.
3.	Incubate at RT for 5 minutes.
4.	Add 1 drop of the appropriate RBC suspension to each tube and mix gently.
5.	Centrifuge all tubes as for hemagglutination tests.
6.	Examine the RBCs macroscopically; grade and record the results.
7.	Interpret the reactions as follows:

If tests with anti-B + GalNH$_2$-HCl are...	And tests with anti-B + PBS are...	Then...
positive	positive	B antigen is normal.
negative	positive	B antigen is acquired.

Reference

Beck ML, Kirkegaard J, Korth J, Judd WJ. Monoclonal anti-B and the acquired-B phenotype (letter). Transfusion 1993;33:623-4.

**Effective
Date**

Approved by:	Printed Name	Signature	Date
Laboratory Management			
Medical Director			
Quality Officer			

XIV-G. Testing RBCs with Acidified Anti-B

Purpose	To provide instructions for confirming the acquired-B status of RBCs:

- Studies on acquired-B.
- ABO typing problem resolution.

Background Information	Group A_1 RBCs may acquire B-like antigens in vivo by the action of bacterial deacetylases that convert α-N-acetylgalactosamine (α-GalNAc, blood group A immunodominant sugar) into α-galactosamine (α-GalNH$_2$). The latter is similar in structure to α-galactose (α-Gal, blood group B immunodominant sugar) and cross-reacts with anti-B reagents. These acquired-B antigens are extremely susceptible to changes in pH and, in contrast to normal B antigens, may not be detectable with anti-B at pH 6.0, where GalNH$_2$ becomes protonated to GalNH$_3^+$.

Operational Policy	Use this procedure in preference to reacetylation for confirmation of acquired-B phenotype.

Limitations	Incorrect Results:

- Improper storage of reagents.
- Use of incorrect technique.
- Use of wrong reagent.

Sample Requirements	Test RBCs: washed three times and diluted to a 5% suspension with normal saline.

Equipment/ Materials	Acidified anti-B: either monoclonal (eg, ES4) anti-B or human polyclonal anti-B, at pH 6.0 to 6.2.
	Neutral anti-B (from same source as above).
	Normal group B RBCs: washed three times and diluted to a 5% suspension with normal saline.

Quality Control	The procedure includes a control with normal group B RBCs.

Procedure   Use the following steps to perform the procedure:

Step	Action
1.	Mix 1 drop of each RBC sample with 1 drop of acidified anti-B in appropriately labeled 10 or 12 × 75-mm test tubes.
2.	Set up similar tests with the neutral anti-B.
3.	Centrifuge all tubes as for hemagglutination tests.
4.	Examine the RBCs macroscopically; grade and record the results.
5.	Interpret the reactions as follows:

If acidified anti-B...	And neutral anti-B	Then B antigen is...
agglutinates RBCs	agglutinates RBCs	normal.
does not agglutinate RBCs	agglutinates RBCs	acquired.

References   Cheng MS. Two similar cases of weak agglutination with anti-B reagent. Lab Med 1981;12:506-7.

Judd WJ, Annesley T, Kirkegaard J, Beck ML. Know your monoclonals: An absolute must for the effective resolution of ABO grouping discrepancies (abstract). Transfusion 1992;32(Suppl):18S.

Effective Date

	Printed Name	Signature	Date
Approved by			
Laboratory Management			
Medical Director			
Quality Officer			

Section XV. Miscellaneous Methods

This final section contains methods that do not properly belong elsewhere in this book. Some have limited clinical utility but may be of value in research laboratories. Others, such as the Ham's test and sucrose lysis test, are hematologic procedures that are useful in the diagnosis of hemolytic anemias that do not necessarily have an immune basis and cannot, therefore, be placed in Section XI. However, blood group serologists may be asked to perform these procedures because the reagents and necessary equipment are readily available to them.

Procedures for differentiating between IgM and IgG are also included in this section, and these general methods can be applied in a number of situations—eg, in prenatal testing to determine if an agglutinating antibody has an IgG component and, therefore, could cross the placenta and cause HDFN, or in antibody identification studies to denature IgM autoantibodies and detect underlying IgG alloantibodies.

Still other methods provide means of predicting the in-vivo survival of serologically incompatible RBCs.

XV-A. Testing for PNH: Acid Hemolysis (Ham's) Test

Purpose

To provide a method for performing a Ham's test:

- Investigation of paroxysmal nocturnal hemoglobinuria (PNH).

Background Information

RBCs from patients with PNH are susceptible to lysis by complement without prior sensitization by immunoglobulins. This non-antibody-induced, complement-mediated hemolysis is associated with deficiency of phosphatidylinosyl-linked proteins, notably CD55 (decay accelerating factor, or DAF) and CD59 (membrane inhibitor of reactive lysis, or MIRL), and is enhanced at an acidic pH. This procedure is used in the differential diagnosis of hemolysis, particularly when tests for immune hemolysis and other (nonimmune) hemolytic anemias are not informative.

Note: Flow cytometric tests using antibodies to CD55 and CD59 provide a more sensitive test for PNH than the Ham's test, but such tests are beyond the scope of this book.

Operational Policy

Use Procedure XV-B for the investigation of HEMPAS.

Limitations

Unwanted Positive Reactions:

- Incorrect technique.
- Addition of wrong reagent.
- Failure to inactivate complement.

Unwanted Negative Reactions:

- Incorrect technique.
- Omission of serum or HCl.
- Use of inactive complement.

Sample Requirements

RBCs: from defibrinated blood or blood anticoagulated with heparin, sodium citrate, or ACD; washed three times and diluted to a 50% suspension with saline; 0.6 mL.

Serum: preferably collected within 24 hours of testing; 2 mL.

Equipment/
Materials

AET-treated RBCs (see Section VII): washed and diluted to a 50% suspension with saline.

Control group O RBCs: from defibrinated blood or blood anticoagulated with heparin, sodium citrate, or ACD; washed three times and diluted to a 50% suspension with saline.

Sheep RBCs (eg, Pel-Freez Biologicals, Rogers, AR).

Fresh normal serum (FNS) lacking unexpected antibodies: as a source of complement; either group AB or ABO-compatible with the patient's RBCs; 2 mL.

0.2 N HCl.

Heat-inactivated serum (to destroy complement): prepared by incubating 0.6 mL FNS at 56 C for 30 minutes.

Quality
Control

AET-treated RBCs should show lysis when tested with acidified autologous or acidified homologous serum.

The procedure includes internal controls.

Before use, each batch of human complement should be shown to lyse sheep RBCs: use 1 drop of 3%-5% washed sheep RBCs in saline, 3 drops of human complement, and 15 minutes incubation at 37 C; centrifuge as for hemagglutination tests and examine the supernate for hemolysis.

Procedure

Use the following steps to perform the procedure:

Step	Action
1.	Label 10 × 75-mm tubes 1-7 and place them in numerical order at 37 C.
2.	Using volumes of 9 drops of serum and 1 drop (≈0.05 mL per drop) each of HCl and RBCs, set up tests as shown in Table XV-A-1.
3.	Mix the contents within each tube and incubate at 37 C for 1 hour.
4.	Centrifuge all tubes to pack the RBCs.
5.	Examine the supernates in each tube for evidence of hemolysis against a white illuminated background.

6.	Interpret the reactions as follows:	
	If hemolysis is...	**Then the test result for PNH is...**
	seen only in tubes 2 and 5	positive.
	not observed in any tube	negative.
	seen only in tubes 2 and 7 (or only in tubes 1, 2, 6, and 7)	invalid for PNH: • Consider a warm-reactive hemolysin.
	seen only in tubes 2, 3, and 5	invalid for PNH: • Consider spherocytosis.
	See Table XV-A-1.	

Reference Henry JB. Clinical diagnosis and management by laboratory methods. 16th ed. Philadelphia, PA: WB Saunders, 1979.

Effective Date

Approved by:	Printed Name	Signature	Date
Laboratory Management			
Medical Director			
Quality Officer			

Table XV-A-1. Acid Hemolysis Test Procedure

Tube	Reactants			Expected Results	
	RBCs*	Serum	HCl	PNH	HEMPAS
1	Patient	Patient	No	0	0
2	Patient	Patient	Yes	H	0
3	Patient	Normal[†]	Yes	0	0
4	Patient	Normal	No	0	0
5	Patient	Normal	Yes	H	H
6	Normal	Patient	No	0	0
7	Normal	Patient	Yes	0	0

*50% suspension when testing for PNH; 10% suspension when testing for HEMPAS.

[†]Heat inactivated serum.

RBCs = red cells; PNH = paroxysmal nocturnal hemoglobinuria; HEMPAS = hereditary erythroblastic multinuclearity with a positive acidified serum; O = no agglutination; H = hemolysis.

Judd's Methods in Immunohematology
Testing for HEMPAS: Modified Acid Hemolysis (Ham's) Test
Page 1 of 3

XV-B. Testing for HEMPAS: Modified Acid Hemolysis (Ham's) Test

Purpose
To provide instructions for performing a modified Ham's test:

- Investigation of hereditary erythroblastic multinuclearity with a positive acidified serum test (HEMPAS).

Background Information
Like PNH RBCs, the RBCs from patients with HEMPAS, also known as congenital dyserythropoietic anemia type II, are hemolyzed by acidified serum. However, hemolysis of HEMPAS RBCs is associated with an RBC membrane glycosylation abnormality recognized by naturally acquired complement-binding antibodies present in about one-third of adult human sera. A modified Ham's test is required for optimal demonstration of this abnormality.

Operational Policy
Use Procedure XV-A for the investigation of PNH.

Do not proceed if screening tests with acidified ABO-compatible sera are nonreactive (see below); report the test result as negative.

Limitations
Unwanted Positive Reactions:

- Incorrect technique.
- Addition of wrong reagent.
- Failure to inactivate complement.

Unwanted Negative Reactions:

- Incorrect technique.
- Omission of serum or HCl.
- Selection of serum lacking activity against HEMPAS RBCs.

Sample Requirements
RBCs: from defibrinated blood or blood anticoagulated with heparin, sodium citrate or ACD; washed three times and diluted to a 10% suspension with saline; 0.6 mL.

Serum: preferably collected within 24 hours of testing; 2 mL.

Equipment/
Materials

Control group O RBCs: from defibrinated blood or blood anticoagulated with heparin, sodium citrate or ACD; washed three times and diluted to a 10% suspension with saline.

Fresh normal serum (FNS) lacking unexpected antibodies: as a source of complement; either group AB or ABO-compatible with patient RBCs; 2 mL.

Note: Screen 6-12 ABO-compatible, acidified sera for activity against patient RBCs by mixing 9 drops of serum, 1 drop of 0.2 N HCl, and 1 drop of 10% RBCs (ie, tube 5 in Table XV-A-1), followed by incubation on melting ice for 30 minutes, then at 37 C for 1 hour. Centrifuge and select the sample(s) showing the most hemolysis for use in the controlled procedure.

0.2 N HCl.

Heat-inactivated serum (to destroy complement): prepared by incubating 0.6 mL FNS at 56 C for 30 minutes.

Quality
Control

The procedure includes internal controls.

Procedure

Use the following steps to perform the procedure:

Step	Action
1.	Label 10 × 75-mm tubes 1-7 and place them in numerical order in melting ice.
2.	Using volumes of 9 drops of serum and 1 drop (≈0.05 mL per drop) each of HCl and RBCs, set up tests as shown in Table XV-A-1.
3.	Mix the contents within each tube and incubate on melting ice for 30 minutes.
4.	Mix the contents within each tube and incubate at 37 C for 1 hour.
5.	Centrifuge all tubes to pack the RBCs.
6.	Examine the supernates in each tube for evidence of hemolysis against a white illuminated background.

7.	Interpret the reactions as follows:	
	If hemolysis is…	**Then the test result for HEMPAS is…**
	seen only in tube 5	positive.
	not observed in any tube	negative.
	seen only in tubes 2 and 7 (or only in tubes 1, 2, 6, and 7)	invalid for HEMPAS: • Consider a warm-reactive hemolysin.
	seen only in tubes 2, 3, and 5	invalid for HEMPAS: • Consider spherocytosis.
	See Table XV-A-1.	

Reference　　Rosse WF, Logue GL, Adams J, Crookston JH. Mechanisms of immune lysis of the red cells in hereditary erythroblastic multinuclearity with a positive acidified serum test and paroxysmal nocturnal hemoglobinuria. J Clin Invest 1974;53:31-43.

Effective Date

Approved by:	**Printed Name**	**Signature**	**Date**
Laboratory Management			
Medical Director			
Quality Officer			

XV-C. Converting IgG Antibodies to Direct Agglutinins

Purpose

To provide instructions for converting IgG-coating antibodies to agglutinins:

- Phenotyping by direct agglutination using IgG antibodies.

Background Information

IgG molecules consist of two heavy (γ) chains and two light chains that are linked by interchain disulfide (S-S) bonds. Mild reduction of S-S bonds linking the two heavy chains enhances flexibility at the hinge region of IgG. This increases the distance between antigen-binding sites at the NH_2-terminal of each Fab portion and allows the modified immunoglobulins to agglutinate RBCs in a saline (low-protein) test medium.

Operational Policy

Consider this procedure for phenotyping samples with a positive DAT that cannot be rendered DAT-negative by Procedures IV-P and IV-Q.

Limitations

Unwanted Positive Reactions:

- Use of wrong reagent.
- Improper storage of reagents.
- Use of incorrect technique.

Unwanted Negative Reactions:

- Use of low-titer antibody.
- Use of wrong reagent.
- Omission of DTT.
- Improper storage of reagents.
- Use of incorrect technique.

Sample Requirements

IgG antibody: titer ≥ 32.

Equipment/ Materials

0.01 M DTT.

pH 7.3 PBS.

Pipettors with disposable tips to deliver 1 mL (eg, VWR, Batavia, IL).

Procedure   Use the following steps to perform the procedure:

Step	Action
1.	Dispense 1 mL of serum into each of 2 appropriately labeled 12 × 75-mm test tubes.
2.	To 1 tube, add 1 mL of 0.01 M DTT (label "test").
3.	To the other tube, add 1 mL of pH 7.3 PBS (label "control").
4.	Mix and incubate at RT for 30 minutes.
5.	Immediately test both samples against a reagent RBC panel using the saline agglutination procedure described in Section II.
6.	Interpret the reactions as follows:

If direct agglutination is...	And specificity is...	Then...
observed	confirmed	conversion was successful: • Use for direct testing.
not observed	(not applicable)	conversion was not successful: • Try antibody of higher titer

Reference   Romans DG, Tilley CA, Crookston MC, et al. Conversion of incomplete antibodies to direct agglutinins by mild reduction: Evidence for segmental flexibility within the Fc fragment of immunoglobulin G. Proc Natl Acad Sci U S A 1977;74:2531-5.

**Effective
Date**

Approved by:	Printed Name	Signature	Date
Laboratory Management			
Medical Director			
Quality Officer			

XV-D. Assessing RBC Survival Using ^{51}Cr-Labeled RBCs

Purpose

To provide instructions for performing RBC survival studies using radio-labeled RBCs:

- Assessing the clinical significance of RBC alloantibodies.
- Demonstrating the efficacy of RBC preservative solutions.

Background Information

RBCs may be labeled with a radioactive isotope and injected into a patient with antibodies to RBC antigens. The percent-survival of these RBCs is calculated from radioactivity measurements of postinjection blood samples. The procedure may be used to evaluate the outcome of transfusion of incompatible blood to patients for whom compatible blood cannot be obtained. Alternatively, a 1-hour postsurvival determination can be used to demonstrate the efficacy of anticoagulants used to preserve RBCs intended for transfusion.

Operational Policy

Consult with Nuclear Medicine Department personnel and obtain their assistance when performing these studies.

Because this is an invasive procedure, informed consent must be obtained.

All precautions applicable to the handling of radionucleotides must be taken.

RBCs must be administered under the direction of a licensed physician.

Limitations

Incorrect Results:

- Use of incorrect technique.
- Use of wrong donor RBCs.
- Use of wrong isotope or inactive ^{51}Cr.
- Inadequate washing of RBCs after labeling.
- Inadequate mixing of labeled RBCs in vivo.
- Extravasation at the injection site.

Sample Requirements

Donor unit or blood samples for survival study: a fresh, sterile, anticoagulated sample (not heparinized) or an ACD/CPD/CPD-A1-anticoagulated unit is preferred. Ensure that the results of hepatitis, HIV, and other infectious disease testing are satisfactory.

Patient for study: normally, patients will be those for whom compatible blood is unobtainable because of potentially significant unexpected serum alloantibodies (ie, antibodies reactive at 37 C and/or by the IAT). There should be no clinical signs of bleeding. Determine the height (in meters) and weight (in kilograms) of the patient on the day of study.

Equipment/ Materials

^{51}Cr sodium chromate solution: $Na_2{}^{51}CrO_4$ (eg, Perkin-Elmer, Waltham, MA) with a specific activity such that less than 2 μg of chromium is added per mL of packed RBCs. The solution should have a minimum volume of 0.2 mL, being diluted with sterile normal saline.

Gamma counter: in Nuclear Medicine Department.

Spinal needles: 3 inches long (for sterile aspiration of supernates).

Sterile normal saline (SNS): pyrogen-free, sterile saline (NaCl, 9 g/L).

Sterile tubes: 10-mL size.

Syringes: 2-mL and 10-mL sizes.

Quality Control

The procedure includes checks for inadequate washing of RBCs after labeling, inadequate mixing of labeled RBCs in vivo, extravasation at the injection site, and rapid hemolysis.

Procedure

Use the following steps to perform the procedure:

Step	Action
1.	Using sterile technique, withdraw 1-2 mL of donor whole blood (0.5 to 1.0 mL RBCs) and transfer to a sterile tube. Centrifuge to pack the RBCs, and remove the supernatant plasma.
2.	With continuous mixing, slowly add 20 μCi ^{51}Cr and incubate on a rotary mixer for 30 minutes at RT.
3.	Using sterile technique, wash the RBCs by gently suspending them in 6-8 mL of SNS and centrifuging to pack the RBCs. Discard the supernate into radioactive waste.

4.	Repeat Step 3 once.
5.	Gently suspend the RBCs in approximately 10 mL of SNS and mix well.
6.	Using a volumetric pipette, withdraw exactly 1 mL for preparation of a standard solution. Dilute, using a volumetric flask, to 250 mL with distilled water.
7.	Withdraw exactly 8 mL for infusion into the patient. Infuse the 8-mL sample into a freely flowing antecubital vein. Aspirate a small amount of venous blood back into the syringe and re-inject.
8.	Collect 3 mL anticoagulated (EDTA/heparin) blood samples from the contralateral antecubital vein at 3 minutes, 7 minutes, 10 minutes, 60 minutes, and 24 hours after injection.
9.	Determine radioactive counts, using a gamma counter, in exactly 1 mL of well-mixed whole blood. Subtract background counts and correct the 24-hour count for elution (counts × 1.03). **Note:** A minimum of 4000 counts should be recorded per sample.
10.	Count 1 mL standard solution prepared in Step 6.

11.	Count 1 mL of plasma from the 3-minute sample:

If plasma counts are...	Then...
<5% of total counts in the 3-minute sample	proceed.
>5% of total counts in the 3-minute sample	consider very rapid hemolysis or inadequate washing of the labeled sample.

Note: Proceed if plasma counts are <5% of total counts in the 3-minute sample. If >5%, consider very rapid hemolysis or inadequate washing of the labeled sample.

12.	Predict the patient's blood volume (predicted blood volume = PBV) using the following calculations:

If patient is...	Then use the formula (PBV in liters)...
male	$(0.3669 \times$ height in meters$^3) + (0.03219 \times$ weight in kilograms$) + 0.6041$.
female	$(0.3561 \times$ height in meters$^3) + (0.03308 \times$ weight in kilograms$) + 0.1833$.

13.	Calculate the patient's blood volume (calculated blood volume = CBV) from the standard solution and the 3-minute sample using the following formula: CBV in liters = (counts/1 mL standard × 8 × 0.25) ÷ counts/1 mL 3-minute sample
14.	Interpret the results as follows:

If the CBV...	Then...
does not exceed the PBV by more than 10%	assume the 3-minute sample equates with 100% survival: • Compare subsequent sample counts to the 3-minute count to determine RBC survival. • Determine survival curve and percentages. In an emergency, the study may be terminated at 60 minutes. It is preferable, however, to extend the study to 24 hours, when possible.
exceeds the PBV by more than 10%	• Suspect inadequate mixing secondary to splenomegaly or congestive heart failure. • Plasma counts should be low.
calculated from the 7-minute sample more closely approximates the PBV	use the 7-minute count to represent 100% survival.
calculated from all subsequent counts is elevated and plasma counts are low	suspect extravasation at injection site: • To confirm, check site with Geiger counter.
and plasma counts are high	suspect rapid hemolysis.

Reference   Davey RJ. Mechanisms of premature red cell destruction. In: Judd WJ, Barnes A. Clinical and serologic aspects of transfusion reactions. Arlington, VA: AABB, 1982:1-35.

**Effective
Date**

Approved by:	Printed Name	Signature	Date
Laboratory Management			
Medical Director			
Quality Officer			

XV-E. Differentiating IgM from IgG Antibodies Using DTT

Purpose

To provide instructions for distinguishing IgM from IgG antibodies to RBC antigens using dithiothreitol (DTT):

- Assessing the potential of an alloantibody encountered in pregnancy to cause HDFN.

- Detection of IgG alloantibodies in samples containing IgM autoantibodies.

Background Information

IgM molecules consist of five radially arranged subunits linked by inter-subunit disulphide (S-S) bonds. Each subunit consists of two heavy chains and two light chains that are linked by interchain S-S bonds. The intersubunit S-S bonds are susceptible to cleavage by thiol reagents, whereas interchain S-S bonds are resistant to such cleavage. Similarly, the interchain S-S bonds of IgG and IgA, which have a structure similar to that of IgM subunits, are not readily cleaved by thiol reagents such as dithiothreitol.

This procedure may be used to determine the immunoglobulin class (IgG or IgM) of antibody molecules, or it may be used specifically to inactivate IgM antibodies.

Operational Policy

Dialysis is not required after treatment of serum with DTT.

Limitations

Incorrect Results:

- Improper storage of reagents.
- Use of incorrect technique.
- Inadequate treatment of serum with DTT.

Sample Requirements

Test serum or plasma: 2 mL.

Equipment/ Materials

0.01 M DTT.

pH 7.3 PBS.

Pipettors with disposable tips to deliver 1 mL (eg, VWR, Batavia, IL).

Quality Control

Test the treated serum for "naturally occurring" antibodies other than those under investigation. For example, if treatment is undertaken to determine the immunoglobulin class of an anti-M, test treated serum for inactivation of the expected anti-A and/or anti-B using A_1 and/or B RBCs that are M–. There should be inactivation of the expected antibody. For AB samples, treat an A, B, or O plasma sample in parallel and test for inactivation of the expected anti-A and/or B.

The procedure includes a control for antibody dilution.

Procedure

Use the following steps to perform the procedure:

Step	Action
1.	Dispense 1 mL of serum into each of 2 appropriately labeled 12 × 75-mm test tubes.
2.	To 1 tube, add 1 mL of 0.01 M DTT (label "test").
3.	To the other tube, add 1 mL of pH 7.3 PBS (label "control").
4.	Mix and incubate at 37 C for 2 hours.
5.	Test the antibody activity in each sample against the appropriate RBCs by titration analysis (eg, the method used for determining the specificity of cold antibodies described in Section XI).
6.	Interpret the reactions as follows:

If the DTT-treated sample...	Then...
has the same titer as the untreated (control) sample	the antibody is IgG.
is nonreactive, yet the control sample does react	the antibody is IgM.
has a lower titer than the control sample	IgM and IgG antibodies are present.
has the same titer as the control sample	the procedure did not work: • Consider inactive DTT.
and the control sample are both nonreactive	the antibody was subject to dilution.

Note: See Table XV-E-1.

Reference

Pirofsky B, Rosner ER. A new method to differentiate IgM and IgG erythrocyte antibodies. Vox Sang 1974;27:480-8.

**Effective
Date**

Approved by	Printed Name	Signature	Date
Laboratory Management			
Medical Director			
Quality Officer			

Table XV-E-1. Interpretation of 2-ME/DTT Studies to Determine Immunoglobulin Class of Antibody

Sample	Serum Dilutions					Interpretation*
	1 in 2	1 in 4	1 in 8	1 in 16	1 in 32	
Untreated	4+	3+	3+	2+	1+	IgG
Treated	4+	3+	3+	2+	1+	
Untreated	4+	3+	3+	2+	1+	IgM
Treated	0	0	0	0	0	
Untreated	4+	3+	3+	2+	1+	IgM + IgG
Treated[†]	3+	2+	1+	0	0	

*Provided "natural" agglutinins are inactivated by 2-ME.

[†]Titer may vary depending on the different proportions of IgG and IgM.

XV-F. Differentiating IgM from IgG Antibodies Using 2-ME

Purpose

To provide instructions for distinguishing IgM from IgG antibodies to RBC antigens using 2-mercaptoethanol (2-ME):

- Assessing the potential of an alloantibody encountered in pregnancy to cause HDFN.

- Detection of IgG alloantibodies in samples containing IgM autoantibodies.

Background Information

IgM molecules consist of five radially arranged subunits linked by inter-subunit disulphide (S-S) bonds. Each subunit consists of two heavy chains and two light chains that are linked by interchain S-S bonds. The intersubunit S-S bonds are susceptible to cleavage by thiol reagents, whereas interchain S-S bonds are resistant to such cleavage. Similarly, the interchain S-S bonds of IgG and IgA, which have a structure similar to that of IgM subunits, are not readily cleaved by thiol reagents, such as 2-ME.

This procedure may be used to determine the immunoglobulin class (IgG or IgM) of antibody molecules, or it may be used specifically to inactivate IgM antibodies. Specific situations where this method may be helpful are prenatal testing (to determine if an agglutinating antibody has an IgG component and, therefore, could cross the placenta and cause HDN) and antibody identification studies (to denature IgM autoantibodies and detect underlying IgG alloantibodies).

Operational Policy

Because of the obnoxious odor of 2-ME, it is preferable to perform the 37-C incubation step under a chemical hood.

Limitations

Incorrect Results:

- Improper storage of reagents.

- Use of incorrect technique.

- Inadequate treatment of serum with 2-ME.

Sample Requirements

Test serum or plasma: 2 mL.

Equipment/ Materials

Dialysis tubing: 10-mm-ID cellulose-membrane tubing with MW cutoff ≈12,400 (eg, Sigma-Aldrich, St Louis, MO).

1 M 2-ME.

pH 7.3 PBS.

Pipettors with disposable tips to deliver 0.1-1 mL (eg, VWR, Batavia, IL).

1-L beaker (eg, VWR, Batavia, IL).

Quality Control

Test the treated serum for "naturally occurring" antibodies other than those under investigation. For example, if treatment is undertaken to determine the immunoglobulin class of an anti-M, test treated serum for inactivation of the expected anti-A and/or anti-B using A_1 and/or B RBCs that are M–. There should be inactivation of the expected antibody. For AB samples, treat an A, B, or O plasma sample in parallel and test for inactivation of the expected anti-A and/or B.

The procedure includes a control for antibody dilution.

Procedure

Use the following steps to perform the procedure:

Step	Action
1.	Dispense 1 mL of serum into each of 2 appropriately labeled 12 × 75-mm test tubes.
2.	To 1 tube, add 0.1 mL of 2-ME and 0.9 mL pH 7.3 PBS (label "test").
3.	To the other tube, add 1 mL of pH 7.3 PBS (label "control").
4.	Mix and incubate at 37 C for 2 hours.
5.	Cut two 10-inch lengths of dialysis tubing and knot one end of each length.
6.	Open the free end of each piece of tubing (a splintered wooden applicator stick is ideal for this).
7.	Fill one dialysis bag with 2-ME-treated serum and knot the free end.
8.	Attach a tail from the knotted dialysis bag with a rubber band to a 10 or 12 × 75-mm test tube (label "test").
9.	Fill the second dialysis bag with the control serum/PBS mixture.
10.	Attach a tail from the knotted dialysis bag with a rubber band to a 10 or 12 × 75-mm test tube (label "control").

11.	Fill both test tubes with pH 7.3 PBS and immerse in a large volume (eg, 1 L) of pH 7.3 PBS.
12.	Allow to dialyze overnight against several changes of PBS.
13.	Remove the dialysis tubing and blot dry. Cut the tubing and transfer the contents into clean test tubes.
14.	Test the antibody activity in each sample against the appropriate RBCs by titration analysis (eg, the method used for determining the specificity of cold antibodies described in Section XI).
15.	Interpret the reactions as follows:

If the 2-ME-treated sample…	Then…
has the same titer as the untreated (control) sample	the antibody is IgG.
is nonreactive, yet the control sample does react	the antibody is IgM.
has a lower titer than the control sample	IgM and IgG antibodies are present.
has the same the titer as the control sample	the procedure did not work: • Consider inactive 2-ME.
and the control sample are both nonreactive	the antibody was subject to dilution.

Note: See Table XV-E-1.

Reference   Klein HG, Anstee DJ. Mollison's blood transfusion in clinical medicine. 11th ed. Oxford, UK: Blackwell Publishing, 2005.

**Effective
Date**

Approved by	Printed Name	Signature	Date
Laboratory Management			
Medical Director			
Quality Officer			

XV-G. Performing Dosage Studies Using the Enzyme-Linked Antiglobulin Test

Purpose

To provide instructions for performing dosage studies using the enzyme-linked antiglobulin test (ELAT):

- To determine if apparent phenotype represents true genotype by a non-molecular method.

Background Information

In the ELAT, RBCs precoated with alloantibody are washed as for the DAT. The coated RBCs are then incubated with an anti-IgG plus alkaline phosphatase conjugate (IgG-AP). Unbound anti-IgG-AP is removed by washing, and a substrate is added that interacts with AP to produce a yellow color, the intensity of which is measured at 405 nm. The amount of color produced is directly proportional to the amount of alloantibody bound to the RBCs, which—within certain limits—is proportional to the antigen site density of the coated RBCs. This procedure has been developed to determine antigen dosage, which is a reflection of the zygosity of the RBC donor.

Operational Policy

Because of the complexities of Rh antigen expression, do not attempt to determine *RHD* zygosity by serologic means.

Limitations

Incorrect Results:

- Improper storage of reagents.
- Use of incorrect technique, including failure to wash RBCs free of unbound globulins and improper transfer of supernates.
- Use of wrong reagent.
- Omission of a test component.
- Use of inactive or contaminated reagents.

Sample Requirements

RBCs: from anticoagulated blood collected within the preceding 24 hours, washed three times in saline. Centrifuge to pack the RBCs. Remove the buffy coat and upper portion of the RBCs by vacuum aspiration. Wash once with BSA-LISS and dilute to a 2% suspension with BSA-LISS; a minimum of 1 mL of each RBC suspension is required.

Note: Accuracy is essential when preparing RBCs for the direct ELAT. Prepare approximate 2% suspensions and check counts with an electronic particle counter; adjust to 2×10^8 RBCs/mL before use.

Equipment/ Materials

Anti-IgG conjugate: AP-conjugated antihuman IgG (eg, Jackson Immu-noResearch Laboratories, West Grove, CA). Determine the appropriate dilution for the anti-IgG-AP from titration studies (using serial twofold dilutions in BSA-PBS) with Rh-positive RBCs precoated with a 1000× dilution of commercially prepared modified-tube (high-protein) anti-D. Plot the OD values against the anti-IgG-AP dilution on linear graph paper. Choose a dilution of anti-IgG-AP that gives an OD value with Rh-positive RBCs on the straight part of the curve yet gives a low OD with Rh-negative RBCs.

Carbonate buffer: 0.05 M; pH 9.8.

Laboratory film (eg, Parafilm, VWR, Batavia, IL).

ρ-nitrophenol phosphate (PNP) substrate: PNP (eg, Sigma-Aldrich, St Louis, MO), diluted to 2 mg/mL with 0.05 M carbonate buffer just before use.

Three examples of RBCs carrying single-dose expression and three examples of RBCs carrying presumed double-dose expression of the antigen under investigation: washed and prepared to a 2% suspension in BSA-LISS, as described above.

Antigen-negative RBCs: washed and prepared to a 2% suspension in BSA-LISS, as described above.

1 N NaOH.

Pipettors with disposable tips to deliver 0.2-0.5 mL (eg, VWR, Batavia, IL).

Spectrophotometer (eg, Spectronic 200, VWR, Batavia, IL, or equivalent): at wavelength of 405 nm.

Test tubes: glass, 12 × 75-mm. Prepare for ELAT by filling with BSA-PBS, discarding BSA-PBS after a few minutes and inverting to drain.

BSA-PBS.

BSA-NS.

BSA-LISS.

Quality Control

The procedure uses RBCs from presumed homozygotes and known heterozygotes; several examples of each are included in the assay.

Procedure   Use the following steps to perform the procedure:

Step	Action
1.	For each RBC sample to be tested, dispense 0.5 mL of dilute antibody (in BSA-PBS) into duplicate sets of appropriately labeled, precoated 12 × 75-mm glass test tubes. **Note:** In order to avoid erroneous values from using too little or too much antibody, precoat each RBC sample with different dilutions of antiserum. See Wilson et al in the reference list for a detailed discussion.
2.	Prepare a "hemolysis control" for each RBC sample tested by dispensing 0.5 mL of BSA-PBS in an appropriately labeled, precoated 12 × 75-mm test tube.
3.	Add 0.5 mL of 2% RBCs in BSA-LISS to the duplicate tubes containing antibody and to the "hemolysis control tube."
4.	Incubate all tubes at 37 C for 15 minutes.
5.	Wash the RBCs six times with BSA-PBS and aspirate the final supernate.
6.	Add 0.2 mL of anti-IgG-AP (at working concentration) to each tube.
7.	Cover the tubes with Parafilm and incubate at 37 C for 1 hour; mix periodically by gentle agitation during this time.
8.	Wash the RBCs three times with BSA-PBS and aspirate the supernates.
9.	Resuspend the RBCs in BSA-NS and transfer to clean, appropriately labeled 12 × 75-mm test tubes.
10.	Centrifuge to pack the RBCs and aspirate the supernate.
11.	Add 0.2 mL BSA-NS and 0.2 mL PNP to the RBC buttons.
12.	Mix well, cover the tubes with Parafilm and incubate at 37 C for 60 minutes.
13.	Remove Parafilm and centrifuge to pack the RBCs.
14.	Transfer the supernates into clean test tubes and add 0.5 mL of 1 N NaOH (to stop the enzyme reaction).
15.	Using 1-cm cuvettes, read the OD of each supernate at 405 nm. **Note:** Read against a reagent blank consisting of: PNP, 0.2 mL; BSA-NS, 0.2 mL; and 1 N NaOH, 0.5 mL.

16.	For each test, determine the corrected OD as follows: [(OD TAg+) – (OD CAg+)] – [(OD Tag–) – (OD Cag–)] where T = test; C = hemolysis control; Ag+ = antigen-positive RBCs; Ag– = antigen-negative RBCs.
17.	Take the average of the two corrected OD values for each sample and compare with the OD values for the controls.
18.	Express the antigen content of unknown and known single-dose samples as a percentage of the antigen content of known double-dose samples.
19.	Interpret the reactions as follows:

If the percentage of antigen content of the test sample best matches that of…	Then the test sample is likely from…
the double-dose RBCs	a homozygote.
the single-dose RBCs	a heterozygote.
neither the double-dose nor the single-dose RBCs	an individual of indeterminate zygosity.

References

Leikola J, Perkins HA. Enzyme-linked antiglobulin test: An accurate and simple method to quantitate red cell antibodies. Transfusion 1980;20:138-44.

Postoway N, Nance SJ, Garratty G. Variables affecting the enzyme-linked antiglobulin test when detecting and quantitating IgG red cell antibodies. Med Lab Sci 1985;42:11-19.

Wilson L, Wren MR, Issitt PD. Enzyme linked antiglobulin test: Variables affecting the test when measuring levels of red cell antigens. Med Lab Sci 1985;42:20-25.

**Effective
Date**

Approved by	Printed Name	Signature	Date
Laboratory Management			
Medical Director			
Quality Officer			

XV-H. Predicting Clinical Significance Using the Monocyte Monolayer Assay

Purpose	To provide a method for performing a monocyte monolayer assay (MMA): • Assessing the clinical significance of an alloantibody.
Background Information	Antibody-coated RBCs are incubated in vitro with mononuclear cells. The ability of monocytes to adhere and phagocytose these sensitized RBCs is an index of the antibody's potential to decrease the survival of transfused RBCs. This procedure was developed as a means of predicting the clinical significance of antibodies to RBC antigens.
Operational Policy	Confirm expected rise in hematocrit and measure markers of hemolysis (eg, haptoglobin, unconjugated bilirubin) when a low percentage of reactivity is encountered with serologically incompatible units.
Limitations	Incorrect Results: • Improper storage of reagents. • Use of incorrect technique, including failure to wash RBCs free of unbound globulins. • Use of wrong reagent. • Omission of a test component, especially fresh normal serum as specified. • Use of inactive or contaminated reagents.
Sample Requirements	Serum, not plasma: minimum volume of 2 mL.

**Equipment/
Materials**

Anti-D: commercially prepared modified-tube polyclonal anti-D, diluted 1 in 50 with human complement (see below).

Culture chamber: Lab-Tek tissue culture chamber slides (eg, VWR, Batavia, IL).

Sheep RBCs (eg, Pel-Freez Biologicals, Rogers, AR).

Human complement: freshly collected normal human serum known to lack unexpected antibodies.

Mononuclear cell suspension: prepared as described in Section V.

Note: Prepare homologous monocytes from normal donors and autologous monocytes, if available.

Mounting medium (eg, Permount, VWR, Batavia, IL).

Phosphate buffer for Romanowsky stains: pH 7.2 at 25 C (eg, #P3288, Sigma-Aldrich, St Louis, MO).

pH 7.3 PBS.

RBCs: as described in Step 1 of Procedure.

Tissue culture medium: Roswell Park Memorial Institute 1640 medium (eg, Sigma-Aldrich, St Louis, MO); supplement with 10% (vol/vol) fetal bovine serum (eg, Sigma-Aldrich, St Louis, MO).

Wright-Giemsa stain (eg, Sigma-Aldrich, St Louis, MO).

Pipettors with disposable tips to deliver 0.2 mL (eg, VWR, Batavia, IL).

**Quality
Control**

The procedure includes internal controls.

Before use, each batch of human complement should be shown to lyse sheep RBCs: use 1 drop of 3%-5% washed sheep RBCs in saline, 3 drops of human complement, and 15 minutes incubation at 37 C; centrifuge as for hemagglutination tests and examine the supernate for hemolysis.

Procedure   Use the following steps to perform the procedure:

Step	Action
1.	Prepare 3%-5% suspensions of washed, antibody-coated RBCs in tissue culture medium: incubate 1 drop of 3%-5% RBCs with 3 drops of serum for 60 minutes at 37 C; wash four times with saline before dilution with tissue culture medium. **Note:** Use at least two examples of RBCs that lack and two examples that carry antigens to which the test serum manifests specificity. Include the following reaction mixtures for RBC coating: a) Test serum + antigen-positive RBCs. b) Test serum + antigen-positive RBCs + complement. c) Complement + antigen-positive RBCs. d) PBS + antigen-positive RBCs. e) Test serum + antigen-negative RBCs. f) Test serum + antigen-negative RBCs + complement. g) Complement + antigen-negative RBCs. h) PBS + antigen-negative RBCs. i) Anti-D + Rh-positive RBCs.
2.	Add 0.2 mL of the mononuclear cell suspension ($3\text{-}6 \times 10^6$/mL) to each well of a tissue culture slide.
3.	Incubate at 37 C for 60 minutes.
4.	Carefully aspirate nonadherent cells (lymphocytes) with a Pasteur pipette and discard.
5.	Add 0.2 mL of each sensitized RBC sample to appropriately labeled wells.
6.	Incubate at 37 C for 60 minutes.
7.	Aspirate the supernate and discard.
8.	Break off the plastic chambers and remove gaskets.
9.	Gently rinse the slide three times with saline.
10.	Blot the edge of the slide with a paper towel and immediately place in Wright's stain for 3 minutes.
11.	Blot the edge of the slide with a paper towel and place in Giemsa stain for 20 minutes.

12.	Blot the edge of the slide with a paper towel and wash in Romanowsky buffer for 3 minutes.
13.	Rinse with distilled water.
14.	Blot the edge of the slide with a paper towel, wipe the back of the slide clean, and air dry.
15.	Cover with a coverslip using Permount (Thermo Fisher Scientific, Waltham, MA) and allow to dry.
16.	Examine microscopically for reactive monocytes (RBC adherence and/or phagocytosis).
17.	Count 600 monocytes (200 if reactivity >20%).
18.	Express the results in terms of the percentage of reactive monocytes.
19.	Interpret the reactions as follows:

If the percentage of reactivity with antigen-positive RBCs is...	And the percentage of reactivity with antigen-negative RBCs is ...	Then...
<5%	<5	accelerated RBC destruction is unlikely.
5-20	<5	antibody is likely to cause accelerated RBC destruction in vivo.
>20	<20	antibody is likely to cause rapid RBC destruction in vivo.

References   Arndt P, Garratty G. A retrospective analysis of the value of monocyte monolayer assay results for predicting the clinical significance of blood group alloantibodies. Transfusion 2004;44:1273-81.

Garratty G. Predicting the clinical significance of alloantibodies and determining the in vivo survival of transfused red cells. In: Judd WJ, Barnes A, eds. Clinical and serological aspects of transfusion reactions. Arlington, VA: AABB, 1982:91-119.

**Effective
Date**

Approved by	Printed Name	Signature	Date
Laboratory Management			
Medical Director			
Quality Officer			

XV-I. Screening for PNH: Sucrose Hemolysis Test

Purpose

To provide instructions for the sucrose hemolysis test:

- Screening test for paroxysmal nocturnal hemoglobinuria (PNH).

Background Information

Normal RBCs agglutinate in iso-osmotic, low-ionic-strength solutions of sucrose; less than 5% of the normal RBCs will hemolyze. In contrast, RBCs from patients with PNH first agglutinate and then hemolyze (10%-80% hemolysis) when suspended in such low-ionic media in the presence of active complement.

Operational Policy

Confirm adequate treatment of positive control (AET-treated) RBCs in tests with anti-k.

Limitations

Incorrect Results:

- Immune-mediated hemolysis.
- Mechanical hemolysis.
- Use of wrong reagent.
- Use of wrong reagent.
- Use of incorrect technique.

Sample Requirements

Washed test RBCs: 50% suspension in pH 7.3 PBS.

Equipment/ Materials

AET-treated group O, k+ RBCs and group O, k+ untreated RBCs: 50% suspensions in pH 7.3 PBS.

Anti-k.

Colorimeter: at 550 nm wavelength (eg, VWR, Batavia, IL).

Drabkin's solution (eg, Sigma-Aldrich, St Louis, MO).

Fresh normal serum (FNS): ABO compatible with test sample and lacking unexpected antibodies.

Sugar water, prepared immediately before use.

pH 7.3 PBS.

Pipettors with disposable tips to deliver 0.1-0.2 mL, and graduated pipettes to deliver 1.0-3.0 mL (eg, VWR, Batavia, IL).

Quality Control

Normal and AET-treated k+ RBCs serve as negative and positive controls, respectively.

Procedure

Use the following steps to perform the procedure:

Step	Action
1.	Dispense 1.7 mL of sugar water into seven 10 or 12 × 75-mm test tubes labeled A-G.
2.	Add 0.1 mL FNS to each tube and mix well.
3.	Add 0.2 mL of test RBCs to tubes A and B and mix promptly.
4.	Add 0.2 mL of untreated normal RBCs to tubes C and D and mix promptly.
5.	Add 0.2 mL of AET-treated normal RBCs to tubes E and F and mix promptly.
6.	Incubate tubes A, C, and E at 37 C for 30 minutes. **Note:** Mix by gentle inversion after 10 minutes and again after 20 minutes incubation.
7.	Centrifuge tubes A, C, and E to pack intact RBCs and harvest the supernates.
8.	Dilute 1 mL of each supernate with 3 mL of Drabkin's solution and mix well.
9.	Mix tubes B, D, and F well; do not centrifuge. Dilute 1 mL of each RBC suspension with 3 mL of Drabkin's solution and mix well.
10.	Similarly, dilute the sugar water + serum mixture in tube G with Drabkin's solution.
11.	Measure the percentage of transmission of dilutions A-F at 550 nm using dilution G as a zero blank.
12.	Determine the percentage of hemolysis in the test supernate, using the percentage of transmission of dilution B as 100% hemolysis.

13.	Interpret the reactions as follows:		
	If hemolysis in test sample is...	**And controls...**	**Then...**
	≥10%	react as expected	test is positive: • Perform Ham's test (Procedure XV-A).
	≤5%	react as expected	test is negative.
	5%-10%	do not react as expected	test is invalid.

Reference   Henry JB. Clinical diagnosis and management by laboratory methods. 16th ed. Philadelphia, PA: WB Saunders, 1979.

Effective Date

Approved by

Printed Name	Signature	Date
Laboratory Management		
Medical Director		
Quality Officer		

XV-J. Isolating Genomic DNA from Blood

Purpose

To provide instructions for isolating genomic DNA from blood and buffy coat samples:

- Blood group genotype determination.

Background Information

Genomic DNA can be readily isolated from any population of nucleated cells and used in many downstream techniques for the analysis of blood group and other genes. High-salt solutions will precipitate cellular components, leaving DNA in solution, which may be readily precipitated with ethanol.

Operational Policy

For optimal results:

- Use samples for DNA isolation that are no more than 1 week old.
- Use only molecular-biology-grade chemicals.
- Prepare all reagents in nuclease-free distilled water.
- Wear gloves throughout the procedure.
- Avoid cross-contamination of samples and reagents; use fresh pipette tip for each sample/reagent addition.
- Work in a clean area—eg, an ethanol-treated bench top.
- Do not create a vortex when mixing.

Limitations

Incorrect Results:

- DNA is insufficiently dissolved.
- DNA pellet was lost in transfer.
- Protein contamination indicates that insufficient 6 M NaCl was used.

Sample Requirements

5-10 mL ACD or EDTA-anticoagulated blood sample.

**Equipment/
Materials**

95% ethanol (eg, Sigma-Aldrich, St Louis, MO).

70% ethanol (eg, Sigma-Aldrich, St Louis, MO).

Proteinase K: 20 mg/mL (eg, #P2308, Sigma-Aldrich, St Louis, MO).

Lysing buffer.

6 M NaCl.

Nuclease-free distilled water (eg, Qiagen, Valencia, CA).

SET-buffer.

20% sodium dodecyl sulphate (SDS).

TE-buffer.

50-mL centrifuge tubes (eg, #62.548.004, Sarstedt, Numbrecht, Germany).

15-mL centrifuge tubes (eg, #62.554.001, Sarstedt, Numbrecht, Germany).

1.5-mL Eppendorf centrifuge tube (eg, LabScientific, Livingston, NJ).

Hybridization oven (eg, model 5400, with multi-tube carousel, #47746-114, VWR, Batavia, IL).

Spectrophometer (eg, Eppendorf BioPhotometer, Thermo Fisher Scientific, Waltham, MA).

Pipettors with disposable tips to deliver 2 µL, 100 µL, 175 µL, and graduated pipettes to deliver 5 mL (eg, VWR, Batavia, IL).

**Quality
Control**

Quantify the DNA by measuring the OD at 260 nm.

Assess purity by calculating the 260/280 nm ratio: values between 1.6 and 2.0 are acceptable.

Procedure

Use the following steps to perform the procedure:

Step	Action
1.	Mix the blood sample gently and transfer to a 50-mL plastic centrifuge tube.
2.	Add lysing buffer to 50 mL and mix to hemolyze the RBCs.
3.	Centrifuge at 1500 × g for 15 minutes.
4.	Discard the supernate and resuspend the pellet in 20 mL of SET buffer.

5.	Centrifuge at 1500 × *g* for 15 minutes.
6.	Discard the supernate, resuspend in 4.7 mL of SET buffer, and transfer to a 15-mL centrifuge tube.
7.	Add 175 μL of 20% SDS and 50 μL of proteinase K.
8.	Mix the tube in a hybridization oven at 55 C for 1 to 2 hours until the pellet is completely dissolved.
9.	Add 2.5 mL of 6 M NaCl and mix gently. A precipitate should form. If no precipitate forms, add 1-mL volumes of NaCl until a precipitate is seen.
10.	Centrifuge at 1600 × *g* for 15 minutes.
11.	Transfer the supernate to a new 50-mL centrifuge tube and add 2 volumes of 95% ethanol. Mix gently until the DNA precipitates.
12.	Using a transfer pipette, carefully transfer the DNA precipitate to a labeled 1.5-mL Eppendorf centrifuge tube.
13.	Centrifuge at 15,000 × *g* for 1 minute.
14.	Discard supernate and add 1 mL of 70% ethanol to wash the pellet.
15.	Centrifuge at 15,000 × *g* for 1 minute.
16.	Discard the supernate and carefully dry the sides of the tube with a cotton bud.
17.	Allow the pellet to dry at RT for 1-2 hours.
18.	Add 100 μL of TE buffer to the pellet and allow to dissolve overnight at RT. **Note:** If DNA is not to be quantified immediately after dissolving, refrigerate until required. Alternatively, if DNA is required sooner, incubate sample at 37 C for 2 hours.
19.	Dilute 2 μL DNA with 98 μL distilled water.
20.	Measure the OD at 260 nm and calculate the DNA concentration using the equation: Concentration in ng/μL = $OD_{260} \times 50 \times 50$
21.	Determine purity by calculating the OD_{260}/OD_{280} ratio.

22.	Evaluate the results as follows:		
	If concentration is...	**And/or ratio is...**	**Then DNA is...**
	≥20 ng/μL	≥1.6	suitable for PCR.
	any level	<1.6	unsuitable for PCR: • Obtain a fresh sample and repeat isolation. • Consider preparing new reagents.
23.	Store at 4 C. For long term storage, store below –20 C.		

Reference   Miller SA, Dykes DD, Polesky HF. A simple salting out procedure for extracting DNA from human nucleated cells. Nucleic Acids Res 1988;16: 1215.

Effective Date

Approved by

	Printed Name	**Signature**	**Date**
Laboratory Management			
Medical Director			
Quality Officer			

XV-K. Converting Plasma to Serum

Purpose	To provide instructions for converting plasma to serum:
	• Preparation of typing reagents from blood donors with useful antibody.

Background Information	This procedure uses thrombin and calcium chloride to convert donor plasma to serum. The intended application of this procedure is to convert antibody-containing donor plasma to serum for reagent use.

Operational Policy	Donor blood should be nonreactive in tests for infectious diseases.

Limitations	Incorrect Results:
	• Improper storage of reagents.
	• Use of incorrect technique.
	• Use of wrong reagent.

Sample Requirements	Donor plasma: anticoagulated with ACD/CPD/CPD-A1.

Equipment/ Materials	Bovine thrombin: 1000 NIH units/mg of protein (eg, #82040, MP Biomedicals, Irvine, CA): reconstitute to 500 units/mL with distilled water.
	Calcium chloride: 10% wt/vol; use within 7 days of preparation.
	Sampling site couplers (eg, #4C2405, Fenwal, Lake Zurich, IL).
	Syringes: 2 mL with needles.
	Transfer pack: 300 mL (eg, #4R2014, Fenwal, Lake Zurich, IL).

Quality Control	Check for adequate coagulation by performing serologic tests with recalcified plasma.
	Reconfirm specificity and reactivity of antibody; ideal titer is ≥ 8.

Procedure   Use the following steps to perform the procedure:

Step	Action
1.	Weigh the unit of plasma: assume 1 g = 1 mL of plasma.
2.	Insert a sampling site coupler into the bag.
3.	Draw $CaCl_2$ solution into the syringe (0.25 mL per 100 mL of plasma).
4.	Clean the injection site with an alcohol swab and inject the $CaCl_2$ solution into the plasma.
5.	Flush the syringe three times with plasma, withdraw the needle, and mix well.
6.	Draw thrombin into the syringe (0.4 mL per 100 mL of plasma).
7.	Clean the injection site with an alcohol swab, inject the thrombin into the bag, and mix well.
8.	Allow fibrin clot to form at RT for at least 1 hour. Maintain at RT for at least 4 hours.
9.	Freeze the converted plasma at below –20 C overnight.
10.	Thaw the plasma at RT and centrifuge at $5000 \times g$ for 5 minutes (or equivalent).
11.	Transfer the recalcified plasma into the transfer pack, leaving the fibrin in the original bag.
12.	Weigh the recalcified unit and determine the volume.
13.	Label the unit as "Recalcified Plasma, NOT FOR TRANSFUSION"; also include the donor number, antibody specificity, ABO type, date of collection, volume, and results of tests for infectious diseases.
14.	Perform antibody identification studies to confirm specificity.
15.	Interpret the results as follows:

If specificity is...	And fibrin formation is...	Then...
confirmed	absent	perform titer.
confirmed	present	repeat recalcification procedure.
not confirmed	absent	consider removing unwanted antibody by adsorption/elution.

16.	Determine titer by Procedure X-D if coating antibody, or test doubling dilutions by Procedure II-H if aggutinating antibody. **Note:** Use single-dose RBCs, if available, when determining titer.	
17.	Interpret the results as follows:	
	If titer is…	**Then…**
	≥8	antibody is suitable for reagent purposes: • Dispense into convenient aliquots and store below −20 C.
	<8	consider concentrating antibody by adsorption/elution.

Effective Date

	Printed Name	**Signature**	**Date**
Approved by			
Laboratory Management			
Medical Director			
Quality Officer			

Appendices

Supplemental information is contained in the following appendices:

A.   Reagent Preparation and Storage

B.   Reagent Preparation Documentation Form

C.   Incidental Spill Response

D.   Directions for Managing Hazardous Chemical Spills

E.   Sources of Reagents and Equipment

Appendix A. Reagent Preparation and Storage

This appendix contains the formulae for the preparation of the majority of reagents used in procedures throughout this book. Included are group AB serum for use in the investigation of polyagglutination or as an antibody diluent, and buffer solutions that are widely used in the preparation of clinical laboratory reagents. Specific applications of these reagents are to be found among the outlines of individual procedures.

Documentation

Any time a reagent is prepared, it is important to document on the reagent vial, tube, or bottle the date of expiration, the name of the reagent (product), and its concentration (when applicable). In a separate book or file, a record of the specific ingredients (manufacturer, lot number, etc) should be maintained, together with the name or initials of the person preparing the product and the date the product was put into routine use (see Appendix B).

Storage

The storage temperatures and times given for each reagent are somewhat arbitrarily derived. Laboratories are at liberty to modify the recommendations based on institutional needs and experiences. The following times and temperatures are suggested:

Reagent RBCs: Up to 72 hours in saline/PBS refrigerated, 4 weeks in Alsever's solution refrigerated in stoppered bottles, or until visible signs of hemolysis occur.

Proteolytic Enzymes: Up to 1 year at –20 C (or below) for stock enzyme solutions. Once thawed, use within 1 hour; DO NOT REFREEZE. Discard diluted enzyme solutions immediately after use.

Frozen RBCs/Sera: Indefinite storage, provided control tests verify reactivity.

All Other Reagents: Up to 1 year, unless otherwise indicated. Discard if visible signs of bacterial contamination (eg, turbidity) occur.

Chemical Hazards

Before preparing any reagent, the manufacturer's safety data sheet (MSDS) for each ingredient should be obtained and reviewed by all staff involved in preparing and using that reagent. Warnings about the hazardous nature of certain chemicals (eg, organic solvents used in elution methods) are given in the specific procedures. Such hazards, the recommended personal protective equipment, and the appropriate responses to chemical spills are summarized in Appendices C and D.

Reagent	Materials/Instructions	Amount/Time
AB serum	AB serum from whole blood that has been allowed to clot before being refrigerated overnight	10 mL
	Note: Donor should lack unexpected antibodies.	
	Adsorb twice at 2-8 C with 5-mL aliquots of ficin-treated A_1 RBCs	30 minutes each aliquot
	Adsorb twice at 2-8 C with 5-mL aliquots of ficin-treated B RBCs	30 minutes each aliquot
	Test vs A1, B, and O RBCs by Procedure II-H	
	If tests are positive, repeat adsorption	
	When tests are negative, dispense into convenient aliquots and store frozen	Indefinitely
Acidified anti-B	0.1 N HCl	0.5 mL
	ES-4 monoclonal anti-B or human polyclonal anti-B	4.5 mL
	Check if pH is below 6.2 and adjust, if necessary, with additional 0.1 N HCl	
	Store refrigerated	1 year
AET 6% wt/vol	2-aminoethylisothiouronium bromide hydrobromide, $C_3H_{11}Br_2N_3SN_3$, Sigma-Aldrich	0.6 g
	Dissolve in 6-8 mL of distilled water and dilute	to 10 mL
	Adjust pH to 8.0 with 5 N NaOH	
	Dispense into convenient aliquots and store frozen	1 year
Alsever's solution	Citric acid, monohydrate, $C_6H_8O_7.H_2O$	0.55 g
	Dextrose, $C_6H_{12}O_6$	20.5 g
	Inosine	2.0 g
	Chloramphenicol	0.33 g
	Neomycin sulphate	0.5 g
	NaCl	4.2 g
	Dissolve in 600-800 mL distilled water and dilute	to 1 liter
	Check pH	6.8 ±0.2
	Check mOsm/kg	340 ±10
	Store refrigerated	1 year
Barbital buffer pH 9.6	Barbital sodium, $C_8H_{11}N_2NaO_3$, Sigma-Aldrich	20.6 g
	Distilled water	600 mL
	Adjust to pH 9.6 with 0.1 N HCl	
	Distilled water	to 1 liter
	Store refrigerated	1 year

Reagent	Materials/Instructions	Amount/Time
Boric acid buffer	Boric acid, H_3BO_3	5.16 g
	KCl	2.2 g
	Distilled water	600 mL
	Adjust to pH 9.8 with 0.1 N NaOH	
	Distilled water	to 1 liter
	Store refrigerated	1 year
0.1% BSA-LISS	Bovine serum albumin, 22% wt/vol	4.5 mL
	OR bovine serum albumin, 30% wt/vol	3.3 mL
	Dilute with LISS	to 1 liter
	Store refrigerated	1 year
1% BSA-PBS	Bovine serum albumin, 22% wt/vol	45.5 mL
	OR bovine serum albumin, 30% wt/vol	33.3 mL
	NaN_3	1 g
	Dilute with pH 7.3 PBS	to 1 liter
	Store refrigerated	1 year
2% BSA-NS	Bovine serum albumin, 22% wt/vol	91 mL
	OR bovine serum albumin, 30% wt/vol	66.6 mL
	NaN_3	1 g
	Dilute with normal saline	to 1 liter
	Store refrigerated	1 year
2% BSA-PBS	Bovine serum albumin, 22% wt/vol	91 mL
	OR bovine serum albumin, 30% wt/vol	66.6 mL
	NaN_3	1 g
	Dilute with pH 7.3 PBS	to 1 liter
	Store refrigerated	1 year
2% BSA-LISS	Bovine serum albumin, 22% wt/vol	91 mL
	OR bovine serum albumin, 30% wt/vol	66.6 mL
	NaN_3	1 g
	Dilute with LISS	to 1 liter
	Store refrigerated	1 year
3% BSA	Bovine serum albumin, 22% wt/vol	136 mL
	OR bovine serum albumin, 30% wt/vol	100 mL
	NaN_3	1 g
	Dilute with pH 7.3 PBS	to 1 liter
	Store refrigerated	1 year

Reagent	Materials/Instructions	Amount/Time
6% BSA	Bovine serum albumin, 22% wt/vol	2.7mL
	OR bovine serum albumin, 30% wt/vol	2 mL
	Dilute with pH 7.3 PBS	to 10 mL
	Store refrigerated	1 month
6% BSA + Tween 20	6% BSA	100 mL
	Add Tween 20	100 μL
	Store refrigerated	1 year
11% BSA + Tween 20	Bovine serum albumin, 22% wt/vol	50 mL
	Dilute with pH 7.3 PBS	to 100 mL
	Add Tween 20	100 μL
	Store refrigerated	1 year
Bromelain 1% wt/vol	Bromelain, MP Biomedicals	1 g
	Note: Protect eyes, mouth, nose, and hands when weighing dry enzyme. Powder may damage mucous membranes if inhaled; the solution is less hazardous.	
	Agitate in pH 7.3 PBS for 15 minutes at room temperture	100 mL
	Centrifuge to remove particulate matter	
	Dispense into 1-mL aliquots	
	Store below −20 C	1 year
	Use within 1 hour after thawing; do not refreeze	
Buffered formalin 20% wt/vol	150 mM KH_2PO_4	40 mL
	150 mM Na_2HPO_4	60 mL
	Formaldehyde, 37% wt/vol, Sigma-Aldrich	200 mL
	Distilled water	To 1 liter
	Store at room temperature	1 year
Calcium chloride 10% wt/vol	$CaCl_2$	1 g
	Distilled water	to 10 mL
	Store refrigerated	1 week
Carbonate buffer 0.05 M	0.05 M $NaHCO_3$, 4.2 g/L	400 mL
	Adjust pH to 9.8 with 0.05 M Na_2CO_3, 5.3 g/L	
	Add 1 M $MgCl_2$, 9.52 g/100 mL, to final concentration of 0.001M	
	Store refrigerated	1 year
Chloroquine diphosphate	Chloroquine diphosphate: $C_{18}H_{32}ClN_3O_8P_2$, Sigma-Aldrich	20 g
	Dissolve in 60-80 mL normal saline and dilute	to 100 mL
	Adjust to pH 5.1 with 1 N NaOH	
	Store refrigerated	1 year

Reagent	Materials/Instructions	Amount/Time
Chromic chloride	$CrCl_3.6H_2O$, 98% pure, Sigma-Aldrich	1.0 g
	Dissolve in distilled water	100 mL
	Store at room temperature in a dark, acid-washed bottle	1 year
α-chymo-trypsin	α-chymotrypsin Type VII; TLCK-treated, Sigma-Aldrich	25 mg
5 mg/mL	Dissolve in pH 8.0 PBS	5 mL
	Dispense into 1 mL aliquots	
	Store below -20 C	1 year
	Use within 1 hour after thawing; do not refreeze	
Citric acid	Citric acid (monohydrate) $C_6H_8O_7.H_2O$	21 g
0.1 M	Dissolve in 600-800 mL distilled water and dilute	to 1 liter
	Store refrigerated	1 year
Citric acid	KH_2PO_4	1.3 g
Eluting Solution	Citric acid (monohydrate) $C_6H_8O_7.H_2O$	0.65g
	Dissolve in 60-80 mL normal saline and dilute with saline	to 100 mL
	Store refrigerated	1 year
Citric acid	Na_3PO_4	13 g
Neutralizing	Dissolve in 60-80 mL distilled water and dilute	to 100 mL
solution	Store refrigerated	1 year
L-cysteine	L-cysteine hydrochloride, $C_3H_7NO_2S.HCl$, Sigma-Aldrich	0.88 g
hydrochloride	Dissolve in distilled water	10 mL
0.5 M	Prepare on day of use	
Dextran	Normal serum (lacking unexpected antibodies)	2.5 mL
4% in normal	70,000 MW dextran, Sigma-Aldrich	0.1 g
serum	Store refrigerated	1 month
Dextrose	Dextrose, $C_6H_{12}O_6$	40 g
20% wt/vol	Dissolve in distilled water	100 mL
	Autoclave at 10 lb/in^2	10 minutes
	Adjust to pH 7.0 with 1 N NaOH	
	Dilute with 9% NaCl	to 200 mL
	Dispense into 8-mL aliquots	
	Store below −20 C	

Reagent	Materials/Instructions	Amount/Time
DIDS	4,4′-diisothiocyanatostilbene-2,2′-disulfonic acid (DIDS), $C_{16}H_8N_2O_6S_4Na_2$, Sigma-Aldrich	5 mg
	Note: DIDS is moist and light sensitive; store desiccated, in the dark at 4 C.	
	Normal saline	to 100 mL
	Prepare fresh daily in a dark glass bottle wrapped in aluminium foil.	
Digitonin 0.5% wt/vol	$C_{56}H_{92}O_{29}$	0.5 g
	Dissolve in 60-80 mL distilled water and dilute	to 100 mL
	Store refrigerated	1 year
	Note: Digitonin is an irritant and may cause death if swallowed or adsorbed through the skin. In case of contact, immediately flush eyes or skin with large amounts of water for at least 15 minutes and remove contaminated clothing. If inhaled, remove to fresh air; if breathing is difficult, give oxygen. Wash contaminated clothing before reuse.	
Dithiothreitol (DTT) 0.2 M	DTT (Cleland's reagent)	1 g
	pH 7.3 PBS	32.4 mL
	Dispense into 2.5-mL aliquots for ZZAP preparation	
	Store below −20 C	1 year
Dithiothreitol (DTT) 0.01 M	DTT (Cleland's reagent)	0.154 g
	Dissolve in pH 7.3 PBS	100 mL
	Store refrigerated	1 year
Drabkin's solution	Potassium cyanide, KCN	0.2 g
	Potassium ferricyanide, $K_3Fe(CN)_6$	0.2 g
	Sodium bicarbonate, $NaHCO_3$	1g
	Dissolve in 600-800 mL distilled water and dilute	to 1 liter
	Store refrigerated	1 year
EDTA-saline	$K_2EDTA.2H_2O$	500 g
	NaOH	40 g
	Dissolve in normal saline	20 L
	Note: EDTA-saline should inhibit the hemolysis of 1 drop of 20% sheep RBCs (Pel-Freez) by 9 drops of fresh normal serum after 15 minutes incubation at room temperature.	
	Store at room temperature	1 year

Reagent	Materials/Instructions	Amount/Time
EDTA-glycine-acid solutions	**A. 10% wt/vol Na_2EDTA**	
	$Na_2EDTA.2H_2O$	10 g
	Dissolve in 60-80 mL distilled water and dilute	to 100 mL
	Store at room temperature	1 year
	B. 0.1 M glycine at pH 1.5	
	Glycine: $H_2NCH_2CO_2H$	3.754 g
	NaCl	2.922 g
	Dissolve in 300-400 mL distilled water and dilute	to 500 mL
	Adjust to pH 1.5 with 12 N HCl	
	Store at 4 C	1 year
	C. Tris base, 1 M	
	$C_4H_{11}NO_3$, (TRIZMA base, Sigma-Aldrich)	12.1 g;
	Dissolve in 60-80 mL distilled water and dilute	to 100 mL
	Store at room temperature	1 year
EDTA-LISS	$K_2EDTA.2H_2O$	2.7 g
	Dissolve in 0.125 N NaOH	50 mL
	Dilute with LISS	to 500 mL
	Store refrigerated	1 year
Erythrosin B 0.5% wt/vol	Erythrosin B, Sigma-Aldrich	0.5 g
	Distilled water	to 100 mL
	Store at room temperature	4 months
Ethanol 80% vol/vol	Ethyl alcohol, C_2H_5OH, 80 mL	80 mL
	Distilled water	to 100 mL
	Store in an explosion-proof cabinet	1 year
Ficin 1% wt/vol	Ficin, MP Biomedicals	1 g
	Note: Protect eyes, mouth, nose, and hands when weighing dry enzyme. Powder may damage mucous membranes if inhaled; the solution is less hazardous.	
	Add pH 7.3 PBS	100 mL
	Agitate at room temperature	15 minutes
	Centrifuge to remove particulate matter	
	Dispense into 1-mL aliquots	
	Store below –20 C	1 year
	Use within 1 hour after thawing; do not refreeze	

Reagent	Materials/Instructions	Amount/Time
Ficin 4% wt/vol	Ficin, MP Biomedicals	4 g
	Note: Protect eyes, mouth, nose, and hands when weighing dry enzyme. Powder may damage mucous membranes if inhaled; the solution is less hazardous.	
	Add pH 7.3 PBS for 15 minutes at room temperature	100 mL
	Agitate at room temperature	15 minutes
	Centrifuge to remove particulate matter	
	Dispense into 1-mL aliquots	
	Store below –20 C	1 year
	Use within 1 hour after thawing; do not refreeze	
Freezing solution For freezing RBCs in liquid N_2	Glucose	54 g
	sucrose, $C_{12}H_{22}O_{11}$	154 g
	NaCl	2.9 g
	Distilled water	to 1 liter
	Store refrigerated	1 year
D-galactosamine-HCl 0.1 M GalNH$_2$-HCl	D-galactosamine hydrochloride, Sigma-Aldrich	215 mg
	Dissolve in distilled water	10 mL
	Store refrigerated	1 year
Glycine 0.1 M (acidic)	$H_2NCH_2CO_2H$	3.754 g
	NaCl	2.922 g
	Dissolve in distilled water	300-400 mL
	Adjust to pH 3.0 with 12 N HCl	
	Dilute	to 500 mL
	Store at 4 C	1 year
HCl 0.1 N	Hydrochloric acid (concentrated), 12 N	0.1 mL
	Distilled water	11.9 mL
	Store at room temperature	1 year
HCl 0.2 N	Hydrochloric acid (concentrated), 12 N	0.1 mL
	Distilled water	5.9 mL
	Store at room temperature	1 year
Human milk I substance	Obtain via breast pump from lactating mothers	
	Centrifuge immediately after collection and discard cream	
	Place in a boiling tube, and place tube in a beaker of boiling water	10 minutes
	Dispense in convenient aliquots	
	Store below –20 C	Indefinitely

Reagent	Materials/Instructions	Amount/Time
Human saliva ABH/Le substance	Collect saliva into a centrifuge tube	≈2 mL
	Note: Adults should rinse their mouths thoroughly with water. Women should remove lipstick. Do not promote salivation by chewing gum (sugars may inhibit reagent antisera). Use cotton swab to collect saliva from infants and express swab into 0.5 mL pH 7.3 PBS.	
	Centrifuge immediately after collection to remove particulate matter	
	Dilute saliva with an equal volume of pH 7.3 PBS	
	Transfer to a boiling tube, and place tube in a beaker of boiling water	10 minutes
	Centrifuge to remove precipitate	
	Dispense into convenient aliquots	
	Store below −20 C	Indefinitely
Hydatid cyst fluid (HCF) P_1 substance	Harvest HCF from sheep infested with live protoscalices of the tapeworm *Echinococcus granulosus*.	
	Note: Material is highly infectious. Wear double rubber gloves when handling.	
	Neutralize with 1 N HCl	
	Filter through 0.45-μ filter	
	Dilute 1 in 20 with pH 7.3 PBS	
	Dispense into convenient aliquots	
	Store below −20 C	Indefinitely
Hypotonic saline 0.3% NaCl	NaCl	0.3 g
	Distilled water	to 100 mL
	Store refrigerated	1 year
Hyaluronidase	Type I-S (EC 3.2.1.35) hyaluronidase, from bovine testes, Sigma-Aldrich.	10mg
	Note: Store lyophilized, desiccated, and below 0 C	
	Normal saline	to 10 mL
	Dispense into 0.2-mL aliquots	
	Store below −20 C	1 year
K_2EDTA 4.45% wt/vol	$K_2EDTA.2H_2O$	4.45 g
	Distilled water	80 mL
	Adjust pH to 7.0 with 1 N NaOH	
	Distilled water	to 100 mL
	Store refrigerated	1 year

Reagent	Materials/Instructions	Amount/Time
LISS wash solution	150 mM Na_2HPO_4	8.7 mL
	150 mM KH_2PO_4	11.3 mL
	Glycine: NH_2CH_2COOH	18 g
	NaCl	1.75 g
	Distilled water	to 1 liter
	Methyl paraben	0.6 g
	Propyl paraben	0.1 g
	Check pH = 6.7 ±0.1; osmolarity = 289 ±10 mOsm/kg	
	Store refrigerated	1 year
Low-ionic medium (LIM)	Dextrose, $C_6H_{12}O_6$	25 g
	$Na_2EDTA.2H_2O$	1 g
	Distilled water	to 500mL
	Adjust to pH 6.4 with 3 N NaOH	
	Store refrigerated	1 year
Lysing buffer pH 7.4	Sucrose, $C_{12}H_{22}O_{11}$	110 g
	$MgCl_2.6H_2O$	5 g
	Tris, VWR	1.2 g
	Triton X-100 (molecular biology grade), Sigma-Aldrich	10 mL
	Distilled water	to 1 liter
	Store refrigerated	1 year
Magnesium chloride 0.63 M	$MgCl_2.6H_2O$	1.281 g
	Distilled water	to 10 mL
	Store refrigerated	1 year
2-mercapto-ethanol (2-ME) 1 M	1.12 g/mL 2-ME, Sigma-Aldrich	0.7 mL
	pH 7.3 PBS	9.3mL
	Store refrigerated in dark glass container	1 year
NaCl 6 M	NaCl	32.0 g
	Nuclease-free distilled water, Qiagen	to 100 mL
	Store refrigerated	1 year
NaCl 2.5% wt/vol	NaCl	12.5 g
	Distilled water	to 500 mL
	Store refrigerated	1 year
NaCl 9.0% wt/vol	NaCl	45.0 g
	Distilled water	to 100 mL
	Store refrigerated	1 year

Reagent	Materials/Instructions	Amount/Time
NaClO 0.001%	Clorox (domestic bleach), 5% Normal saline Discard immediately after use	0.1 mL 500 mL
Na$_2$HPO$_4$ 0.2 M	Na$_2$HPO$_4$.2H$_2$O Dissolve in 600-800 mL distilled water and dilute Store refrigerated	28.4 g to 1 liter 1 year
NaOH 0.1 N	Sodium hydroxide pellets, anhydrous Distilled water Dissolve by mixing at room temperature Store at room temperature	0.4 g 100 mL 1 year
NaOH 0.125 N	Sodium hydroxide pellets, anhydrous Distilled water Store at room temperature	0.5 g 100 mL 1 year
NaOH 3 N	Sodium hydroxide pellets, anhydrous Distilled water Dissolve by mixing at room temperature Store at room temperature	12 g 100 mL 1 year
NaOH 5 N	Sodium hydroxide pellets, anhydrous Distilled water Dissolve by mixing at room temperature Store at room temperature	20 g 100 mL 1 year
Neutral-buffered formalin (NBF) 10% wt/vol	NaH$_2$PO$_4$ Na$_2$HPO$_4$ Formaldehyde (37 % wt/vol) Distilled water Store at room temperature **Note:** To prepare formal saline, dilute 1 part NBF with 9 parts pH 7.3 PBS	3.5 g 6.5 g 100 mL to 1 liter 1 year
Normal saline	NaCl Distilled water Store refrigerated	9.0 g to 1 liter 1 year
ρ-nitrophenol phosphate (PNP)	PNP, disodium salt, Sigma-Aldrich Dilute to 2 mg/mL with 0.05 M carbonate buffer Prepare immediately before use **Note:** Volumes required will depend upon number of assays to perform.	

Reagent	Materials/Instructions	Amount/Time
Papain 1% wt/vol	Papain, crude powder, Sigma-Aldrich	2 g
	Note: Protect eyes, mouth, nose and hands when weighing dry enzyme. Powder may damage mucous membranes if inhaled; the solution is less hazardous.	
	Phosphate buffer, pH 5.4	100 mL
	Agitate at room temperature	15 minutes
	Filter through Whatman #1 filter paper	
	Add L-cysteine hydrochloride	10 mL
	Incubate at 37 C	1 hour
	Dilute with pH 5.4 phosphate buffer	to 200 mL
	Dispense into 1-mL aliquots	
	Store below –20 C	1 year
	Use within 1 hour after thawing; do not refreeze	
Polyethylene glycol (PEG) 20% wt/vol	3350 MW PEG, $H(OCH_2CH_2)_nOH$, Sigma-Aldrich	20 g
	pH 7.3 PBS	to 100 mL
	Store refrigerated	1 year
Percoll-Renografin	Percoll, Sigma-Aldrich	35 mL
	Renografin, x-ray contrast medium: Meglumine diatrizoate, $C_{11}H_9I_3N_2O_4 \cdot C_7H_{17}NO_5$, Sigma-Aldrich	15 mL
	0.9% NaCl	25 mL
	Distilled water	25 mL
	Check SG = 1.095; osmolarity = 300 ±10 mOsm/kg	
	Store refrigerated	1 year
Phosphate buffers Stock solutions	67 mM KH_2PO_4	9.1 g/L
	67 mM Na_2HPO_4	9.5 g/L
	100 mM KH_2PO_4	13.6 g/L
	100 mm Na_2HPO_4	14.2 g/L
	150 mM KH_2PO_4	20.4 g/L
	150 mM Na_2HPO_4	21.3 g/L
	Store refrigerated	1 year

Reagent	Materials/Instructions			Amount/Time
Phosphate buffers	Prepare phosphate buffer at desired pH level using the volumes of stock solutions according to the following table:			
Stock solutions and pH level	**pH**	**mL KH$_2$PO$_4$**	**mL Na$_2$HPO$_4$**	
	5.29	97.5	2.5	
	5.40	96.5	3.5	
	5.59	95.0	5.0	
	5.91	90.0	10.0	
	6.24	80.0	20.0	
	6.47	70.0	30.0	
	6.64	60.0	40.0	
	6.81	50.0	50.0	
	6.98	40.0	60.0	
	7.17	30.0	70.0	
	7.30	23.6	76.4	
	7.38	20.0	80.0	
	7.73	10.0	90.0	
	8.04	5.0	95.0	
	Adjust pH level with 0.1 N HCl or 0.1 N NaOH			
	Store refrigerated			1 year
Phosphate buffer 0.5 M, pH 8.5	Na$_2$HPO$_4$			7.1 g
	Distilled water			to 100 mL
	Store refrigerated			1 year
Phosphate buffer 0.8 M, pH 8.2	Na$_2$HPO$_4$			109.6 g
	KH$_2$PO$_4$			2.922 g
	Distilled water			to 500 mL
	Adjust to pH 8.2 with 1 N HCl or 1 N NaOH			
	Store refrigerated			1 year

Reagent	Materials/Instructions	Amount/Time
Phosphate buffer Hendry's isosmotic	Na_2HPO_4 (dibasic)	17.92 g/L
	$NaH_2PO_4.H_2O$ (acidic)	22.16 g/L
	These buffers are about 0.14 M and have an osmolarity of 289 mOsm/kg	
	Prepare iso-osmotic phosphate buffers at desired pH level using the following volumes of solutions:	

pH	mL KH_2PO_4	mL Na_2HPO_4
6.6	50	50
6.8	40	60
7.2	20	80
7.4	15	85
7.6	10	90

Reagent	Materials/Instructions	Amount/Time
	Check pH and adjust as necessary with acid or base.	
	Store refrigerated	1 year
Phosphate-buffered saline (PBS)	For 6.7 mM, 10 mM, or 15 mM PBS, mix:	
	Phosphate buffer of appropriate molar concentration (eg, 100 mM for 10 mM PBS) and desired pH	1 part
	Normal saline	9 parts
	Note: For pH 7.3 PBS (10 mM), use 100 mM buffer.	
	For 67 mM, 100 mM, or 150 mM PBS, mix:	
	NaCl	0.9 g
	Phosphate buffer of appropriate molar concentration and desired pH	to 100 mL
	Store refrigerated	1 year
Phosphate-buffered saline/glycerol 0.2 M, pH 8.5	Na_2HPO_4	2.84 g
	NaCl	0.85 g
	Glycerol	2 mL
	Distilled water	to 100 mL
	Store refrigerated	1 year
Phosphate-NaOH buffer pH 7.4	KH_2PO_4	14.52 g
	1 N NaOH	87.5 mL
	Distilled water	to 1 liter
	Store refrigerated	1 year

Reagent	Materials/Instructions	Amount/Time
Phthalate ester mixtures	Dibutyl phthalate, C_6H_4-1,2-$[CO_2(CH_2)_3CH_3]_2$, Sigma-Aldrich Dimethyl phthalate, C_6H_4-1,2-$(CO_2CH_3)_2$, Sigma-Aldrich Prepare mixtures of decreasing specific gravity by volume as follows:	

Specific Gravity	Dibutyl Phthalate	Dimethyl Phthalate
1.110	4.8 mL	4.2 mL
1.106	5.1 mL	3.9 mL
1.102	5.3 mL	3.7 mL
1.098	5.6 mL	3.4 mL
1.094	5.8 mL	3.2 mL
1.090	6.0 mL	3.0 mL
1.086	6.3 mL	2.7 mL
1.082	6.5 mL	2.5 mL
1.078	6.8 mL	2.2 mL
1.074	7.0 mL	2.0 mL

Alternative volumes:

Specific Gravity	Dibutyl Phthalate	Dimethyl Phthalate
1.110	5.676 g	5.424 g
1.106	5.960 g	5.100 g
1.102	6.244 g	4.775 g
1.098	6.528 g	4.453 g
1.094	6.811 g	4.129 g
1.090	7.095 g	3.806 g
1.086	7.379 g	3.481 g
1.082	7.663 g	3.156 g
1.078	7.947 g	2.833 g
1.074	8.230 g	2.510 g

Store ester mixtures in the dark at room temperature	2 years

Reagent	Materials/Instructions	Amount/Time
Pigeon egg white P_1 substance	Separate egg white from yolk	
	Test 1/100 to 1/10,000 dilutions in pH 7.3 PBS to determine optimal dilution to inhibit potent anti-P_1	
	Dilute as required	
	Dispense into convenient aliquots	
	Store below −20 C	Indefinitely
Piperazine-buffered saline 0.27 M	Piperazine hydrate, $C_4H_{10}N_2.6H_2O$, Sigma-Aldrich	5.44 g
	Distilled water	100 mL
	Adjust to pH 6.5 with 1 N HCl	≈33 mL
	Normal saline	to 200 mL
	Store refrigerated	1 year
Polybrene Stock solution 10% wt/vol	Hexadimethrine bromide, $(C_{13}H_{30}Br_2N_2)_x$, Sigma-Aldrich	10 g
	Normal saline	100 mL
	Store refrigerated in a plastic container	1 year
Polybrene Working solution	Stock Polybrene solution	1 mL
	Normal saline	199 mL
	Store refrigerated in a plastic container	1 month
Polybrene neutralizing reagent	Trisodium citrate, $Na_3C_6H_5O_7.2H_2O$	3.53 g
	Dextrose, $C_6H_{12}O_6$	2 g
	Distilled water	to 100 mL
	Store refrigerated	1 year
Pronase 2.5 mg/mL	Pronase, Roche Applied Science	0.25 g
	pH 8.0 PBS	100 mL
	Dissolve by gentle mixing	
	Dispense into 1-mL aliquots	
	Store below −20 C	1 year
	Use within 1 hour after thawing; do not refreeze	
Proteinase K 20 mg/mL	Proteinase K (molecular biology grade), Sigma-Aldrich	200 mg
	Nuclease-free distilled water, Qiagen	to 10 mL
	Store refrigerated	1 year
Salt-EDTA-Tris (SET) Buffer pH 8.2	Tris-HCl, VWR	1.6 g
	NaCl	23.4 g
	$Na_2EDTA.2H_2O$	0.75 g
	Nuclease-free distilled water, Qiagen	to 1 liter
	Store refrigerated	1 year

Reagent	Materials/Instructions	Amount/Time
Sodium dodecyl sulphate (SDS) 20% wt/vol	SDS (molecular biolograde), Sigma-Aldrich	2 g
	Nuclease-free distilled water, Qiagen	to 10 mL
	Store at room temperature	1 year
Sucrose K$_3$EDTA	Sucrose, C$_{12}$H$_{22}$O$_{11}$	10 g
	K$_3$EDTA	150 mg
	Distilled water	to 100 mL
	Store refrigerated	1 month
Sucrose reagent A	NaH$_2$PO$_4$.H$_2$O	345 mg
	Na$_2$EDTA.2H$_2$O	789 mg
	Sucrose, C$_{12}$H$_{22}$O$_{11}$	46.2 g
	Distilled water	to 500 mL
	Store refrigerated	1 month
Sucrose Reagent B	Na$_2$HPO$_4$	355 mg
	Na$_2$EDTA.2H$_2$O	789 mg
	Sucrose, C$_{12}$H$_{22}$O$_{11}$	46.2 g
	Distilled water	to 500 mL
	Store refrigerated	1 month
Sucrose sensitizing diluent	Sucrose reagent A	500 mL
	Adjust to pH 5.1 with sucrose reagent B ($\approx$30-50 mL)	
	Store refrigerated	1 month
Sugar water 10% wt/vol	Sucrose, C$_{12}$H$_{22}$O$_{11}$	10 g
	Dissolve in 60 mL distilled water and dilute	to 100 mL
	Use immediately	
Tris-EDTA (TE) Buffer pH 7.5	Tris-HCl	1.6 g
	Na$_2$EDTA.2H$_2$O	0.075g
	Nuclease-free distilled water, Qiagen	to 1 liter
	Store refrigerated	1 year
Trypsin (crude) 1% wt/vol	1:250 trypsin, Difco Brand, BD Diagnostic Systems	1 g
	Note: Protect eyes, mouth, nose, and hands when weighing dry enzyme. Powder may damage mucous membranes if inhaled; the solution is less hazardous.	
	0.05 N HCl	100 mL
	Agitate at room temperature	15 minutes
	Refrigerate	Overnight
	Store refrigerated	1 year
	Centrifuge to remove insoluble matter before use	

Reagent	Materials/Instructions	Amount/Time
Trypsin (pure) 180,000 BAEE units/mL	Purified type IX trypsin, from porcine pancreas, Sigma-Aldrich	See note
	Note: As supplied, BAEE units of activity per mg of protein are indicated on the vial. The amount of protein supplied is also given together with the total weight of solids present. The required concentration of trypsin is 180,000 BAEE units/mL. One unit equals Δ_{253} of 0.00l per minute with N-benzoyl-<u>L</u>-arginine ethyl ester (BAEE) as substrate at pH 7.6 at 25 C (reaction volume = 3.2 mL; light path = 1 cm).	
	Determine the milligrams of solid required to prepare 20 mL of purified trypsin solution. Multiply the units of activity/mg by the weight of protein/vial, then divide by the weight of solid/vial. Divide this figure into 180,000 and multiply by 20. The calculation can be written as follows: [180,000 ÷ (BAEE units/mg × mg protein/vial ÷ mg solid/vial)] × 20.	20 mL
	Dissolve the required amount of trypsin in 100 mM pH 7.7 PBS	
	Dispense into 1-mL aliquots	1 year
	Store below −20 C	
	Use within 1 hour after thawing; do not refreeze	
Trypsin for CrCl$_3$ coupling method	NaCl	8.0 g
	KCl	0.4 g
	Na$_2$PO$_4$ (anhydrous)	0.12 g
	Glucose	1.0 g
	Phenol red	10 mg
	Trypsin (Difco Grade 1, 1:250)	2.5 g
	Stir in distilled H$_2$O to dissolve	to 1 liter
	Filter, aliquot and store at −20 C	1 year
	Adjust pH to 7.0 with 1N NaOH before use (by observing color change in indicator).	
	Use within 1 hour after thawing; do not refreeze	
Trypsin inhibitor 2.5 mg/mL	Trypsin inhibitor type 1 S, Sigma-Aldrich	25 mg
	Distilled water	10 mL
	Store refrigerated	3 years

Reagent	Materials/Instructions	Amount/Time
Urea	CH_4N_2O	120.12 g
2 M	NaCl	4 g
	Dissolve in distilled water	600 mL
	100 mM KH_2PO_4 (see phosphate buffers)	23.6 mL
	100 mM Na_2HPO_4 (see phosphate buffers)	76.4 mL
	Distilled water	to 1 liter
	Store refrigerated	1 year
ZZAP	0.2 M DTT	2.5 mL
	1% ficin	1 mL
	pH 7.3 PBS	1.5 mL
	Prepare immediately before use	

Appendix B. Reagent Preparation Documentation Form

Reagent		Lot #	
Date Prepared		Expiration Date	
Prepared by		Date in Use	
Ingredient:	Amount:	Source:	Outdate:
Storage:	Time:		Location:
QC Check:	Tested by:		Date:

Appendix C. Incidental Spill Response*

Chemicals	Hazards	PPE	Control materials
Acids Acetic Hydrochloric Nitric Perchloric Sulfuric Photographic chemicals (acid)	Severe irritant if inhaled Contact causes burns to skin and eyes Corrosive Fire or contact with metal may produce irritating or poisonous gas Nitric, perchloric, and sulfuric acids are water-reactive oxidizers	Acid-resistant gloves Apron and coveralls Goggles and face shield Acid-resistant foot covers	Acid neutralizers/absorbent Absorbent boom Absorbent pillow Drain mat Leakproof containers Shovel or paddle
Bases and caustics Potassium hydroxide Sodium hydroxide Photographic chemicals (basic)	Corrosive Fire may produce irritating or poisonous gas	Gloves Impervious apron or coveralls Goggles or face shield Impervious foot covers	Base control/neutralizer Absorbent boom Absorbent pillow Drain mat Leakproof container Shovel or paddle
Chlorine Bleach Sodium hypochlorite	Inhalation can cause respiratory irritation Liquid contact can produce irritation of eyes or skin Toxicity due to alkalinity, possible chlorine gas generation, and oxidant properties	Gloves (double set 4H undergloves and butyl or nitrile overgloves) Impervious apron or coveralls Goggles or face shield Impervious foot covers (neoprene boots for emergency response releases) Self-contained breathing apparatus (emergency response releases)	Chlorine control powder Absorbent Absorbent boom Absorbent pillow Drain mat Leakproof container Shovel or paddle Vapor barrier

Chemicals	Hazards	PPE	Control materials
Cryogenic gases Carbon dioxide Nitrous oxide Liquid nitrogen	Contact with liquid nitrogen can produce frostbite Asphyxiation (displaces oxygen) Anesthetic effects (nitrous oxide)	Gloves (insulated to protect from the cold) Full face shield or goggles Neoprene boots	Hand truck (to transport cylinder outdoors if needed) Putty (to stop minor pipe and line leaks) Soap solution (to check for leaks)
Flammable gases Acetylene Oxygen gases Butane Propane	Simple asphyxiate (displaces air) Anesthetic potential Extreme fire and explosion hazard Release can create an oxygen-deficient atmosphere	Gloves (double set) Coveralls with hood and feet Goggles and face shield Neoprene boots	Hand truck (to transport cylinder outdoors if needed) Soap solution (to check for leaks)
Flammable liquids Acetone Xylene Methyl alcohol-toluene Ethyl alcohol Other alcohols	Vapors harmful if inhaled (central nervous system depressants) Harmful via skin absorption Extreme flammability Liquid evaporates to form flammable vapors	Gloves (double set 4H undergloves and butyl or nitrile overgloves) Impervious apron or coveralls Goggles or face shield Impervious foot covers	Absorbent Absorbent boom Absorbent pillow Drain mat Leakproof containers Shovel or paddle (nonmetal, nonsparking)
Formaldehyde and glutaraldehyde 4% formaldehyde 37% formaldehyde 10% formalin 2% glutaraldehyde	Harmful if inhaled or absorbed through skin Irritation to skin, eyes, and respiratory tract Formaldelyde is a suspected human carcinogen Keep away from heat, sparks, and flame (37% formaldehyde)	Gloves (double set 4H undergloves and butyl or nitrile overgloves) Impervious apron or coveralls Goggles Impervious foot covers	Aldehyde neutralizer/absorbent Absorbent boom Absorbent pillow Drain mat Leakproof container Shovel or pallet (nonsparking)

Chemicals	Hazards	PPE	Control materials
Mercury Cantor tubes Thermometers Barometers Sphygmomanometers Mercuric chloride	Mercury and mercury vapors are rapidly absorbed in respiratory tract, GI tract, and skin Short-term exposure may cause erosion of respiratory/GI tract, nausea, vomiting, bloody diarrhea, shock, headache, and metallic taste Inhalation of high concentrations can cause pneumonitis, chest pain, dyspnea, coughing stomatitis, gingivitis, and salivation	Gloves (double set 4H underglove and butyl or nitrile overgloves) Impervious apron or coveralls Goggles Impervious foot covers	Absorbent Aspirator Disposable towels Hazardous waste containers Mercury indicator powder Mercury vacuum or spill kit Scoop Spatula Sponge with amalgam Vapor suppressor **Note:** Avoid evaporation of mercury from tiny globules by quick and thorough cleaning

*This list of physical and health hazards is not intended as a substitute for the specific material safety data sheet (MSDS) information. In the case of a spill, or if any questions arise, always refer to the chemical-specific MSDS for more complete information.

PPE = personal protective equipment; GI = gastrointestinal.

Appendix D. Directions for Managing Hazardous Chemical Spills

Actions	Instructions for Hazardous Liquids, Gases, and Mercury
De-energize	Liquids: • For 37% formaldehyde, de-energize and remove all sources of ignition within 10 ft of spilled hazardous material. • For flammable liquids, remove all sources of ignition. Gases: • Remove all sources of heat and ignition within 50 ft for flammable gases. • Remove all sources of heat and ignition for nitrous oxide release.
Isolate, evacuate, and secure the area	Isolate the spill area and evacuate everyone from the area surrounding the spill except those responsible for cleaning up the spill. (For mercury, evacuate within 10 ft for small spills; 20 ft for large spills.) Secure the area.
Have the appropriate PPE	See Appendix C for recommended personal protective equipment.
Contain the spill	Liquids or mercury: Stop the source of spill if possible. Gases: Assess the scene; consider the circumstances of the release (quantity, location, and ventilation): • If circumstances indicate it is an emergency response release, make appropriate notifications. • If the release is determined to be incidental, contact the supplier for assistance.
Confine the spill	Liquids: Confine the spill to the initial spill area using appropriate control equipment and material. For flammable liquids, dike off all drains. Gases: Follow the supplier's suggestions or request outside assistance. Mercury: Use appropriate materials to confine the spill (see Appendix C). Expel mercury from the aspirator bulb into a leakproof container, if applicable.

Actions	Instructions for Hazardous Liquids, Gases, and Mercury
Neutralize the spill	<u>Liquids:</u> Apply appropriate control materials to neutralize the chemical (see Appendix C). <u>Mercury:</u> Use mercury spill kit if needed.
Clean up the spill area	<u>Liquids:</u> Scoop up solidified material, booms, pillows, and any other materials. Put used materials into a leakproof container. Label the container with the name of the hazardous material. Wipe up residual material. Wipe the spill area surface three times with detergent solution. Rinse areas with clean water. Collect supplies used (goggles, shovels, etc) and remove gross contamination; place them in a separate container for equipment to be thoroughly washed and decontaminated. <u>Gases:</u> Follow supplier's suggestions or request outside assistance. <u>Mercury:</u> Vacuum spill using a mercury vacuum, or scoop up mercury paste after neutralization and collect it in a designated container. Use a sponge and detergent to wipe and clean the spill surface three times to remove absorbent. Collect all contaminated disposal equipment and put into a hazardous waste container. Collect supplies and remove gross contamination; place them in a separate container for equipment to be thoroughly washed and decontaminated.
Disposal	<u>Liquids:</u> • For material that was neutralized, dispose of it as solid waste. Follow the facility's procedures for disposal. • For flammable liquids, check with the facility safety officer for appropriate waste determination. <u>Gases:</u> The manufacturer or supplier will instruct the facility on disposal if applicable. <u>Mercury:</u> Label container with the appropriate hazardous waste label and Department of Transportation diamond label.
Report	Follow appropriate spill documentation and reporting procedures. Investigate the spill; perform root-cause analysis if needed. Act on opportunities for improving safety.

Appendix E. Sources of Reagents and Equipment

Note: Listing of sources of chemicals, reagents, and equipment in this book should not be construed as an endorsement of a specific company's products. Alternative sources may be equally acceptable.

Company	Address	Telephone	Web site
BD (formerly Becton Dickinson and Company)	1 Becton Drive Franklin Lakes, NJ 07417	201.847.6800	www.bd.com
BD Diagnostic Systems	7 Loveton Circle Sparks, MD 21152	410.316.4000	www.bd.com/ds
Beckman Coulter	4300 N Harbor Blvd PO Box 3100 Fullerton, CA 92834	800.742.2345	www.beckmancoulter.com
Bracco Diagnostics	107 College Road East Princeton, NJ 08540	609.514.2200	www.bracco.com
DiaMed AG	Pra Rond 26 1785 Cressier-sur-Morat Switzerland	+41.26.674.51.11	www.diamed.com
Elkay Laboratory Products (UK)	Unit E Lutyens Industrial Ctr Bilton Road Basingstoke Hampshire RG24 8LJ United Kingdom	+44.1256.811118	www.elkay.uk.co.uk
EMD Biosciences	EMD Biosciences 10394 Pacific Center Ct San Diego, CA 92121	800.854.3418	www.emdbiosciences.com
E-Y Laboratories	107 N. Amphlett Blvd San Mateo, CA 94401	800.821.0044	www.eylabs.com
Fenwal	3 Corporate Drive Lake Zurich, IL 60047	800.333.6925	www.fenwalinc.com
Friedrich and Dimmock	2127 Wheaton Ave PO Box 230 Millville, NJ 08332	800.524.1131	www.fdglass.com
GE Healthcare	800 Centennial Ave PO Box 1327 Piscataway, NJ 08855	800.526.3593	www.gehealthcare.com
Immucor	3130 Gateway Drive PO Box 5625 Norcross, GA 30091	800.829.2553	www.immucor.com

Company	Address	Telephone	Web site
Jackson ImmunoResearch Laboratories	PO Box 9 872 West Baltimore Pike West Grove, PA 19390	800.367.5296	www.jacksonimmuno.com
J. L. Hudson, Seedsman	PO Box 337 La Honda, CA 94020	—	www.jlhudsonseeds.net
LabScientific	114 W Mt Pleasant Ave Livingston, NJ 07039	800.886.4507	www.labscientific.com
Lake Charles Manufacturing	4905 Common St Lake Charles, LA 70607	866.739.4600	www.testtubesonline.com
MP Biomedicals	15 Morgan Irvine, CA 92618	800.833.2500	www.mpbio.com
National Institute for Biological Standards and Control	Blanche Lane South Mimms Potters Bar Hertfordshire EN6 3QG United Kingdom	+44.1707.641000	www.nibsc.ac.uk
Pall Corporation	2200 Northern Blvd East Hills, NY 11548	516.484.5400	www.pall.com
Park Seed Company	1 Parkton Ave Greenwood, SC 29647	800.213.0076	www.parkseed.com
Pel-Freez Biologicals	291 N Arkansas St Rogers, AR 72756	800.643.3426	www.pelfreez.bio.com
Perkin-Elmer	940 Winter Street Waltham, MA 02481	800.762.4000	www.perkinelmer.com
Praxair	39 Old Ridgebury Road Danbury, CT 06810	800.772.9247	www.praxair.com
QA Supplies	1185 Pineridge Road Norfolk, VA 23502	800.472.7205	www.qasupplies.com
Qiagen	27220 Turnberry Lane Suite 200 Valencia, CA 91355	800.426.8157	www.qiagen.com
Roche Applied Science	PO Box 50414 9115 Hague Road Indianapolis, IN 46250	800.428.5433	www.roche-applied-science.com
Sanquin Reagents	Plesmanlaan 125 1055 CS Amsterdam The Netherlands	+31.2051.23553	www.sanquinreagents.com

Company	Address	Telephone	Web site
Sigma-Aldrich Corporation	PO Box 14508 St Louis, MO 63718	800.325.3010	www.sigma-aldrich.com
Spectrocell	143 Montgomery Ave Oreland, PA 19075	215.572.7605	www.spectrocell.com
Starstedt	Postfach 12 20 D-51582 Numbrecht Germany	+48.229.33050	www.starstedt.com
Ted Pella	PO Box 492477 Redding, CA 96049	800.237.3526	www.tedpella.com
Thermo Fisher Scientific	81 Wyman Street Waltham, MA 02454	800.678.5599	www.thermofisher.com
VWR Labshop	800 East Fabyan Pkwy Batavia, IL 60510	866.360.7522	www.vwrlabshop.com
Whatman PLC	Springfield Mill James Whatman Way Maidstone Kent ME14 2LE United Kingdom	+44.1622.676670	www.whatman.com

Index

Blood group substances, antibody inhibition by, 323-325, *326*
Blood samples
    with negative autocontrol, identification of, *290*
    with positive autocontrol, identification of, *291*
Blood selection, for patients with alloantibodies, 304-307, *308*
B(A) phenotype, ABO typing problems related to, 517
Bromelain one-stage method, in antibody detection, 77-79
Buffer(s)
    boric acid, 630
    carbonate, 631
    Hendry's iso-osmotic, 641
    lysing, 637
    phosphate, 639-641
    phosphate-NaOH, 641
    SET, 643
    TE, 644
Buffered gel columns
    in antibody detection, 237-239
    preparation of, 229-232

C

C3b/C4b-coated RBC preparation, 250-253
C3b-coated RBC preparation, Fruitstone method, 257-259
C4, allogeneic, 354-356
C4b-coated RBC preparation, 260-262
Capillary methods
    for albumin one-layer procedure, 198-200
    for albumin two-layer procedure, 201-203
    for ficin one-stage procedure, 207-209
    general considerations, 243
    for IAT on precoated RBCs procedure, 210-212
    for papain one-stage procedure, 204-206
    for precoating RBCs for IAT, 213-215
    saline agglutination procedure, 195-197
Carbimazole, immune hemolysis due to, *476*
Caustics spills, response measures for, 648
Cell panel, evaluation of results of, 298-299, *300*
Cell separation methods, 173-192
    described, 173
    harvesting autologous RBCs by direct centrifugation, 174-176
    harvesting autologous RBCs in hemoglobin S or sickle cell disease, 184-186
    harvesting autologous RBCs with phthalate esters, 177-180
    mononuclear, 190-192

    Percoll-Renografin procedure, 181-183
    separating mixed-cell populations with antibodies, 187-189
Centrifugation, 174-176
Cephalosporin(s), reacting with drug-treated RBCs, 490-495
Cephalothin-dependent antibodies, detection of, 500-502
Chemical(s), effects on reactions of antibodies to high-prevalence antigens, *343*
Chemical spills, management of, 651-652
Chlorine spills, response measures for, 648-650
Chloroform, in eluting IgG auto- and alloantibodies from RBCs, 116-119
Chloroform/trichloroethylene, 120-123
Chloroquine diphosphate
    in dissociation of IgG from RBCs, 170-172
    in stripping residual HLA antigens from RBCs, 351-353
α-Chymotrypsin, treating RBCs with, 80-82
Citric acid, in eluting IgG auto- and alloantibodies from RBCs, 124-127
Cold acid solution in eluting antibodies from RBCs, 128-131
Cold agglutinins, management of samples and patients with, 294-297
Cold autologous adsorption, procedure for, 444-446
Cold-reactive antibodies, 68-70
Cold-reactive autoantibodies, 407-408
    adsorption with autologous RBCs, 444-446
    adsorption with heterologous (rabbit) RBCs, 447-450
    specificity of, *411*
    testing thermal amplitude of, 435-437
    titration in diagnostic testing of, 438-440
    titration in specificity determination of, 441-443
Complement-fixing antibodies, 333-335
Cord blood
    prenatal and perinatal testing, 365
    serum, AB blood group and, 561-563
    testing in infants of Rh-negative mothers, 365
    treatment of, 404-405
[51]Cr-Labeled RBCs, 594-598
Crossmatching
    by immediate-spin, 21-24
    by LISS antiglobulin, 11-14
Crude extracts of lectins, 564-566
Cryogenic gases, 649
Cyst(s), hydatid, 636